100 Years of Human Chorionic Gonadotropin

100 Years of Human Chorionic Gonadotropin

Reviews and New Perspectives

Edited by

Laurence A. Cole, PhD

USA hCG Reference Service
Angel Fire, New Mexico
United States

Stephen A. Butler, PhD

SAB Scientific Consultancy Ltd
Flitton, Bedfordshire
United Kingdom

ELSEVIER

Elsevier
Radarweg 29, PO Box 211, 1000 AE Amsterdam, Netherlands
The Boulevard, Langford Lane, Kidlington, Oxford OX5 1GB, United Kingdom
50 Hampshire Street, 5th Floor, Cambridge, MA 02139, United States

Notices
Knowledge and best practice in this field are constantly changing. As new research and experience broaden our understanding, changes in research methods, professional practices, or medical treatment may become necessary.

Practitioners and researchers must always rely on their own experience and knowledge in evaluating and using any information, methods, compounds, or experiments described herein. In using such information or methods they should be mindful of their own safety and the safety of others, including parties for whom they have a professional responsibility.

To the fullest extent of the law, neither the Publisher nor the authors, contributors, or editors, assume any liability for any injury and/or damage to persons or property as a matter of products liability, negligence or otherwise, or from any use or operation of any methods, products, instructions, or ideas contained in the material herein.

Library of Congress Cataloging-in-Publication Data
A catalog record for this book is available from the Library of Congress

British Library Cataloguing-in-Publication Data
A catalogue record for this book is available from the British Library

ISBN: 978-0-12-820050-6

For information on all Elsevier publications visit our website at
https://www.elsevier.com/books-and-journals

Publisher: Stacy Masucci
Acquisitions Editor: Tari K. Broderick
Editorial Project Manager: Anna Dubnow
Production Project Manager: Kiruthika Govindaraju
Cover Designer: Alan Studholme

Typeset by TNQ Technologies

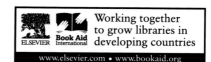

Working together
to grow libraries in
developing countries

www.elsevier.com • www.bookaid.org

Contents

SECTION 1 Genes and structure

SECTION 2 Detection and quantitation

SECTION 3 Pregnancy and fertility

CHAPTER 3.8   Evaluation of delivery systems for active immunization with synthetic peptides of hCG as a fertility control method: A collection of study data and discussion by the World Health Organization task force on the Regulation of Human Reproduction 1999—2007 227

Vernon C. Stevens and Stephen A. Butler

SECTION 4 Cancer and therapy

SECTION 5 Conclusion

Contributors

Thommas Kwenko Abban
Kratos Analytical Ltd, Manchester, United Kingdom

Robert C. Baxter
Hormones and Cancer Group, Kolling Institute, Royal North Shore Hospital, University of Sydney, St Leonards, NSW, Australia

Giulia Brigante
Unit of Endocrinology, Department of Biomedical, Metabolic and Neural Sciences, University of Modena and Reggio Emilia, Modena, Italy; Unit of Endocrinology, Department of Medical Specialties, Azienda Ospedaliero-Universitaria, Modena, Italy

Stephen A. Butler
SAB Scientific Consultancy Ltd, Bedfordshire, United Kingdom

Livio Casarini
Unit of Endocrinology, Department of Biomedical, Metabolic and Neural Sciences, University of Modena and Reggio Emilia, Modena, Italy; Center for Genomic Research, University of Modena and Reggio Emilia, Modena, Italy

Laurence A. Cole
USA hCG Reference Service, Angel Fire, NM, United States

Jemma Evans
Centre for Reproductive Health, The Hudson Institute of Medical Research, Clayton, VIC, Australia

Mazen R. Founay
Department of Obstetrics & Gynecology, UPMC Cole, Assistant Professor Lock Haven University, Coudersport, PA, United States

Thierry Fournier
Université de Paris, INSERM, U1139, 3PHM, Paris, France; PremUp Foundation, Paris, France

Nicholas Gibbons
Center for Investigative and Diagnostic Oncology, Middlesex University, London, United Kingdom

Jagdish C. Gupta
Talwar Research Foundation, New Delhi, India

Trine Grønhaug Halvorsen
Section of Pharmaceutical Chemistry, Department of Pharmacy, University of Oslo, Oslo, Norway

Ilpo T. Huhtaniemi
Research Center for Integrative Physiology and Pharmacology, Institute of Biomedicine and Turku Center for Disease Modeling, University of Turku, Turku, Finland; Institute of Reproductive and Developmental Biology, Department of Surgery & Cancer, Hammersmith Campus, Imperial College London, London, United Kingdom

Ray K. Iles
MAP Diagnostics Ltd, Bedfordshire, United Kingdom; College of Health Sciences, Abu Dhabi University, Abu Dhabi, United Arab Emirates

Anna Jankowska
Department of Cell Biology, Poznan University of Medical Sciences, Poznan, Poland

Sarah Johnson
Clinical Research Director, SPD Development Company Ltd., Bedfordshire, United Kingdom

R.S. Kabeer
Talwar Research Foundation, New Delhi, India

Hannu K. Koistinen
Department of Clinical Chemistry, University of Helsinki and Helsinki University Central Hospital, Helsinki, Finland

Clara Lazzaretti
Unit of Endocrinology, Department of Biomedical, Metabolic and Neural Sciences, University of Modena and Reggio Emilia, Modena, Italy; International PhD School in Clinical and Experimental Medicine (CEM), University of Modena and Reggio Emilia, Modena, Italy

Jameel Luttoo
Center for Investigative and Diagnostic Oncology, Middlesex University, London, United Kingdom

Deborah J. Marsh
Hormones and Cancer Group, Kolling Institute, Royal North Shore Hospital, University of Sydney, St Leonards, NSW, Australia; University of Technology Sydney, Translational Oncology Group, School of Life Sciences, Faculty of Science, Ultimo, NSW, Australia

Ricardo J. Pais
MAP Diagnostics Ltd, Bedfordshire, United Kingdom

Elia Paradiso
Unit of Endocrinology, Department of Biomedical, Metabolic and Neural Sciences, University of Modena and Reggio Emilia, Modena, Italy; International PhD School in Clinical and Experimental Medicine (CEM), University of Modena and Reggio Emilia, Modena, Italy

Matti Poutanenn
Research Center for Integrative Physiology and Pharmacology, Institute of Biomedicine, and Turku Center for Disease Modeling, University of Turku, Turku, Finland

Shilpi Puruswani
Qiagen Sciences Inc , Germantown, MD, United States

Léon Reubesat
Section of Pharmaceutical Chemistry, Department of Pharmacy, University of Oslo, Oslo, Norway

Susana B. Rulli
Instituto de Biología y Medicina Experimental- Consejo Nacional de Investigaciones Científicas y Técnicas, Buenos Aires, Argentina

Daniele Santi
Unit of Endocrinology, Department of Biomedical, Metabolic and Neural Sciences, University of Modena and Reggio Emilia, Modena, Italy; Unit of Endocrinology, Department of Medical Specialties, Azienda Ospedaliero-Universitaria, Modena, Italy

Fady I. Sharara
Virginia Center for Reproductive Medicine, Reston, VA, United States; Department of Obstetrics and Gynecology, George Washington University, Washington, DC, United States

Manuela Simoni
Unit of Endocrinology, Department of Biomedical, Metabolic and Neural Sciences, University of Modena and Reggio Emilia, Modena, Italy; Center for Genomic Research, University of Modena and Reggio Emilia, Modena, Italy; Unit of Endocrinology, Department of Medical Specialties, Azienda Ospedaliero-Universitaria, Modena, Italy; Biology and Bioinformatics of Signaling Systems Group, Unité Mixte de Recherche 85, Unité Physiologie de la Reproduction et des Comportements, Institut National de la Recherche Agronomique, Nouzilly, France; Centre National de la Recherche Scientifique, Unité Mixte de Recherche 7247, Nouzilly, France; Université François Rabelais, Nouzilly, France

Snega M. Sinnappan
Hormones and Cancer Group, Kolling Institute, Royal North Shore Hospital, University of Sydney, St Leonards, NSW, Australia

Ulf-Håkan Stenman
Department of Clinical Chemistry, University of Helsinki and Helsinki University Central Hospital, Helsinki, Finland

Vernon C. Stevens
Professor, Department of Obstetrics and Gynecology, The Ohio State University Research Foundation, Ohio State University, Columbus, OH, United States

Anna Szczerba
Department of Cell Biology, Poznan University of Medical Sciences, Poznan, Poland

G.P. Talwar
Talwar Research Foundation, New Delhi, India

Hemant K. Vyas
Department of Virology and Immunology, Biomedical Research Institute, San Antonio, TX, United States

Raminta Zmuidinaite
MAP Diagnostics Ltd, Bedfordshire, United Kingdom

About the editors

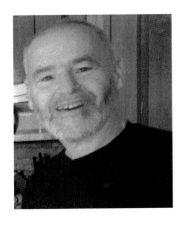

Dr. Laurence A. Cole, PhD
The USA hCG Reference Service
Angel Fire, New Mexico, USA
lachcglab@gmail.com
Larry@hCGLab.com

In 1971, Larry Cole began academic life studying medicine in England. A stroke in 1974 put him in a coma for 3 months and left him with amnesia and severe brain damage, and he was forced to abandon his medical degree. After a year in hospital, he moved to Israel in 1976, then to the United States in 1977. He learned to "program" the other side of his brain, and he began to learn again. In 1978, he attended the Medical College of Wisconsin, Milwaukee, for a PhD in Biochemistry, studying cancer cell hCG with Robert Hussa, and graduated in 1981. During this time, Larry also worked with Roland Pattillo on gestational trophoblastic disease and attended the first international symposium on GTD which he has attended ever since.

In 1983, Larry completed a postdoctoral fellowship with Raymond Ruddon, PhD, at the University of Michigan. He continued to specialize in hCG and was inspired by Raymond to study hCG carbohydrate structure and joined the faculty of the University of Michigan.

In 1984, Larry took a position at Yale University, where he spent 15 years as part of the Obstetrics and Gynecology team. He advanced at Yale University from Assistant Professor to Associate Professor, then to Full Professor. While at Yale University, Larry's research purely focused on hCG, investigating hCG and gestational trophoblastic disease, hCG as a tumor marker, and oligosaccharide structure and hCG. It was at this time that Stephen Butler joined Larry as a Postdoc Fellow at Yale School of Medicine. During this time, Larry studied the structure of choriocarcinoma hCG, which ultimately led to his discovery of hyperglycosylated hCG and to new diagnostic protocols in gestational trophoblastic diseases.

In 1999, Larry moved to the University of New Mexico as a tenured Full Professor and Chief of the new division and Center for Women's Health Research. While at the University of New Mexico, he started the US government CLIA—endorsed program called the USA hCG Reference Service, which globally advises scientists who research hCG, physicians who treat gestational trophoblastic disease, and patients with persistent low levels of hCG. In 2004, he received an endowment of the Howard and Friedman Distinguished Professor of Obstetrics and Gynecology which was set up and funded by grateful reference service patients.

Today, 38 years after receiving his PhD, Dr. Cole still specializes in hCG research. Larry's research interest now centers on cancer biology and treatment, building on his hypothesis that hyperglycosylated hCG and its free ß-subunit controls malignancy in all or most human cancers. In 1987, Larry's PhD advisor, Robert Hussa, wrote the first book on hCG. Now, together with Stephen, Larry has written and edited two editions of *Human Chorionic Gonadotrophin*, and it is with great dignity that Larry follows in the footsteps of his advisor and edits this fourth text on hCG, celebrating 100 years of this fascinating molecule.

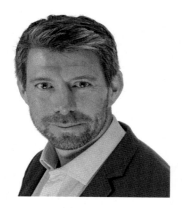

Dr. Stephen Butler, PhD
SAB Scientific Consultancy Ltd
Flitton, Bedfordshire, UK
ButlerSA1@gmail.com
Stephen.Butler@ScientificConsultancy.co.uk

It was in 1994 that Stephen was first introduced to hCG as an undergraduate biochemistry student on work placement in the Williamson Laboratory for Molecular Oncology which was founded by Dr. Ray Iles, in the Department of Reproductive Physiology under Professor Tim Chard. Stephen ran immunoassays for hCG and hCGβ which, back then, were all radioactive RIAs and IRMAs to study disorders of early pregnancy and cancer. He also had his first exposure to reverse transcriptase PCR, investigating the complex expression of the CGB gene cluster. After his placement, during his final year at university, Stephen carried on working with hCG at the laboratory and graduated in 1996. It was in this year he met Larry Cole, and they conducted a study on stability of hCG with variable glycosylation. In 1998, Stephen published his first paper on hCG based on this study.

Already hooked on hCG, Stephen immediately started a PhD, with Ray as his supervisor, on the structure and function of hCGβ in epithelial carcinoma. During his PhD, he demonstrated the role of hCGβ in carcinoma and postulated it's function in apoptosis and as growth factor modulator. It was here that Stephen first observed hCG and hCGβ by MALDI-ToF MS and first studied the effect of hCG vaccines as a potential treatment for hCGβ expressing cancers.

In 1999, Stephen started his Postdoc fellowship at Yale University School of Medicine with Professor Larry Cole. It was during these first few weeks in New Haven that Stephen and Larry discussed the commonality of their work, and they were struck by the similarity in what they had separately discovered; Larry on hyperglycosylated hCG in GTD and pregnancy and Stephen on the free β-subunit of hCG in carcinoma. It was from these early discussions that their work together developed and featured at the heart of the last two books on hCG which they coedited; their collaboration and discussion on hCG continues to this day.

Stephen moved with Larry to the University of New Mexico where he became Assistant Professor in the Center for Women's Health Research and, with Larry, set up the hCG reference service resolving the problems of phantom hCG and immunodetection of hCG. Stephen returned to the UK after 2.5 years in the United States and took positions in Italy and London and his last academic post was Reader in Biomedical Diagnostics at the Centre for Investigative and Diagnostic Oncology, Middlesex University, London. In 2014, he left higher education and cofounded a diagnostic company with Ray Iles specializing in MALDI-ToF analysis.

Most recently Stephen founded SAB Scientific Consultancy where carries out hCG based consultancy work in cancer, pregnancy and fertility and collaborates on hCG projects around the world; 25 years after his first introduction to hCG. He is privileged to be involved with this project to celebrate 100 years of a molecule which has influenced so many, not least himself.

Foreword—100 Years of hCG

In 2019, it is difficult to ignore the effect that our understanding of hCG has had on the lives of millions of people worldwide. The hCG immunoassay, in one form or another, is now one of the most common tests conducted and is often the first indication that a mother-to-be is pregnant. 100 years ago, in 1919, a Japanese physician, Toyoichi Hirose [1], was demonstrating the gonadotropic function of a chorionic factor by stimulating ovarian function in rabbits by implanting fragments of human placenta into the peritoneum in his *experimentalle histologische studie zur genese corpus luteum* (experimental histological study on the genesis of the corpus luteum). This is the earliest, well-defined study on the effect of a chorionic gonadotropin being described; although there were studies on pituitary gonadotropins and more general effects of placental extracts a few years earlier [2,3] and the Egyptians were urinating on wheat and spelt 4000 years ago to use germination as a test for pregnancy.

The chorionic factor with gonadotropic functions described by Hirose was later defined as a gonadotropic hormone in the experiments of Aschheim and Zondek, who demonstrated that pregnant women produce a gonad-stimulating substance [4]. They showed that injecting this substance subcutaneously into intact immature female mice produced follicular maturation, luteinization, and hemorrhaging into the ovarian stroma. These findings were confirmed by others [4,5,6] and the first hCG pregnancy tests were born [4—6].

Hundred years of hCG is not an attempt to recount the history of every publication on hCG but rather a collection of reviews and new perspectives by some of the "hCG-ologists," as Hussa [7] referred to us, who are still working in the field today. Some of them have been around a while, some not so long, but others are just beginning their journey with a most fascinating molecule.

Stephen A. Butler
Laurence A. Cole

REFERENCES

[1] Hirose T. Experimentalle histologische studie zur genese corpus luteum. Mitt Med Fakultd Univ ZU 1919;23:63—70.

[2] Aschner B. Ueber die function der hypophyse. Pflug Arch Gest Physiol 1912;146:1—147.

[3] Fellner OO. Experimentelle untersuchungen uber die wirkung von gewebsextrakten aus der plazenta und den weiblichen sexualorganen auf das genital. Arch Gynakol 1913;100: 641.

[4] Aschheim S, Zondek B. Das Hormon des hypophysenvorderlappens: testobjekt zum Nachweis des hormons. Klin Wochenschr 1927;6:248—52.

[5] Zondek B, Aschheim S. The Zondek-Ascheimpregnancy test. Can Med Assoc J 1930;22: 251—3.
[6] Friedman MH, Lapham MEA. Simple, rapid procedure for the laboratory diagnosis of early pregnancies. Am J Obstet Gynecol 1931;21:405—10.
[7] Hussa RO. The Clinical Marker-hCG. New York: Praeger; 1987xvii.

Acknowledgments

We would simply like to acknowledge the hCG-ologists in the world who have been touched by this intriguing molecule enough to carry out at least one experiment and write about it. These scientists and clinicians are too numerous to mention but it is on their shoulders that we continue to explore the structures and functions of human chorionic gonadotropin.

Genes and structure

hCG anecdote 1 extracting C5 and creating the antibody B152—the birth of hyperglycosylated hCG

1.1

Laurence A. Cole

Since I started my research into hCG, the variability in structure had been at the root of my investigations, and by 1989 I had become extremely curious about the structure of choriocarcinoma hCG. If the structure of hCG had variable glycosylations in pregnancy, then would the hCG seen in choriocarcinoma be any different? If it was different, how different?

Choriocarcinoma was, and still is, very rare in America, occurring in 1 in 30,000 pregnancies. I had contacts and collaborators working on GTD all over the world but the incidence is very similar, in the UK and Europe, for example. However, I was fortunate in having a research fellow from China, Dr. Wang Yixun, who reliably informed me that her hospital back in China, the Liaoning Tumor Institute, sees up to 40 cases at any one time with choriocarcinoma. I immediately made arrangements to fly to China and visit her Tumor Institute hospital. I flew directly to Beijing, then proceeded by train to Shenyang in Manchuria in Northern China. The train journey was an arduous 10 hour trip, but I was pleasantly surprised and somewhat taken aback to be greeted at the station by a parade of 50 doctors, all wearing white coats and lined up along the platform at the station.

During the visit I managed to collect large volumes of urine from some of the most serious cases at the tumor hospital, in total, 5 L from six different patients with choriocarcinoma, all before they had received any therapy. Each 5 L urine sample was concentrated by tangential flow dialysis and concentrated down to 100 mL and then frozen for transport back to the United States. I returned, by train and plane back home to begin the extraction of hCG.

Using a combination of acetone precipitation, ethanol precipitation, Sephacryl S = 200 gel filtration, DEAE-Sepharose ion exchange chromatography, Sephacryl S-100 gel filtration, and reverse phase HPLC, we purified each hCG from each of the six choriocarcinoma urine samples. At the same time, we also purified hCG from six first trimester pregnancy urine samples, from three complete hydatidiform mole urine samples, and from two other abnormal pregnancy urine samples,

100 Years of Human Chorionic Gonadotropin. https://doi.org/10.1016/B978-0-12-820050-6.00001-1

gestational diabetes, I recall. Eight years later the complete carbohydrate and peptide structure of α-subunit and β-subunit of hCG in pregnancy, hydatidiform mole, and choriocarcinoma was published [1].

One particular hCG from the series of purifications, choriocarcinoma hCG named C5 (Choriocarcinoma 5), was particularly interesting for two reasons. C5 was 100% nicked in loop 2 of the beta subunit, and it had 100% type 2 O-linked oligosaccharides (4 of 4). Working with Stephen Birken, PhD, and Alex Krichevsky, PhD, at Columbia University, we were all interested in a monoclonal antibody which was exclusively able to bind nicked hCG, and C5 was the perfect antigen. Several antibodies were made against C5 hCG, but one stood out. That monoclonal antibody was called B152, and ironically it was no good at recognizing nicked hCG but rather good at binding those O-linked sugars on the carboxy terminal peptide. It was using this antibody that hyperglycosylated hCG was discovered and opened an entirely new field of research on hCG in early pregnancy and GTD. B152 binds the autocrine hyperglycosylated hCG and extravillous cytotrophoblast hCG, but not the hormone hCG. This antibody was recently found to bind cancer hCG, it can inhibit cancer cell growth and, as such, is now believed to be a potential cure for cancer.

References

[1] Elliott MM, Kardana A, Lustbader JW, Cole LA. Carbohydrate and peptide structure of the alpha-and beta-subunits of human chorionic gonadotropin from normal and aberrant pregnancy and choriocarcinoma. Endocrine 1997;7(1):15−32.

Evolutionary, structural, and physiological differences between hCG and LH

1.2

Livio Casarini, Clara Lazzaretti, Elia Paradiso, Daniele Santi, Giulia Brigante, Manuela Simoni

Introduction

Luteinizing hormone (LH) and the primate-specific chorionic gonadotropin (CG) are two glycoprotein hormones regulating gonadal functions and gamete development. LH regulates steroidogenesis both in males and females, while hCG is essential to sustain pregnancy and fetal development. For a long time, they have been considered equivalent due to their action on the same receptor (LHCGR) [1], despite their different physiological roles [2]. In the last decade, in vitro studies demonstrated that different structure and carbohydrate structures linked to the two hormones may be source of hormone-specific LHCGR binding and activation of intracellular signaling cascades. In the gonads, LH mainly mediates the phosphorylation of kinases triggering androgen synthesis. Besides this well-known steroidogenic effect, LH is linked to follicular growth and luteinization through activation of proliferative and anti-apoptotic signals in ovarian cells. hCG is produced in pregnancy, when progesterone synthesis is required to support the rescue of the corpus luteum, angiogenesis, and fetal development. These functions are exerted via preferential activation of the cAMP/protein kinase A (PKA) pathway, which is linked to pro-apoptotic signals in ovarian cells in vitro [3,4]. Although the issue is still debated, clinical data overall suggest that LH- and hCG-specific signals emerging by in vitro studies may reflect different assisted reproduction technique (ART) outcomes [2] (Santi et al. 2018).

Evolution of LH and hCG in primates and humans

Gonadotropins are glycoprotein hormones belonging to the superfamily of cystine-knot growth factors. These molecules share a common structure featured by six disulfide-linked cystine residues and the typical "knot" conformation is essential

100 Years of Human Chorionic Gonadotropin. https://doi.org/10.1016/B978-0-12-820050-6.00002-3

to guarantee an extremely selective interaction between the different glycoproteins and their receptors, as well as a different biological activity [5]. Gonadotropins are heterodimers, encoded by specific genes, consisting of a common α subunit and a specific β subunit determining receptor binding [6]. LH and hCG exert their function, thanks to the interaction with LHCGR, a member of the rhodopsin-like G protein-coupled receptors (GPCRs) [2]. These receptors are located in the Leydig, theca, and granulosa cell membranes and are characterized by seven transmembrane segments, a C-terminal intracellular region, and a relatively long N-terminal region, exposed to the extracellular environment [7].

LHCGR structure is overall similar to that of other glycoprotein hormone receptors, suggesting common evolutionary determinants of their gene sequences. It was estimated that the first appearance of glycoprotein hormones and their receptor was at the basal metazoans, becoming increasingly critical for regulating growth, development, and endocrine functions across evolution [8]. Structure-function relationship of glycoprotein hormones and their receptors would be linked to the specialization of systems, as a result of a selective pressure leading to environmental adaptation and optimization of the reproductive success [2]. Hormone receptor systems are supposed to have maintained their signaling mechanisms, indicating conservation of the molecular machinery in spite of functional diversification [9]. In basal vertebrates, gametogenesis is regulated by the action of a unique hormone. This is a glycoprotein consisting of an α and a β subunit, namely thyrostimulin, which is produced and secreted by the pituitary gland of the sea lamprey [10]. The evolutionary appearance of different hormones selectively regulating gametogenesis occurred around 927 millions of years ago, after the duplication of the gene encoding the thyrostimulin β subunit, generating the LH β subunit. Subsequent duplications of this gene gave rise to the thyroid-stimulating hormone (TSH) and follicle-stimulating hormone (FSH) β molecules [11]. In light of evolutionary similarities of the ligand-GPCR systems in vertebrates [12], it was supposed that LHβ and hCGβ subunits originated from duplication of an ancestral gene in primates, although retaining LHCGR binding capability and production by trophoblast instead of pituitary gonadotrope cells [13]. Independent evolutionary pathways occurred depending upon species [11]. For instance, a peculiarly glycosylated form of LH β is highly expressed in the chorion of equids, consisting in the gonadotropin of pregnancy in this organism. This role is exerted by the choriogonadotropin in higher primates [7].

In anthropoid primates, separation between CG and LH β subunit-encoding genes (*CGBs*) likely occurred 55—35 million years ago by repeated duplications, leading to a variable numbers of gene copies among species. Moreover, loss of the original *LHB* stop codon produced an additional encoded sequence of *CGB* genes, resulting in a hCG-specific C-terminal peptide (CTP). The highest complexity of the *LHB/CGB* gene cluster is achieved in humans, where six copies of tandem CGB genes and two pseudogenes are mapped [14]. This genetic locus is located on chromosome 19q13.32 and is characterized by the presence of sequence inversions, typically derived from a high crossover activity, resulting in palindromic genes [13] (Table 1.2.1). Transcription of *CGB* genes results in a variety of hCG isoforms, moreover encountering specific posttranslational modifications, producing differently glycosylated molecules assumed to be required for regulating the complexity of processes underlying hemochorial placentation in the human [2]. In particular, hyperglycosylated forms of hCG would be produced during the first days of pregnancy to support trophoblast cell implantation and early angiogenesis [15], as well as tumorigenesis [16,17], while less glycosylated hCG isoforms would be deputed to progestational functions exerted later during the first trimester of the fetal development [18]. Among the six *CGB* genes, *CGB1* and *CGB2* are thought to exert a crucial role in implantation and placental development as they are highly conserved in humans and great apes [19].

Table 2.1 Genetic, structural and physiological differences between LH and hCG in Homo sapiens.

	Luteinizing hormone (LH)	Human chorionic gonadotropin (hCG)
Genes	1 LHB gene	6 HCGβ genes
β amino acid chain length	121 Amino acids	145 Amino acids
Molecular weight	~26-32 KDa	~37 kDa
LH/hCG-specific amino acid sequences	Absence of the C-terminal peptide (CTP)	C-terminal peptide (CTP)
Half-life	25 minutes	15–462 hours
Glycosylation	3 (2 N-linked in the α subunit; 1 N-linked in the β subunit)	8 (2 N-linked in the α subunit; 2 N-and 4 O-linked in the β subunit)
Physiological role	LH regulates gametogenesis, both in males and in females, and the ovarian cycle	hCG, present only in females, plays a role in pregnancy maintenance, extending the functional life span of corpus luteum, and supporting progesterone production.
Intracellular pathways activated	LH promotes a more potent activation of anti-apoptotic and proliferative signals, mediated by pERK1/2	hCG mainly activates steroidogenic signals mediated by cAMP/PKA

Beside the evolution of gonadotropins' diversification, LHCGR- and FSHR-encoding genes underwent processes of gene duplication as well, from which the two receptors derived [20]. In support of this hypothesis, they share high similarity at the structural, molecular, genetic, and genomic levels, displaying promiscuous hormone binding in certain fishes, but not in humans [21], suggesting they were involved in the specialization of endocrine functions during the evolution [7].

Structural LHβ and hCGβ subunits

While glycoprotein hormones share the same α subunit, the molecular structure of LHβ and hCGβ subunits achieves 80%–85% of identity [22,23]. The LHβ subunit is a 22-kDa glycoprotein of 121 amino acids [24], while hCGβ subunit consists of 145 amino acids [25]. While the α subunit is characterized by two oligosaccharide structures, the LH β subunit features one N-glycosylation site at position 50. hCGβ subunit is 24 amino acids longer than the LH β, consisting in the CTP, which carries one N- and four additional O-linked glycosylation sites [26]. These modifications, together with sulfonations and sialylations, vary according to the day of pregnancy, phase of the ovarian cycle [27], and age [28]. The hormone half-life may depend on the number and quality of oligosaccharides structures, as well as sulfonations and sialylations joining the gonadotropin backbone. The more LH molecules are sulfonated, the shorter is their half-life. In particular, the presence of two or three N-acetylgalactosamine residues promotes gonadotropin clearance by hepatic cells. Conversely, a highly sialylated LH molecule has a longer half-life [29]. Most importantly, degree of glycosylation highly impacts gonadotropins serum half-lives, resulting in about 20 minutes for LH and more than 1 hour for hCG due to its additional O- and N-linked carbohydrates [2] (Table 1.2.1).

Physiology of LH and hCG

LH and hCG have long been considered equivalent molecules, as it was difficult to identify differences in action at the molecular level and in their ability to activate intracellular signaling cascades, although clear physiological diversification [30,31]. LH is naturally involved in gametogenesis in both sexes, and in the regulation of the ovarian cycle, where it exerts a crucial role for the follicular growth and oocyte maturation [1,3,32]. In contrast, hCG is produced only in females, where it supports pregnancy extending the functional life span and functions of the *corpus luteum* [1,2] (Table 1.2.1).

In women of fertile age, gametogenesis is characterized by dominant follicular growth and selection, and oocyte maturation. These processes are regulated by the concerted action of FSH and LH, both secreted in a pulsatile fashion by the pituitary gland, and by simultaneous action of growth factors and steroid hormones [3]. However, folliculogenesis begins before birth, around the 20th week of gestation, when a pool of about 7 million primordial follicles is generated. Only a small part of these growing follicles undergoes morphological and molecular changes, still independent from the action of gonadotropins, becoming primary and secondary follicles [33]. At puberty, the monthly recruitment of a cohort of follicles takes place, thanks to LH and FSH, acting on their respective receptors, which are differently expressed across the ovarian cycle [34]. Indeed, at the early follicular phase, elevated FSH levels guarantee proliferation and progression in follicle maturation, thanks to high levels of FSHR on granulosa cells surface. In contrast, at this early phase, relatively low LH levels are achieved, but enough to act on LHCGR, mainly expressed on theca cells, where androgen synthesis occurs [35]. During follicular growth, LHCGR expression gradually increases also on the surface of granulosa cells [36], where likely LHCGR and FSHR physically interact [37], forming heterodimeric structures exerting gonadotropin signaling [38,39]. Therefore, gonadotropin production accompanies follicle maturation, guaranteeing the synthesis of steroid hormones and formation of the antrum, as a phase of the follicular maturation characterized by the decline of FSHR expression and a prevalence of LHCGR on the granulosa cell membrane. LH peak following this phase is necessary for inducing the ovulation and, after oocyte collection by the Fallopian tube, the role of LH is to sustain progesterone production by corpus luteum. The trophoblastic production of hCG is required to sustain the production of progesterone during the first 7−10 weeks of gestation [40], while LH production is inhibited because of the negative feedback exerted by the steroid hormone at the pituitary level. hCG is necessary for stimulating maternal/placental androgen production, which are involved in fetal development, pregnancy progression, and modifications at the cervical and myometrium level before and during parturition [41]. Moreover, it is supposed that the role of hCG goes beyond that progestational during pregnancy. This molecule might exert immunosuppressive and angiogenic functions required for trophoblast and placental invasion of maternal tissues and to prevent fetal rejection [42]. Finally, hCG is supposed to exert specific roles in the fetus, likely activating the hypothalamic pituitary-gonadal axis and sex steroid production [43].

In males, gametogenesis is regulated by the two gonadotropins LH and FSH as well, however, acting on two different cell types, while hCG is supposed to be overall absent, apart from the early fetal life. FSH finds its receptor on Sertoli cells surface, while LH regulates the activity of Leydig cells, stimulating testosterone production to sustain both Sertoli cell function and progression of spermatogenesis [2].

Taken together, these two molecules manage a number of physiological functions acting through the same receptor and activating hormone-specific intracellular signaling pathways.

Differences between LH- and hCG-mediated signaling

LH and hCG binding to LHCGR induces a conformational change leading to the switch from the receptor inactive to the active form, activating simultaneously several intracellular signaling pathways. Indeed, this spatial conformation of LHCGR activates signaling cascades which start with G protein activation mediating steroidogenic, pro-apoptotic and proliferative events [44,45]. Some of the most known LH- and hCG-mediated intracellular events consist in the cAMP/PKA-pathway activation and intracellular calcium ion (Ca^{2+}) increase [46,47]. Recruitment of intracellular Ca^{2+} and cAMP occurs within 1–5 minutes after the ligand-receptor binding [48,49] as two early upstream events triggered by specific LHCGR cytoplasmic interactors. While the Ca^{2+} signaling is due to Gq protein activation, dissociation of the Gαs protein from the βγ dimer results in the activation of adenylyl cyclase membrane enzyme, which, in turn, catalyzes the conversion of ATP into cAMP. The intracellular concentration of this second messenger is regulated by the activity of phosphodiesterases (PDEs), which catalyze the conversion of cAMP to AMP. The accumulation of intracellular cAMP leads to activation of protein kinase a (PKA), phosphorylation of the extracellular-regulated kinase (ERK1/2), and of the transcription factor cAMP-responsive element binding protein (CREB), as well as transcription of genes encoding steroidogenic enzymes [50].

In vitro studies demonstrated ligand-specific steroidogenic signals, consisting in more potent cAMP production and pro-apoptotic signals upon cell treatment by hCG than LH [3,4,32,51,52], which are even amplified in the presence of FSH [53] and would rely on intracellular cAMP increase [54]. The higher potency of hCG than LH in inducing cAMP was revealed by comparing the EC50 values of the two hormones (~100 pM for hCG and 500 pM for LH) resulted from dose-response experiments using cultured human granulosa cells, demonstrating that hCG is five times more potent than LH in inducing steroidogenic signals [3]. These results were confirmed by in vitro studies with COS-7 and HEK293 cells [3,52], in the mouse tumor Leydig MLTC1 cell line [52], in goat granulosa cells [4], and in mouse Leydig primary cells [32], and, overall, reflects the progestational role of hCG in human physiology. On the other hand, the regulation of survival, cellular proliferation, and anti-apoptotic processes in ovarian steroidogenic cells relies on the phosphorylation of ERK1/2 [55], which is preferentially activated by LH than hCG [3,51] (Fig. 1.2.1). Moreover, pERK1/2 activation involved GPCR kinases mRNA downregulation [56] and internalization of the receptor by β-arrestins [57], suggesting weak impact of hCG on signal desensitization of steroidogenic signals. On the other hand, LH proliferative and anti-apoptotic role would be relevant for sustaining the follicular development during the antral phase [58,59].

The activation of the phospholipase C (PLC)/Ca^{2+} signaling pathway [60] is involved in LH-dependent granulosa cell differentiation during the preovulatory phase, as well as in hCG-dependent regulation of the cholesterol transport into mitochondria and steroidogenesis during pregnancy [61–63].

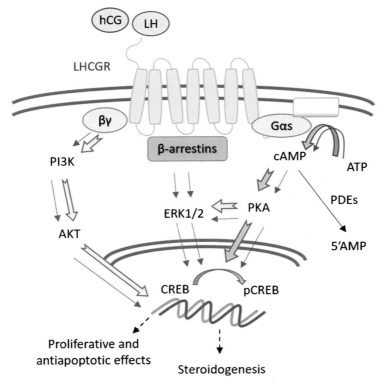

FIGURE 1.2.1

Intracellular signaling pathway mediated by luteinizing hormone (LH) and human chorionic gonadotropin (hCG) in human granulosa lutein cells. LH and hCG bind the extracellular portion of their specific receptor LHCGR inducing a conformational change. Gαs protein activates adenylyl cyclase (AC) enzyme, which converts ATP to cAMP. Intracellular cAMP increase induces CREB phosphorylation and, subsequently, the activation of steroidogenesis. The βγ dimer of G proteins activates PI3K/AKT-pathway inducing proliferative and anti-apoptotic effects. LH promotes a more potent activation of anti-apoptotic and proliferative signals, mediated by pERK1/2 and pAKT, while hCG mainly activates the steroidogenic signals mediated by cAMP/PKA pathway.

Applications in assisted reproduction

Gonadotropins are widely used in clinical practice for infertility treatment [40]. In ART, hCG was historically chosen to support FSH in ovarian stimulation due to its relatively high availability as an extractive compound obtained from urine of pregnant women and its steroidogenic activity mediated through LHCGR [2].

Although a unique standardized ART approach does not exist, all protocols provide the administration of FSH to achieve multifollicular growth [64]. Depending on the physician's choice, FSH administration may be accompanied by LH or hCG, and several studies attempted to determine the differential impact of LH or hCG on ART outcomes [65], not achieving, however, clear conclusions. Indeed, although different ART protocols are used so far, no definitive indications were achieved in single clinical studies due to highly variable, individual responses to treatments, and lack of standardization of drugs and dosages. LH- and hCG-specific effects emerged by meta-analyzing published data, allowing the inclusion of large dataset in the analysis [66]. In this context, hormone-specific effects demonstrated by in vitro studies are reflected in vivo. This analysis demonstrated that hCG addition during the follicular phase is associated with higher number of oocyte retrieved than what observed by LH addition, which in turn, is linked to higher pregnancy rate when data were corrected for the number of oocytes [66]. These differences would reflect the high steroidogenic potential of hCG, which results in a relatively high number of growing follicles at the expenses of oocyte quality.

hCG is administered in ART cycles to trigger ovulation, although this role is physiologically assigned to LH [67]. An alternative way for clinically triggering oocytes consists in administrating gonadotropin-releasing hormone (GnRH) agonists in a GnRH antagonist downregulated cycle, resulting in LH release by pituitary and ovulation [2,68−70]. Overall, the physiological hCG production is finalized to progesterone production, a required action for supporting intrauterine modifications, embryo implantation and fetus development [71,72]. Therefore, it is growing opinion that hCG may benefit the individualization of luteal phase support in ART [73].

Conclusions

After being considered as equivalent for long time, in vitro studies highlighted differences between LH and hCG, reflecting their physiological functions. LH mediates preferentially proliferative and anti-apoptotic signals crucial for oocyte growth and maturation, while hCG supports pregnancy through its steroidogenic potential. These features may be relevant for assisted reproduction, where hormone-specific functions of the two molecules may be linked to different ART outcome and considered for improving personalized stimulation protocols.

Acknowledgments

This study was supported by the Departments of Excellence Programme of the Italian Ministry of University and Research to the Department of Biomedical, Metabolic, and Neural Sciences, University of Modena and Reggio Emilia, Modena, Italy. This study was also supported by the International Ph.D. School in Clinical and Experimental Medicine (CEM), University of Modena and Reggio Emilia, Modena, Italy. Prof. Manuela Simoni, is an LE STUDIUM Research Fellow, Loire Valley Institute for Advanced Studies, Orleans & Tours, France,

INRA—Centre Val de Loire, 37380 Nouzilly, France, receiving funding from the European Union's Horizon 2020 research and innovation programme under the Marie Skłodowska-Curie grant agreement No. 665790.

References

[1] Ascoli M, Fanelli F, Segaloff DL. The lutropin/choriogonadotropin receptor, a 2002 perspective. Endocr Rev 2002;23(2):141−74.

[2] Casarini L, Santi D, Brigante G, Simoni M. Two hormones for one receptor: evolution, biochemistry, actions, and pathophysiology of LH and hCG. Endocr Rev 2018;39(5): 549−92.

[3] Casarini L, Lispi M, Longobardi S, Milosa F, La Marca A, Tagliasacchi D, Pignatti E, Simoni M. LH and hCG action on the same receptor results in quantitatively and qualitatively different intracellular signalling. PLoS One 2012;7(10):e46682.

[4] Gupta C, Chapekar T, Chhabra Y, Singh P, Sinha S, Luthra K. Differential response to sustained stimulation by hCG & LH on goat ovarian granulosa cells. Indian J Med Res 2012;135:331−40.

[5] Sun PD, Davies DR. The cystine-knot growth-factor superfamily. Annu Rev Biophys Biomol Struct 1995;24(1):269−91.

[6] Szkudlinski MW. New frontier in glycoprotein hormones and their receptors structure−function. Front Endocrinol 2015;6:155.

[7] Casarini L, Huhtaniemi IT, Simoni M, Rivero-Müller A. Gonadotrophin receptors. In: Simoni M, Huhtaniemi I, editors. Endocrinology of the testis and male reproduction. Endocrinology. Cham: Springer; 2017. p. 123−68.

[8] Roch GJ, Sherwood NM. Glycoprotein hormones and their receptors emerged at the origin of metazoans. Genome Biol Evol 2014;6(6):1466−79.

[9] Graves J, Markman S, Alegranti Y, Gechtler J, Johnson RI, Cagan R, Ben-Menahem D. The LH/CG receptor activates canonical signaling pathway when expressed in *Drosophila*. Mol Cell Endocrinol 2015;413:145−56.

[10] Sower SA, Decatur WA, Hausken KN, Marquis TJ, Barton SL, Gargan J, Freamat M, Wilmot M, Hollander L, Hall JA, Nozaki M, Shpilman M, Levavi-Sivan B. Emergence of an ancestral glycoprotein hormone in the pituitary of the sea lamprey, a basal vertebrate. Endocrinology 2015;156(8):3026−37.

[11] Li MD, Ford JJ. A comprehensive evolutionary analysis based on nucleotide and amino acid sequences of the alpha- and beta-subunits of glycoprotein hormone gene family. J Endocrinol 1998;156(3):529−42.

[12] Schöneberg T, Hofreiter M, Schulz A, Römpler H. Learning from the past: evolution of GPCR functions. Trends Pharmacol Sci 2007;28(3):117−21.

[13] Hallast P, Nagirnaja L, Margus T, Laan M. Segmental duplications and gene conversion: human luteinizing hormone/chorionic gonadotropin beta gene cluster. Genome Res 2005;15(11):1535−46.

[14] Nagirnaja L, Rull K, Uusküla L, Hallast P, Grigorova M, Laan M. Genomics and genetics of gonadotropin beta-subunit genes: unique FSHB and duplicated LHB/CGB loci. Mol Cell Endocrinol 2010;329(1−2):4−16.

[15] Cole LA, Khanlian SA, Riley JM, Butler SA. Hyperglycosylated hCG in gestational implantation and in choriocarcinoma and testicular germ cell malignancy tumorigenesis. J Reprod Med 2006;51(11):919−29.

[16] Burczynska BB, Kobrouly L, Butler SA, Naase M, Iles RK. Novel insights into the expression of CGB1 & 2 genes by epithelial cancer cell lines secreting ectopic free hCGβ. Anticancer Res 2014;34(5):2239−48.

[17] Cole LA, Butler S. Hyperglycosylated hCG, hCGβ and Hyperglycosylated hCGβ: interchangeable cancer promoters. Mol Cell Endocrinol 2012;349(2):232−8.

[18] Cole LA. hCG and hyperglycosylated hCG in the establishment and evolution of hemochorial placentation. J Reprod Immunol 2009;82(2):112−8.

[19] Hallast P, Rull K, Laan M. The evolution and genomic landscape of CGB1 and CGB2 genes. Mol Cell Endocrinol 2007;260−262:2−11.

[20] George JW, Dille EA, Heckert LL. Current concepts of follicle-stimulating hormone receptor gene regulation. Biol Reprod 2011;84(1):7−17.

[21] Lazzaretti C, Riccetti L, Sperduti S, Anzivino C, Brigante G, De Pascali F, Potì F, Rovei V, Restagno G, Mari C, Lussiana C, Benedetto C, Revelli A, Casarini L. Inferring biallelism of two FSH receptor mutations associated with spontaneous ovarian hyperstimulation syndrome by evaluating FSH, LH and HCG cross-activity. Reprod Biomed Online 2019;38(5):816−24.

[22] Stenman U-H, Tiitinen A, Alfthan H, Valmu L. The classification, functions and clinical use of different isoforms of HCG. Hum Reprod Update 2006;12(6):769−84.

[23] Stenman U-H, Alfthan H. Determination of human chorionic gonadotropin. Best Pract Res Clin Endocrinol Metabol 2013;27(6):783−93.

[24] Stanton PG, Pozvek G, Burgon PG, Robertson DM, Hearn MT. Isolation and characterization of human LH isoforms. J Endocrinol 1993;138(3):529−43.

[25] Cole LA. hCG, five independent molecules. Clin Chim Acta 2012;413(1−2):48−65.

[26] Gabay R, Rozen S, Samokovlisky A, Amor Y, Rosenfeld R, Kohen F, Amsterdam A, Berger P, Ben-Menahem D. The role of the 3′ region of mammalian gonadotropin β subunit gene in the luteinizing hormone to chorionic gonadotropin evolution. Mol Cell Endocrinol 2014;382(2):781−90.

[27] Wide L, Eriksson K. Dynamic changes in glycosylation and glycan composition of serum FSH and LH during natural ovarian stimulation. Upsala J Med Sci 2013;118(3):153−64.

[28] Wide L. Median charge and charge heterogeneity of human pituitary FSH, LH and TSH. II. Relationship to sex and age. Acta Endocrinol 1985;109(2):190−7.

[29] Wide L, Eriksson K, Sluss PM, Hall JE. Serum half-life of pituitary gonadotropins is decreased by sulfonation and increased by sialylation in women. J Clin Endocrinol Metab 2009;94(3):958−64.

[30] Mak SMJ, Wong WY, Chung HS, Chung PW, Kong GWS, Li TC, Cheung LP. Effect of mid-follicular phase recombinant LH versus urinary HCG supplementation in poor ovarian responders undergoing IVF − a prospective double-blinded randomized study. Reprod Biomed Online 2017;34(3):258−66.

[31] Zeleznik AJ. In vivo responses of the primate corpus luteum to luteinizing hormone and chorionic gonadotropin. Proc Natl Acad Sci USA 1998;95(18):11002−7.

[32] Riccetti L, De Pascali F, Gilioli L, Potì F, Giva LB, Marino M, Tagliavini S, Trenti T, Fanelli F, Mezzullo M, Pagotto U, Simoni M, Casarini L. Human LH and hCG stimulate differently the early signalling pathways but result in equal testosterone synthesis in mouse Leydig cells in vitro. Reprod Biol Endocrinol 2017;15(1):2.

[33] Wallace WHB, Kelsey TW. Human ovarian reserve from conception to the menopause. PLoS One 2010;5(1):e8772.

[34] Yung Y, Aviel-Ronen S, Maman E, Rubinstein N, Avivi C, Orvieto R, Hourvitz A. Localization of luteinizing hormone receptor protein in the human ovary. Mol Hum Reprod 2014;20(9):844−9.

[35] Chappel SC, Howles C. Reevaluation of the roles of luteinizing hormone and follicle-stimulating hormone in the ovulatory process. Hum Reprod 1991;6(9):1206−12.

[36] Jeppesen JV, Kristensen SG, Nielsen ME, Humaidan P, Dal Canto M, Fadini R, Schmidt KT, Ernst E, Andersen CY. LH-receptor gene expression in human granulosa and cumulus cells from antral and preovulatory follicles. J Clin Endocrinol Metab 2012; 97(8):E1524−31.

[37] Casarini L, Santi D, Simoni M, Potì F. Spare' luteinizing hormone receptors: facts and fiction. Trends Endocrinol Metab 2018;29(4):208−17.

[38] Ji I, Lee C, Song Y, Conn PM, Ji TH. Cis − and trans -activation of hormone receptors: the LH receptor. Mol Endocrinol 2002;16(6):1299−308.

[39] Jonas KC, Chen S, Virta M, Mora J, Franks S, Huhtaniemi I, Hanyaloglu AC. Temporal reprogramming of calcium signalling via crosstalk of gonadotrophin receptors that associate as functionally asymmetric heteromers. Sci Rep 2018;8(1):2239.

[40] Niederberger C, Pellicer A, Cohen J, Gardner DK, Palermo GD, O'Neill CL, Chow S, Rosenwaks Z, Cobo A, Swain JE, Schoolcraft WB, Frydman R, Bishop LA, Aharon D, Gordon C, New E, Decherney A, Tan SL, Paulson RJ, Goldfarb JM, Brännström M, Donnez J, Silber S, Dolmans MM, Simpson JL, Handyside AH, Munné S, Eguizabal C, Montserrat N, Izpisua Belmonte JC, Trounson A, Simon C, Tulandi T, Giudice LC, Norman RJ, Hsueh AJ, Sun Y, Laufer N, Kochman R, Eldar-Geva T, Lunenfeld B, Ezcurra D, D'Hooghe T, Fauser BCJM, Tarlatzis BC, Meldrum DR, Casper RF, Fatemi HM, Devroey P, Galliano D, Wikland M, Sigman M, Schoor RA, Goldstein M, Lipshultz LI, Schlegel PN, Hussein A, Oates RD, Brannigan RE, Ross HE, Pennings G, Klock SC, Brown S, Van Steirteghem A, Rebar RW, LaBarbera AR. Forty years of IVF. Fertil Steril 2018;110(2). 185-324, e5.

[41] Makieva S, Saunders PTK, Norman JE. Androgens in pregnancy: roles in parturition. Hum Reprod Update 2014;20(4):542−59.

[42] Cole LA. hCG physiology. Placenta 2013;34(12):1257.

[43] Pitteloud N, Dwyer A. Hormonal control of spermatogenesis in men: therapeutic aspects in hypogonadotropic hypogonadism. Ann Endocrinol 2014;75(2):98−100.

[44] Amsterdam G, Hosokawa Y, Sasson J, Kotsuji. Crosstalk among multiple signaling pathways controlling ovarian cell death. Trends Endocrinol Metab 1999;10(7):255−62.

[45] Craig J, Orisaka M, Wang H, Orisaka S, Thompson W, Zhu C, Kotsuji F, Tsang BK. Gonadotropin and intra-ovarian signals regulating follicle development and atresia: the delicate balance between life and death. Front Biosci: J Vis Lit 2007;12:3628−39.

[46] Conti M. Specificity of the cyclic adenosine 3',5'-monophosphate signal in granulosa cell function. Biol Reprod 2002;67(6):1653−61.

[47] Lee PSN, Buchan AMJ, Hsueh AJW, Yuen BH, Leung PCK. Intracellular calcium mobilization in response to the activation of human wild-type and chimeric gonadotropin receptors. Endocrinology 2002;143(5):1732−40.

[48] Ayoub MA, Landomiel F, Gallay N, Jégot G, Poupon A, Crépieux P, Reiter E. Assessing gonadotropin receptor function by resonance energy transfer-based assays. Front Endocrinol 2015;6:130.

[49] Trehan A, Rotgers E, Coffey ET, Huhtaniemi I, Rivero-Müller A. CANDLES, an assay for monitoring GPCR induced cAMP generation in cell cultures. Cell Commun Signal 2014;12(1):70.

[50] Montminy MR, Bilezikjian LM. Binding of a nuclear protein to the cyclic-AMP response element of the somatostatin gene. Nature 1987;328(6126):175−8.

[51] Casarini L, Riccetti L, De Pascali F, Gilioli L, Marino M, Vecchi E, Morini D, Nicoli A, La Sala GB, Simoni M. Estrogen modulates specific life and death signals induced by LH and hCG in human primary granulosa cells in vitro. Int J Mol Sci 2017;18(5):926.

[52] Riccetti L, Yvinec R, Klett D, Gallay N, Combarnous Y, Reiter E, Simoni M, Casarini L, Ayoub MA. Human luteinizing hormone and chorionic gonadotropin display biased agonism at the LH and LH/CG receptors. Sci Rep 2017;7(1):940.

[53] Casarini L, Reiter E, Simoni M. β-arrestins regulate gonadotropin receptor-mediated cell proliferation and apoptosis by controlling different FSHR or LHCGR intracellular signaling in the hGL5 cell line. Mol Cell Endocrinol 2016;437:11−21.

[54] Zwain IH, Amato P. cAMP-induced apoptosis in granulosa cells is associated with up-regulation of P53 and bax and down-regulation of clusterin. Endocr Res 2001;27(1−2): 233−49.

[55] Kayampilly PP, Menon KM. AMPK activation by dihydrotestosterone reduces FSH-stimulated cell proliferation in rat granulosa cells by inhibiting ERK signaling pathway. Endocrinology 2012;153(6):2831−8.

[56] Menon B, Franzo-Romain M, Damanpour S, Menon KMJ. Luteinizing hormone receptor mRNA down-regulation is mediated through ERK-dependent induction of RNA binding protein. Mol Endocrinol 2011;25(2):282−90.

[57] Ren XR, Reiter E, Ahn S, Kim J, Chen W, Lefkowitz RJ. Different G protein-coupled receptor kinases govern G protein and beta-arrestin-mediated signaling of V2 vaso-pressin receptor. Proc Natl Acad Sci USA 2005;102(5):1448−53.

[58] Brown C, LaRocca J, Pietruska J, Ota M, Anderson L, Smith SD, Weston P, Rasoulpour T, Hixon ML. Subfertility caused by altered follicular development and oocyte growth in female mice lacking PKB alpha/Akt1. Biol Reprod 2010;82(2): 246−56.

[59] Qiu M, Quan F, Han C, Wu B, Liu J, Yang Z, Su F, Zhang Y. Effects of granulosa cells on steroidogenesis, proliferation and apoptosis of stromal cells and theca cells derived from the goat ovary. J Steroid Biochem Mol Biol 2013;138:325−33.

[60] Gilchrist RL, Ryu KS, Ji I, Ji TH. The luteinizing hormone/chorionic gonadotropin receptor has distinct transmembrane conductors for cAMP and inositol phosphate signals. J Biol Chem 1996;271(32):19283−7.

[61] Manna PR, Pakarinen P, El-Hefnawy T, Huhtaniemi IT. Functional assessment of the calcium messenger system in cultured mouse Leydig tumor cells: regulation of human chorionic gonadotropin-induced expression of the steroidogenic acute regulatory protein. Endocrinology 1999;140(4):1739−51.

[62] Pezzi V, Clark BJ, Ando S, Stocco DM, Rainey WE. Role of calmodulin-dependent protein kinase II in the acute stimulation of aldosterone production. J Steroid Biochem Mol Biol 1996;58(4):417−24.

[63] Gudermann T, Birnbaumer M, Birnbaumer L. Evidence for dual coupling of the murine luteinizing hormone receptor to adenylyl cyclase and phosphoinositide breakdown and Ca2+ mobilization. Studies with the cloned murine luteinizing hormone receptor expressed in L cells. J Biol Chem 1992;267(7):4479−88.

[64] Edwards RG, Steptoe PC. Induction of follicular growth, ovulation and luteinization in the human ovary. J Reprod Fertil Suppl 1975;(22):121−63.

[65] Ezcurra D, Humaidan P. A review of luteinising hormone and human chorionic gonadotropin when used in assisted reproductive technology. Reprod Biol Endocrinol 2014; 12:95.

[66] Santi D, Casarini L, Alviggi C, Simoni M. Efficacy of follicle-stimulating hormone (FSH) alone, FSH + Luteinizing hormone, human menopausal gonadotropin or FSH + Human chorionic gonadotropin on assisted reproductive technology outcomes in the "personalized" medicine era: a meta-analysis. Front Endocrinol 2017;8:114.

[67] Al-Inany HG, Abou-Setta AM, Aboulghar MA, Mansour RT, Serour GI. HMG versus rFSH for ovulation induction in developing countries: a cost-effectiveness analysis based on the results of a recent meta-analysis. Reprod Biomed Online 2006;12(2): 163−9.

[68] Albano C, Smitz J, Camus M, Riethmüller-Winzen H, Van Steirteghem A, Devroey P. Comparison of different doses of gonadotropin-releasing hormone antagonist Cetrorelix during controlled ovarian hyperstimulation. Fertil Steril 1997;67(5):917−22.

[69] Diedrich K, Diedrich C, Santos E, Zoll C, al-Hasani S, Reissmann T, et al.. Suppression of the endogenous luteinizing hormone surge by the gonadotrophin-releasing hormone antagonist Cetrorelix during ovarian stimulation. Hum Reprod 1994;9(5):788−91.

[70] Nakano R, Mizuno T, Kotsuji F, Katayama K, Wshio M, Tojo S. "Triggering" of ovulation after infusion of synthetic luteinizing hormone releasing factor (LRF). Acta Obstet Gynecol Scand 1973;52(3):269−72.

[71] Berndt S, Perrier d'Hauterive S, Blacher S, Péqueux C, Lorquet S, Munaut C, Applanat M, Hervé MA, Lamandé N, Corvol P, van den Brûle F, Frankenne F, Poutanen M, Huhtaniemi I, Geenen V, Noël A, Foidart J-M. Angiogenic activity of human chorionic gonadotropin through LH receptor activation on endothelial and epithelial cells of the endometrium. FASEB J 2006;20(14):2630−2.

[72] Cole LA. Biological functions of hCG and hCG-related molecules. Reprod Biol Endocrinol 2010;8(1):102.

[73] Lawrenz B, Coughlan C, Fatemi HM. Individualized luteal phase support. Curr Opin Obstet Gynecol 2019. https://doi.org/10.1097/GCO.0000000000000530.

hCG and human evolution—The human master molecule

1.3

Laurence A. Cole

I refer to human chorionic gonadotropin (hCG) in this chapter as "the human master molecule"; Why do I call it the master molecule? This is because hCG is both the hormone hCG, the autocrine hyperglycosylated hCG, and the autocrine extravillous cytotrophoblast hCG which together controlled human evolution; they also control human pregnancy or human child birth, thus control human life, they also play a part in human malignancy or start human cancers and thus have a key role in human death (inferred). They controlled human evolution of how humans came about and human life and death, making them the human master molecules.

hCG, hyperglycosylated hCG, and extravillous cytotrophoblast hCG

It is important to first understand that the two sets of genes, hCG α-subunit on chromosome 6 and the 7 parallel genes coding for hCG β-subunit on chromosome 19 code for three independent molecules, the hormone hCG, the autocrine hyperglycosylated hCG, and the autocrine extravillous cytotrophoblast hCG, all having identical amino acid sequence and varying in carbohydrate structure [1,2]. The hormone hCG binds the hCG/luteinizing hormone (LH) joint hormone receptor on ovarian cells and trophoblast cells [3,4], while hyperglycosylated hCG and extravillous cytotrophoblast hCG bind an autocrine transforming growth factor-β-II (TGFβ-II) receptor on cytotrophoblast cells and cancer cells [5—7]. The whole difference between the hormone and the autocrines is due to just four different O-linked oligosaccharides on the two sets of molecules [1,2]. The whole difference between hyperglycosylated hCG and extravillous cytotrophoblast hCG is due to biantennary and triantennary N-linked oligosaccharides on the β-subunit [1,2].

The hormone hCG codes for generation and maintenance of hemochorial placentation or the fetal feeding system during pregnancy [8,9]. hCG also drives corpus luteal progesterone production during pregnancy [4], suppression of myometrial contractions during pregnancy [10,11], and suppression of maternal macrophage

100 Years of Human Chorionic Gonadotropin. https://doi.org/10.1016/B978-0-12-820050-6.00003-5

destruction of fetal and maternal tissues during pregnancy [12,13]. hCG is also produced by pituitary gonadotrope cells during the course of the menstrual cycle, running ovarian steroidogenesis, ovulation, and luteogenesis [7,14,15].

In contrast, the autocrine hyperglycosylated hCG and the autocrine extravillous cytotrophoblast hCG drive implantation of the blastocyst, assist in generation of hemochorial placentation, drive deep implantation of the hemochorial placentation [7−9,16], and drive placenta growth during pregnancy [17]. Extravillous cytotrophoblast hCG also drives malignancy in cancer cells [18,19].

All told, there are three molecules that derive from the hCG α-subunit and β-subunit genes, all having identical amino acid sequences that together are master molecules running human pregnancy (described in this chapter), driving human cancer [18,19], and driving the evolutionary creation of humans (described in this chapter).

Multiple hCG and hyperglycosylated hCG production sites

In pregnancy, placental cytotrophoblast cells fuse together to make multinuclear fused syncytiotrophoblast cells and highly differentiated villous cytotrophoblast cells and extravillous cytotrophoblast cells (Fig. 1.3.1). The simplistic cytotrophoblast cells

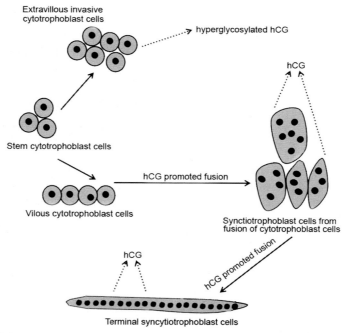

FIGURE 1.3.1

The fusing of placental cytotrophoblast cells to syncytiotrophoblast cells.

process glycoproteins in one way making the autocrine hyperglycosylated hCG and extravillous cytotrophoblast hCG with type 2 pentasaccharide and hexasaccharide O-linked oligosaccharides and triantennary N-linked oligosaccharides on extravillous cytotrophoblast hCG. The fused syncytiotrophoblast cells make glycoproteins in another way making just the hormone hCG with type 1 trisaccharide and tetrasaccharide O-linked oligosaccharide structures and biantennary N-linked oligosaccharides. As explained in the following chapter, the O-linked oligosaccharides alone dictate the final three-dimensional structure of the autocrine hyperglycosylated hCG and extravillous cytotrophoblast hCG and the hormone hCG, and there very different processing upon secretion, leading to three very separate molecules [1].

The hormone hCG is produced by syncytiotrophoblast cells in pregnancy. It is also produced by pituitary gonadotrope cells, hormone pituitary sulfated hCG, produced during the menstrual cycle [14,15], and by kidney and liver cells, of the human fetus, fetal hCG, during pregnancy [20,21].

The autocrine hyperglycosylated hCG is produced by cytotrophoblast cells during pregnancy and the autocrine extravillous cytotrophoblast hCG produced by extravillous cytotrophoblast cells. All cancer cells also produce extravillous cytotrophoblast hCG, it is stolen by all the cancer cells, it is the agent of malignancy, driving malignancy in cancer cells [18,19].

Human evolution

hCG and hyperglycosylated hCG drove the evolution of humans. hCG and hyperglycosylated hCG came into existence or first evolved with early primates, with Callicebus, the early anthropoid primates which evolved 37 million years ago (Table 1.3.1). A primitive form of CG (no h because not human) evolved, pI $= 6.3$, circulating half-life 2.4 hours. This first form of CG and hyperglycosylated CG permitted primates to adopt hemochorial placentation for the first time, a more efficient form of fetal feeding. This allows seven brain growth genes to function for the first time, and for brain growth to start [22,23].

With brain growth, the brain grew from 0.07% of total body weight, found in two ancestors, tarsiers and lemurs (Table 1.3.1), to 0.17% and 0.18% of total body weight in Aotus and Callicebus (2.4X) (Table 1.3.1). Aotus had more advanced hCG β-subunit amino acid sequence than Callicebus, so it is assumed that Callicebus evolved first.

Then, as species evolved, seemingly species by species, CG became more acidic and even more acidic, circulating for longer and longer, gaining more and more biological potency. As the potency of CG increased, it promoted hemochorial placentation more efficiently and even more efficiently. As hemochorial placentation became more and more efficient, it permitted the seven brain growth genes to promote brain growth more and more efficient. As brain growth genes became more potent, they promoted the growth of the brain further and further [22,23]. Looking at species which have been investigated, Callicebus which evolved 37 million years ago had a hCG of pI $= 6.3$ and had a brain of 0.17% (2.4X lemur and tarsier brain) of

Table 1.3.1 The evolution of CG.

Species	Family Evolved ya	Sugar side chains on CG β-subunit	pI	Clearance rate	Depth of implantation	Brain mass % body weight
Homo sapien	200,000 ya	6 sugar chains	pI = 3.5	36 h	30%	2.4% (34X)
Homo heidelbergensis, Hominini	400,000 ya		Extinct	Extinct	Extinct	2.1% (30X)
Homo erectus, Hominini	1,000,000 ya		Extinct	Extinct	Extinct	1.6% (23X)
Homo ergaster, Hominini	1,800,000 ya		Extinct	Extinct	Extinct	1.1% (16X)
Homo habilis, Hominini	2,000,000 ya	5 sugar chains (As)	Extinct	Extinct	Extinct	1.2% (16X)
Australopithecus garhi, Hominini	2,500,000 ya		Extinct	Extinct	Extinct	
Australopithecus africanus, Hominini	2,700,000 ya		Extinct	Extinct	Extinct	0.86% (12X)
Australopithecus afarensis, Hominini	3,500,000 ya		Extinct	Extinct	Extinct	0.83% (12X)
Australopithecus anamensis, Hominini	4,000,000 ya				Extinct	0.74% (11X)
Ardipithecus ramidus, Hominini	4,300,000 ya					
Orrorin tugensis, Hominini	6,000,000 ya					
Sahelanthropus tchadensis, Hominini	7,000,000 ya					
Chimpanzee, Hominidae	6,000,000 ya					
Orangutan, Hominidae	12,000,000 ya	4 sugar chains	pI = 4.9	6.0 h	10%	0.74% (11X)

Hominidae great apes	4–12 mya					
Bonobo, Hominidae	4–12 mya					
Hominidae great apes	4–22 mya					
Hominoidea	12–22 mya					
Colobus, Hominoidea	20,000,000 ya					
Homoinoidea	12–22 mya					
Baboon, Catarrhine	20,000,000 ya	4 sugar chains	pl = 5.6	4.7 h	ND	0.47% (6.7X)
Macaque	24,000,000 ya					
Aotus, anthropoid	37,000,000 ya	3 sugar chains	pl = 6.2	2.6 h	1%	0.18% (2.4X)
Callicebus, anthropoid	37,000,000 ya	3 sugar chains	pl = 6.3	2.4 h	1%	0.17% (2.4X)
Tarsier, Tarsiidae family	45,000,000 ya					
Catarrhine monkeys	45,000,000 ya					
Lemur, Strepsirrhini	55,000,000 ya		pl = 8.0			

Shown in italics are species in which all information is available on CG. Shown in regular text are established evolutionary between links between species for which information is available. Some species like chimpanzee, orangutan, bonobo, and lemur are divergences and not direct lines of human evolution. Human evolution as indicated by species, pl and brain sizes are published data (22,23). Ya, years ago; ND, not determined; As, assumed.

body weight. Aotus had a pI = 6.2 which evolved 37 million years ago and had a brain of 0.18% (2.6X lemur and tarsier brain) of total body weight. Baboons which evolved 20 million years ago produced a hCG of pI 5.6 and had a brain of 0.47% (6.7X) of body weight. Orangutan which evolved 12 million years ago had a hCG of pI = 4.9 and had a brain of 0.74% (11X) of body weight. *Homo habilis* which evolved 2 million years ago had a brain of 1.2% (16X), and humans which evolved 0.2 million years ago have an hCG of pI 3.5 and have a brain size of 2.4% (32X) of body weight [22,23]. This is how the large human brain came about. Fingers evolved as did use of tools and bipedal involvement all evolved parallel to brain size. This is how human evolved, all under the control of CG and acidity of CG.

The hormone hCG, hyperglycosylated hCG, and extravillous cytotrophoblast hCG are the three most acidic protein produced in humans or are an extreme, pI = 3.5. Acidity of a protein is at its limit in humans and cannot go any further than hCG or hyperglycosylated hCG. Further acidity would destabilize a protein and not permit folding. As such, humans are the end or the final end product of this brain expansion pathway, not superhumans or any future evolved species.

The hormone hCG, hyperglycosylated hCG, and extravillous cytotrophoblast hCG first evolved from LH β-subunit in Callicebus (Fig. 1.3.2). LH β-subunit gene underwent duplication, one copy then underwent a deletion mutation leading to read through the termination codon on the LH β-subunit gene, and expansion from coding for 121 amino acids to that coding for 145 amino acids (Fig. 1.3.2). This led to the creation of the first CG β-subunit gene [22,23]. This is where everything started. LH itself evolved directly from TGFβ, thus the reason that hyperglycosylated CG and extravillous cytotrophoblast hCG bind a TGFβ-II receptor.

It is estimated that the changes in CG, Callicebus to human, occurred over approximately 58 species. This is an estimate; 11 species directly linking humans to *Sahelanthropus tchadensis*, all species in between identified, over 7.0 million years, 11/7.0 or 1.57 species per million years. 1.57 X 37 = 58 species per 37 million years or 58 species linking humans to Callicebus. This research indicates that a continuous acidity evolution covering 58 species linked Callicebus to humans.

Table 1.3.2 shows changes in the amino acid sequence of β-subunit Callicebus to humans [22,23]. As shown, 20 amino acids get changed on the β-subunit C-terminal peptide, residues 106—145 and 17 get changed in the balance of the molecule. There are also five amino acids that undergo multiple changes. This is 20 + 17 + 5 or 42 changes total between Aotus and Callicebus and humans. These changes lead to the appearance of two (Callicebus), three (Baboon), and four (*Homo habilis*) acidic O-linked oligosaccharides and one additional N-linked oligosaccharide (humans).

Not every mutation leads to changes in amino acid coding. There are in the genetic code 64 combinations of A, T, C, and G, and just 20 amino acids coded for. There are three codon coding for the termination codon and 61 codons coding for amino acids or 61/20 3.05 codons assigned to each amino acid. Generally speaking, the third nucleotide in each codon has the least effect on changing the amino acid coded for as a result of a point mutation. As such, much more than 42 mutations

Aotus/Callicebus LH ß-subunit, 121 amino acids

CCC **CA**A **C**TC TCA GGC CTC CTC TTC CTC **TAA**   DNA code
Pro Gln Leu Ser Gln Leu Leu Phe Leu   Amino acids
113 114   115 116   117 118   119 120   121 stop

The deletion mutation in Aotus/Callicebus LH ß-subunit

deletion

CCC **CA** **C** TCT CAT CAG GCC TCC TCT TCC TC**T AA**G

The result, Aotus/Callicebus CG ß-subunit, 145 amino acids

CCC **CAC** TCT CAG GCC TCC TCT TCC TC**T AA**G GCC CCT
Pro **Arg** Phe Gln Asp Ser Ser Ser Ser Lys Ala Pro
113 **114** 115 116   117 118   119 120 121 122   123   124

CCC CCC AGC CTT CCA AGT CCA TCC CGA CTC CCG GGG
Pro Pro Ser Leu Pro Ser Pro Ser Arg Leu Pro Gly
125 126   127 128 129   130   131 132 133 134 135   136

CCC TCG GAC ACC CCG ATC CTC CCA CAA **TAA**   DNA code
Pro Ser Asp Thr Pro Ile Leu Pro Gln stop   Amino acids
137 138   139 140 141   142 143   144 145

FIGURE 1.3.2

The deletion mutation of LH β-subunit to create hCG β-subunit.

would be needed for the 42 amino acid changes. It is estimated that all or 58 of 58 species in between Aotus and Callicebus and humans would have had to have point mutation in the CG β-subunit gene to have driven the 42 amino acid changes in CG Aotus/Callicebus to humans.

In conclusion, CG led a massive long evolution pathway involving at least 58 in-between species to drive hemochorial placentation advancement and brain gene promotion in Aotus/Callicebus to humans [22,23].

A total of seven distinct brain growth genes have now been identified coding for brain growth factors in humans and primates. These are the MCPH1 gene also known as microcephalin gene [24–26], WDR62 gene [27], CDK5RAP2 gene [28], CEP152 gene [29], ASPM gene [30], CENPJ gene [28], and STIL gene [31].

Table 1.3.2 Amino acid sequences of CG species. Amino acids which are changed from species to species are shown below the sequence for humans.

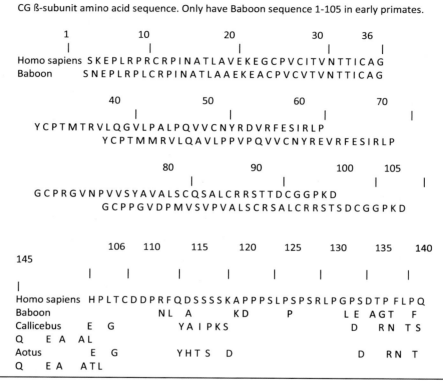

CG ß-subunit amino acid sequence. Only have Baboon sequence 1-105 in early primates.

```
                     1            10          20          30      36
                     |            |           |           |       |
        Homo sapiens S K E P L R P R C R P I N A T L A V E K E G C P V C I T V N T T I C A G
        Baboon       S N E P L R P L C R P I N A T L A A E K E A C P V C V T V N T T I C A G


                     40           50          60          70
                     |            |           |           |
        Y C P T M T R V L Q G V L P A L P Q V V C N Y R D V R F E S I R L P
            Y C P T M M R V L Q A V L P P V P Q V V C N Y R E V R F E S I R L P


                     80           90          100   105
                     |            |           |     |
        G C P R G V N P V V S Y A V A L S C Q S A L C R R S T T D C G G P K D
            G C P P G V D P M V S V P V A L S C R S A L C R R S T S D C G G P K D


                     106  110     115    120    125    130    135    140
              145
               |    |    |        |      |      |      |      |      |
               |
        Homo sapiens H P L T C D D P R F Q D S S S S K A P P P S L P S P S R L P G P S D T P F L P Q
        Baboon                       N L   A        K D          P         L E   A G T     F
        Callicebus         E    G         Y A I P K S                          D     R N   T S
        Q         E A  A L
        Aotus              E    G          Y H T S   D                         D     R N   T
        Q         E A  A T L
```

Amino acids are abbreviated: A, alanine; C, cystine; D, aspartic acid; E, glutamic acid; F, phenylalanine; G, glycine; H, histidine; I, isoleucine; K, lysine; L, leucine; N, asparagine; P, proline; Q, glutamine; R, arginine; S, serine; T, threonine; V, valine; and Y, tyrosine.

Small mutational differences have been noted in MCPH1, ASPM, CD5RAP2, CENPJ genes in early and advanced primates and humans, indicating gene and brain growth factor advancement with evolution [24,25,28,30]. These brain growth genes driven by consistently advancing hemochorial placentation, driven by CG, promoted the evolution of humans.

It has been estimated that CG became more and more acidic between Callicebus and humans because of an accumulation of acidic amino acids, Glu, and Asp, and because of the addition of three acidic sugar side chains, two O-linked and one N-linked. The odds of point mutations adding Glu and Asp, 2 of 20 amino acids are 1 in 10, and the odds of sugar side chains being added involve the presence of specific amino acid in a sequence: Ser in O-linked oligosaccharides and Asn in

N-linked oligosaccharides. The sequence is always proceeded by three amino acids by Pro (Pro-X-X-X-Ser) when O-linked oligosaccharides are added and followed by two amino acids later by Thr when N-linked oligosaccharides are added (Asn-X-Thr), thus two specific amino acids are added making the odds 1 in 400.

Considering 58 species lie in the acidity evolution including three acidic sugars, the odds of the acidity evolution, stepwise increasing acidity over 58 species would be 1 in 64 x 1061. These odds are very extreme, almost impossible that this event just happened naturally in nature. Someone or something had to interfere with nature allowing this evolution, Callicebus to humans, to have occurred, and I like to believe that this was God.

References

[1] Cole LA. The carbohydrate structure of the hormone hCG, the autocrine hyperglycosylated hCG, and the extravillous cytotrophoblast hyperglycosylated hCG. J Glycobiol 2019;7 (in press).

[2] Elliott MM, Kardana A, Lustbader JW, Cole LA. Carbohydrate and Peptide structure of the α- and β-subunits of human chorionic gonadotropin from normal and aberrant pregnancy and choriocarcinoma. Endocrine 1997;7:15−32.

[3] Toth P, Li X, Rao CV, Lincoln SR, Sanfillipino JS, Spinnato JA, Yussman MA. Expression of functional human chorionic gonadotropin/human luteinizing hormone receptor gene in human uterine arteries. J Clin Endocrinol Metab 1994;79:307−15.

[4] Niswender GD. Molecular control of luteal secretion of progesterone. Reproduccion 2002;123:333−9.

[5] Butler SA, Ikram MS, Mathieu S, Iles RK. The increase in bladder carcinoma cell population induced by the free beta subunit of hCG is a result of an anti-apoptosis effect and not cell proliferation. Br J Cancer 2000;82:1553−6.

[6] Berndt S, Blacher S, Munuat C, Detilleux J, Evain-Brion D, Noel A, Fournier T, Foidart JM. Hyperglycosylated human chorionic gonadotropin stimulates angiogenesis through TGF-ß receptor activation. FASEB J 2013;12:213686.

[7] Ahmud F, Ghosh S, Sinha S, Joshi SD, Mehta VS, Sen E. TGF-ß-induced hCG-ß regulates redox homeostasis in glioma cells. Mol Cell Biochem 2015;399:105−12.

[8] Cole LA. In: Nicholson R, editor. hCG and hyperglycosylated hCG, promoters of villous placenta and hemochorial placentation. Placenta: functions, development and disease. Nova Publishers; 2013. p. 155−66.

[9] Cole LA. Chapter 15: the placenta, hemochorial placentation, and implantation. In: Cole LA, editor. The biology and medical dynamics of human reproduction. New York: Nova Science Publishing; 2013.

[10] Eta E, Ambrus G, Rao V. Direct regulation of human myometrial contractions by human chorionic gonadotropin. J Clin Endocrinol Metab 1994;79:1582−6.

[11] Doheny HC, Houlihan DD, Ravikumar N, Smith TJ, Morrison JJ. Human chorionic gonadotrophin relaxation of human pregnant myometrium and activation of the BKCa channel. J Clin Endocrinol Metab 2003;88:4310−5.

[12] Duncan WC, Rodger FE, Illingworth PJ. The human corpus luteum: reduction in macrophages during simulated maternal recognition of pregnancy. Hum Reprod 1998;13:2435−42.

[13] Matsuura T, Sugimura M, Iwaki T, Ohashi R, Kanayama N, Nishihira J. Anti-macrophage inhibitory factor antibody inhibits PMSG-hCG-induced follicular growth and ovulation in mice. J Assist Reprod Genet 2002;19:591−5.

[14] Birken S, Maydelman Y, Gawinowicz MA, Pound A, Liu Y, Stockell Hartree A. Isolation and characterization of human pituitary chorionic gonadotropin. Endocrinology 1996;137:1402−11.

[15] Stenman UH, Alfthan H, Ranta T, Vartiainen E, Jalkanen J, Sepppala M. Serum levels of human chorionic gonadotropin in nonpregnant women and men are modulated by gonadotropin-releasing hormone and sex steroids. J Clin Endocrinol Metab 1987;64: 730−6.

[16] Cole LA. Hyperglycosylated hCG and pregnancy failures. J Reprod Immunol 2012;93: 119−22.

[17] Brennan MC, Wolfe MD, Murray-Krezan C, Cole LA, Rayburn WF. First trimester hyperglycosylated human chorionic gonadotropin and development of hypertension. Prenat Diagn 2013;33:1075−9.

[18] Cole LA. A cure fror cancer. In: Cole LA and Butler SA eds. 100 years of hCG, Elsevier, Oxford U.K.

[19] Cole LA. hCG and cancer. Gynecol Oncol 2019 (in press).

[20] Goldsmith PC, McGregor WG, Raymoure WJ, Kuhn RW, Jaffe RB. Cellular localization of chorionic gonadotropin in human fetal kidney and liver. J Clin Endocrinol Metab 1983;57:54−61.

[21] Abdallah MA, Lei ZM, Li X, Greenwold N, Nakajima ST, Jauniaux E, Rao CV. Human Fetal nongonadal tissues contain human chorionic gonadotropin/luteinizing hormone receptors. J Clin Endocrinol Metab 2004;89:952−6.

[22] Cole LA. hCG and hyperglycosylated hCG in the establishment and evolution of hemochorial placentation. J Reprod Immunol 2009;82:112−8.

[23] Cole LA. The evolution of the primate, hominid and human brain. Primatology 2015;4: 1000124.

[24] Shi L, Li M, Lin Q, Qi X, Su B. Functional divergence of the brain-size regulating gene MCPH1 during primate evolution and the origin of humans. BMC Biol 2013;11:62.

[25] Wang YQ, Su B. Molecular evolution of microcephalin, a gene determining human brain size. Hum Mol Genet 2004;13:1131−7.

[26] Jackson AP, Eastwood H, Bell SM, Adu J, Toomes C, Carr IM, Roberts E, Hampshire DJ, Crow TJ, Mighell AJ, Karbani G, Jafri H, Rashid Y, Mueller RE, Markham AF, Woods CG. Identification of microcephalin, a protein implicated in determining the size of the human brain. Am J Hum Genet 2002;71:136−42.

[27] Nicholas AK, Khurshid M, Désir J, Carvalho OP, Cox JJ, Thorton G, Kauar R, Ansar M, Ahmad W, Verloes A, Passemard S, Misson JP, Lindsay S, Gergely F, Dobyns WB, Roberts E, Abramowicz M, Woods CG. WDR62 is associated with the spindle pole and is mutated in human microcephaly. Nat Genet 2010;42:1010−4.

[28] Bond J, Roberts E, Springell K, Lizarraga SB, Scott S, Higgins J, Hampshire DJ, Morrison EE, Leal GF, ESilva EO, Costa SMR, Baralle D, Raponi M, Karbani G, Rashid Y, Jafri H, Bennett C, Corry P, Walsh CA, Woods CG. A centrosomal mechanism involving CDK5RAP2 and CENPJ controls brain size. Nat Genet 2005;37:353−5.

[29] Guernsey DL, Jiang H, Hussin J, Arnold M, Bouyakdan K, Perry S, Babineau-Sturk T, Beis J, Dumas N, Evans SC, Ferguson M, Matsuoka M, Macgillivray C, Nightingale M, Patry L, Rideout AL, Thomas A, Orr A, Hoffmann I, Michaud JL, Awadalla P,

Meek DC, Ludman M, Samuels ME. Mutations in centrosomal protein CEP152 in primary microcephaly families linked to MCPH4. Am J Hum Genet 2010;87:40–51.

[30] Kouprina N, Pavlicek A, Mochida GH, Solomon G, Gersch W, Yoon YH, Collura R, Ruvolo M, Barrett JC, Woods CG, Walsh CA, Jurka J, Larionov V. Accelerated evolution of the ASPM gene controlling brain size begins prior tohuman brain expansion. PLoS Biol 2004;2:E126.

[31] Kumar A, Girimaji SC, Duvvari MR, Blanton SH. Mutations in STIL, encoding a pericentriolar and centrosomal protein, cause primary microcephaly. Am J Hum Genet 2009;84:286–90.

Human chorionic gonadotropin: different origins, glycoforms, and functions during pregnancy

1.4

Thierry Fournier

Role in pregnancy

After implantation, human chorionic gonadotropin (hCG) is the first trophoblast signal detected in the maternal blood and is used to diagnose pregnancy. hCG and free hCGβ are detected in the maternal blood from the first week of gestation (WG), and their levels increase until reaching a peak at 10−12 WG and then decrease gradually, whereas hCGα levels increase progressively up to term [1]. Maintenance of pregnancy during the first trimester depends on the synthesis of hCG, which prevents regression of the corpus luteum [2] allowing the maintenance of ovarian progesterone secretion [3]. In addition to its well-established endocrine role, hCG has a role in promoting angiogenesis in the uterine endothelium [4], in maintaining the quiescence of the myometrium [5], in contributing to maternal immune tolerance by regulating T cells [6], regulatory T cells (Treg), dendritic cells [7], uNK cells [8,9], and regulatory B cells [10]. hCG also controls the syncytiotrophoblast (ST) formation in an autocrine manner through binding to the LHCGR [11]. Binding of hCG to its receptor activates adenylate cyclase, phospholipase C, and ion channels, which in turn control cellular cAMP, inositol phosphates, and Ca^{2+} [12]. Cyclic AMP, via cyclic-AMP-dependent protein kinases (PKAs), promotes cytotrophoblast fusion in vitro [13] and also elevates mRNA and protein levels of the fusogenic protein syncytin-1 in cultured trophoblasts [14].

Genes and peptides

Specific to the humans and anthropoid primates, hCG is a complex glycoprotein of about 37 kDa composed of two glycosylated subunits, which are noncovalently associated. hCGα subunit is identical to the pituitary gonadotropin hormones

100 Years of Human Chorionic Gonadotropin. **https://doi.org/10.1016/B978-0-12-820050-6.00004-7**

(luteinizing hormone, LH; follicle-stimulating hormone, FSH; thyroid-stimulating hormone, TSH), contains 92 amino acids with two N-glycosylation sites and is encoded by a single gene (CGA) located on chromosome 6q21.1−23 [15]. hCGβ contains 145 amino acids with two sites of N-glycosylation and four sites of O-glycosylation, and is encoded by a cluster of genes that have evolved by duplication from LHβ. The hCGβ subunit is encoded by any one of the six nonallelic genes CGB8, CGB7, CGB5, CGB3, CGB2, and CGB1 present on chromosome 19q13.32 [16,17]. CGB1 and CGB2 are two pseudogenes, whereas the other CGB genes are regrouped in two subtypes: type 1 (CGB7) and type 2 (CGB3, CGB5, CGB8), which correspond to two proteins with a three amino acids' difference [18] (Fig. 1.4.1). It was shown that in first trimester, both type 1 and type 2 CGB were expressed by the villous trophoblast in situ and in vitro [19]. CGB5 is the most actively transcribed in the placenta and contributes to about 65% of the total pool of β-subunit mRNA transcripts in the placenta. CGB8 represents the second most transcribed gene [20,21]. In comparison, CGB3 is less transcribed and CGB7 expression is weak [17,20−23]. Buckberry et al. reported that all seven genes were more expressed in female compared to male placentas [24]. Because hCGα is produced in large excess along pregnancy, hCGβ expression represents a step limiting for hCG synthesis.

Regulation of gene expression

Regulation of hCG gene expression has been studied by analysis of CGA and CGB5 promoters. CGA and CGB expressions are controlled by transcription factors such as AP2 and SP1 that recognize specific response elements in their promoters [25−27].

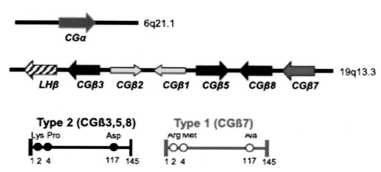

FIGURE 1.4.1

Location and organization of *CGA* gene and *LH-CGB* cluster of genes. *CGB3, CGB5,* and *CGB8* encode for type 2 β-subunit, *CGB7* encodes for type 1 β-subunit, which differs from type 2 by three amino acids.

hCG expression is regulated by hormones (corticoids, progesterone, GnRH), oxygen levels, growth factors, and cytokines such as EGF, TNFα, cAMP [28], and by the homeobox gene DLX3 [29]. The role of oxygen in the regulation of hCG and the implication of HIF remain unclear. hCG expression is decreased in term villous trophoblast cultured in vitro under 9% oxygen level compared to 20% [30]. More recently, it was shown in situ and in vitro that villous trophoblast isolated from early first trimester (8–9 WG) while chorionic villous physiological oxygen environment is about 2% –3%, produced more hCG than cells isolated from 12 to 14 WG when oxygen levels in the intervillous space raised up to 8% due to the entry of unrestricted arterial maternal blood flow after release of endovascular trophoblast plugs [19,31].

Another major regulator of hCG is the nuclear receptor PPARγ [32,33] shown to be essential for placental development, uterine placental vascularization, and fetal growth in vivo in mice [34–36] and in differentiation of both human villous and extravillous trophoblast in vitro [37–39]. Surprisingly, it was reported that secretion of hCG as well as expression of *CGA* and *CGB* transcripts was inversely regulated by PPARγ in endocrine villous compared to invasive extravillous cytotrophoblasts (EVTs) primary cultures obtained from first trimester chorionic villi [33]. In primary villous trophoblast, PPARγ activation increases hCG production in first [33] and third trimesters [40,41], while in primary invasive EVCT, hCG was downregulated at both transcript and protein levels [33] (Fig. 1.4.2).

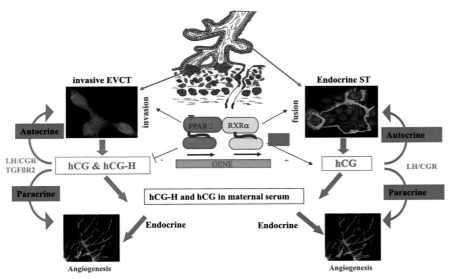

FIGURE 1.4.2

hCG is a PPARG target gene: different sources of production, different glycoforms, and functions. The syncytiotrophoblast (ST in green) secretes hCG that signals through LHCGR. The invasive extravillous cytotrophoblast (EVT in red) secretes both hCG and hCG-H, the latter signaling through TGFβ-RII.

Structure of the glycoprotein

hCG is a highly glycosylated molecule and contains about 30% of carbohydrate in mass. The sugar branches covalently bound to the peptide chains consist of O-linked oligosaccharide containing an N-acetylgalactosamine residue linked to either a serine residue and N-linked oligosaccharide containing an N-acetylglucosamine residue linked to an asparagine residue. The α subunit contains two N glycosylation sites and the β subunit, two N and four O glycosylation sites [42]. The secretion, biological activity, and half-life of hCG are highly dependent on the glycosylated state of the molecule (microheterogeneity due to the variability of oligosaccharide moiety). The sialic acid content of hCG has a major significance in its receptor binding ability, biological activity, and clearance from the maternal circulation [43].

A hyperglycosylated form of hCG (hCG-H) or invasive trophoblast antigen (ITA) has been characterized from urine of a patient with choriocarcinoma [44]. An antibody (B152) was raised against the O-linked oligosaccharides of the β subunit [45]. Hyperglycosylated hCG (hCG-H) is a glycoprotein with the same polypeptide structure as hCG, and much larger N- and O-linked oligosaccharides. The oligosaccharides increase the molecular weight of hCG from 36−37 kDa to 40−41 kDa, depending on the extent of hyperglycosylation. hCG-H has triantennary N-linked oligosaccharides and double molecular size O-linked oligosaccharides (hexasaccharide compared with predominantly trisaccharide structures) [46].

Placental source of production

The ST is the main source of hCG production during pregnancy. The placenta is a transient organ necessary for implantation, adaptation of the mother to pregnancy, fetal development and growth, and pregnancy outcome. The human placenta is characterized by extensive invasion of uterus wall by the trophoblast, allowing direct contact of cytotrophoblasts with maternal blood (hemochorial placenta), by remodeling of uterine vasculature, and by the extent and specificity of its hormonal production. Chorionic villi represent the structural and functional unit of the human placenta and are bathed—from about 12 WG—in maternal blood via the spiral arteries. After the initial phase of nidation, human trophoblasts differentiate along either the villous or EVT pathway [47] (Fig. 1.4.3).

The mononucleated villous cytotrophoblasts (VCTs) form an epithelium that covers the floating chorionic villi containing the fetal-placental vessels. The VCTs aggregate and fuse with the outer layer, a multinucleated ST, allowing the renewal of the ST throughout pregnancy. The ST is in direct contact with maternal blood within the intervillous space and ensures exchanges of gases and nutrients between the mother and the fetus. The ST represents also the hormonal tissue of the placenta, secreting large amounts of steroid and peptide hormones including hCG. Therefore, any anomalies in formation and renewal of the ST by cell-cell fusion

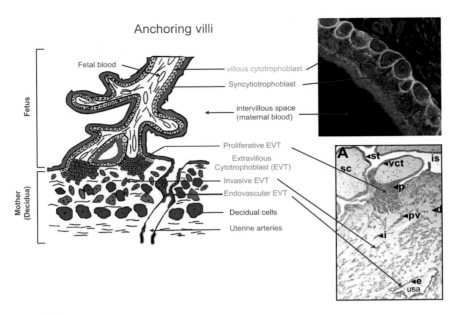

FIGURE 1.4.3

Human trophoblast differentiation. This scheme depicts a chorionic villus anchored in the decidua at the maternal fetal interface. It is composed of a stromal core (sc) containing fetal vessels surrounding by a monolayer of VCT (yellow) that have the ability to fuse to form the ST (green). At the tip of the villus, EVTs (red) are proliférative (p), then undergo EMT, and invade the decidua basalis (i) and the usa (e). Confocal microscopy (yellow = CK7; cyan = DNA; magenta = actin F). Immunohistochemistry: staining of human trophoblasts at the implantation site (CK7).

process will interfere with the main functions of the placenta and directly alter fetal growth and pregnancy outcome.

EVTs are located at the tip of the anchoring chorionic villi in contact with the *decidua basalis*. They are involved in anchoring the placenta within the uterine wall and participate to immune tolerance of the conceptus and to the remodeling of uterine placental vascularization. EVTs proliferate to form multilayered columns of cells, undergo an epithelial mesenchymal transition, exit cell cycle, and invade uterine wall up to the upper third of the myometrium. EVTs also specifically migrate toward and invade uterine arterioles through endovascular or perivascular routes and replace the endothelial lining and most of the musculoelastic tissue, leading to low-resistance vessels that escape to vasomotor molecules. During the early first trimester, blood flow to the placenta is severely restricted, due to obstruction of uterine vessels by migrating trophoblastic cells [31]. During physiologic remodeling of these arteries, trophoblastic plugs disappear, allowing unrestricted flow of maternal blood to the intervillous space. Thus, prior to around 10 weeks of amenorrhea (WG), oxygen concentrations in the intervillous space are approximately 2.5% (pO$_2$ of 20 mmHg), whereas after the onset of maternal blood flow to the placenta (at about 12 WG), oxygen concentrations in the intervillous space rise to approximately 6% $-$8%, corresponding to a pO$_2$ of about 60 mmHg [48,49]. This invasion process and remodeling of the uterine arterioles occur during the first trimester and are essential for placental development and to provide an adequate supply of maternal blood to the developing fetus.

It has been extensively reported that the ST represents the main source of hCG production whose 99% is secreted from the basal side of the ST into maternal blood. Interestingly, it has been reported in situ and in vitro that ST from early first trimester (8$-$9 WG) produce more hCG (transcripts and protein levels and secreted hCG) than trophoblasts from later gestation (12$-$14 WG) when oxygenated arterial maternal blood enter into the intervillous space and bath the chorionic villi [19]. This observation explains in part the maternal plasmatic peak of hCG observed during the first trimester of pregnancy. Other hypothesis have been suggested such as (1) the presence of the truncated form of the LHCG receptor that would block autocrine regulation of hCG synthesis and (2) high levels of GnRH that would upregulate hCG expression through an autocrine/paracrine mechanism [50].

In addition to the ST, it has been shown in situ and in vitro that human invasive extravillous trophoblasts (EVT stained negative for the cell cycle KI67 marker) also produce and secrete hCG, suggesting an autocrine/paracrine function at the maternal-fetal interface [32]. After normalization to trophoblast DNA, it was reported that invasive EVTs secrete in cell supernatant about 50% of hCG in comparison to hCG secreted by the ST differentiated in vitro and isolated from the same first trimester chorionic villi [33]. Interestingly and by contrast to the ST, the α subunit in EVT is not expressed in large excess compared to the beta subunit. Therefore, the ratio hCGα/hCGβ is about 100-fold lower in EVT compared to the ST suggesting that in EVTs the β-subunit might not be the limiting step for hCG synthesis as it is for the ST [33]. These results suggest that hCG from invasive EVT origin is regulated differently thygan hCG from ST origin and target locally at the maternal interface with decidual and immune cells as well as uterine arteries.

Biological activity of hCG from EVT versus ST origin

The biological activity and the role of hCG secreted in vitro by primary cultures of human-invasive EVT in comparison with hCG produced by in vitro differentiated ST have been investigated. The human first trimester and nontumoral EVT cell line (HIPEC65), that do not endogenously secretes hCG and express the luteinizing hormone/choriogonadotropin receptor (LHCGR) [51], were used to study the effect of hCG on the invasion process in vitro [32]. HIPEC65 were incubated in boyden chambers with 1 nM hCG from either EVT or ST supernatants. Only hCG from EVT origin induced a 10-fold increase in cell invasion, as assayed in Matrigel-coated transwells (Fig. 1.4.4). This stimulating effect was strongly decreased

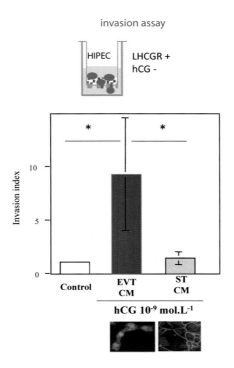

FIGURE 1.4.4

Effect of hCG from ST or EVT origin on trophoblast invasion. The human first trimester EVT cell line (HIPEC) expressing LHCGR but not hCG were incubated in Matrigel-coated transwell with 1 nM hCG from either EVT conditioned medium (CM) or ST CM or medium alone (control). Invasion index was quantified ($*P < .05$).

when hCG was depleted from EVT supernatants by immunoprecipitation before the invasion assay [32]. These results suggest that EVT and ST produce different hCG glycoforms that signal through different pathways.

Hyperglycosylated forms of hCG (hCG-H) are mainly produced by choriocarcinoma and JEG-3 cells and promote choriocarcinoma growth and malignancy, and inhibit apoptosis (for review, see Ref. [46]). hCG-H (using B152 antibody) was quantified in cell supernatants of EVT and ST primary cultures obtained from the same 8—10 WG human chorionic villi. It was found that hCG-H represents about 20% of total hCG in EVT supernatant at these terms, whereas it was almost undetectable in the ST cell cultures. These results offer strong evidence that hCG secreted in vitro by the invasive EVT, likely the hyperglycosylated forms of hCG, but not by the ST, promotes trophoblast invasion and may participate to the control of the trophoblast invasion process in an autocrine manner. Since hCG secreted by the ST has no effect on trophoblast invasion, hCG from EVT origin probably signals through an LHCGR independent pathway. Others reported that hCG modulated the invasion process in an LHCGR independent manner [50,52,53]. In situ, hCG-H immunostaining was found strong in invasive and endovascular EVT from 9-WG placenta tissue sections, weaker in mononucleated villous cytotrophoblasts but negative in the ST. hCG-H was quantified in maternal sera collected between 9 and 19 WG during normal pregnancies and concentrations were found to continuously decrease, while hCG peaks at 11 WG and then decreases as previously showed [54]. These results suggest that circulating hCG-H is from invasive endovascular EVT rather than ST origin and reflect the trophoblast invasion process during first trimester.

It was also demonstrated that like hCG [4,55,56], hCG-H displays a potent angiogenic effect [57]. However, it was reported that hCG-H induced angiogenesis through an LHCGR-independent signaling pathway using LHCGR KO mice. Instead, TGFβ-RII was identified as the hCG-H receptor responsible for its angiogenic effect using coimmunoprecipitation, competitive binding, TGFβ reporter gene assays, inhibitors of Smad signaling, and phosphorylated Smad immunoblotting [57].

Structural data indicate that in hCG-H, the additional sugar chains prevent a complete folding of the heterodimer, allowing the unmasking of the cryptic central cystine knot domain. Such structures have been identified in a number of factors that collectively form the cystine knot growth factor family including TGFβ. The structural similarities between hCG-H and TGFβ led to the suggestion that the exposed cystine knot structure in hCG-H could interact with the TGFβ receptor, resulting in decreased first-trimester trophoblast apoptosis and enhanced invasion associated with secretion of metalloproteinases. All together, these results suggest that the high levels of hCG-H observed in first trimester maternal sera are mainly from invasive EVCT origin, reflecting the early trophoblast invasion process. Furthermore, unlike hCG, hCG-H does not signal through LHCGR but induces trophoblast invasion and displays angiogenic activity via a TGFβ-RII signaling pathway (Fig. 1.4.2).

Together, these results offer evidence that glycoforms of hCG secreted by the invasive EVT and by the ST participate as PPARγ-target genes to the control of trophoblast differentiation and uterine placental vascularization through two different signaling pathways (Fig. 1.4.2).

hCG glycoforms and placental dysfunctions

Many complications of pregnancy and parturition are related to placental or uterine placental interface dysfunctions. The deep invasion of the EVT within the uterine wall, and the important ST hormonal functions (in particular hCG), are specific to humans. Shallow trophoblast invasion and defective uterine arteries remodeling during the first trimester are often associated with fetal growth restriction (FGR) and preeclampsia, which is a pregnancy disease specific to humans. Poor placentation is directly involved in many pregnancy diseases, including FGR, prematurity, and preeclampsia. Preeclampsia is a major and frequent complication of human pregnancy (about 2%—8% world wide) with serious maternal and fetal consequences such as prematurity. To date, there is neither curative nor preventive treatment for preeclampsia, which has been identified as one of the first causes of severe prematurity. As reported in this review, hCG-H represents a good candidate—a serum marker of early physiological EVT trophoblast invasion—to screen pregnancy diseases from placental origin [54]. Quantification of hCG-H in urine of pregnant women about 1 week after conception (hCG > 1 mU/mL) indicated that in all normal term pregnancies, the proportions of hCG-H over total hCG on the day of implantation was greater than 50%. Statistically significant lower proportions of hCG-H were observed in 13 of 20 spontaneous abortions, the others seven complications having normal ratio [58,59]. hCG-H was also reported as an early predictor of pregnancy outcomes after in vitro fertilization [60,61]. More recently, two studies reported that low concentrations of hCG-H in first trimester (8—13 WG) maternal sera are associated with subsequent early onset form of preeclampsia [62]. The same team reported that in the second trimester (14—17 WG), hCG-H in maternal serum is no longer able to predict preeclampsia [63].

Conclusion

hCG is the major pregnancy glycoprotein hormone, whose maternal concentration and glycan structure change throughout pregnancy. Depending on its placental source of production (EVT or ST), glycoforms of hCG display different biological activities and functions that may play a role in determining pregnancy outcome. In early first trimester, hCG-H is produced by the invasive and endovascular EVT that signals through TGFβ-RII, whereas hCG is mainly produced by the ST in large amount at about 10 WG and signals through the LHCGR. hCG glycoforms might provide promising biomarkers for screening of pregnancy diseases from placental origin.

References

[1] Jaffe RB, Lee PA, Midgley Jr AR. Serum gonadotropins before, at the inception of, and following human pregnancy. J Clin Endocrinol Metab 1969;29(9):1281—3.

[2] Hay, Lopata. Placental histology and the production of human choriogonadotrophin and its subunits in pregnancy. Br J Obstet Gynaecol 1988;95:1268—75.

[3] Jameson JL, Hollenberg AN. Regulation of chorionic gonadotropin gene expression. Endocr Rev 1993;14:203—21 [Review].

[4] Zygmunt M, Herr F, Keller-Schoenwetter S, Kunzi-Rapp K, Münstedt K, Rao CV, Lang U, Preissner KT. Characterization of human chorionic gonadotropin as a novel angiogenic factor. J Clin Endocrinol Metab 2002;87:5290—6.

[5] Ambrus G, Rao CV. Novel regulation of pregnant human myometrial smooth muscle cell gap junctions by humn chorionic gonadotropin. Endocrinology 1994;135:2772—9.

[6] Dong M, Ding G, Zhou J, Wang H, Zhao Y, Huang H. The effect of trophoblasts on T lymphocytes: possible regulatory effector molecules—a proteomic analysis. Cell Physiol Biochem 2008;21:463—72.

[7] Schumacher A, Heinze K, Witte J, Poloski E, Linzke N, Woidacki K, Zenclussen AC. Human chorionic gonadotropin as a central regulator of pregnancy immune tolerance. J Immunol 2013;190:2650—8.

[8] Kane N, Kelly R, Saunders PT, Critchley HO. Proliferation of uterine natural killer cells is induced by human chorionic gonadotropin and mediated via the mannose receptor. Endocrinology 2009;150:2882—8.

[9] Bansal AS, Bora SA, Saso S, Smith JR, Johnson MR, Thum MY. Mechanism of human chorionic gonadotrophin-mediated immunomodulation in pregnancy. Expert Rev Clin Immunol 2012;8:747—53.

[10] Muzzio D, Zygmunt M, Jensen F. The role of pregnancy-associated hormones in the development and function of regulatory B cells. Review Front Endocrinol 2014;5:39.

[11] Shi Q, Lei Z, Rao C, Lin J. Novel role of human chorionic gonadotropin in differentiation of human cytotrophoblasts. Endocrinology 1993;132:1387—95.

[12] Gudermann T, Birnbaumer M, Birnbaumer L. Evidence for dual coupling of the murine luteinizing hormone receptor to adenylyl cyclase and phophoinositide breakdown and Ca^{2+} mobilization. Studies with the cloned murine luteinizing hormone receptor expressed in L cells. J Biol Chem 1992;267. 4479e88.

[13] Keryer G, Alsat E, Tasken K, Evain-Brion D. Cyclic AMP-dependent protein kinases and human trophoblast cell differentiation in vitro. J Cell Sci 1998;111. 995e1004.

[14] Frendo JL, Olivier D, Cheynet V, Blond JL, Bouton O, Vidaud M, Rabreau M, Evain-Brion D, Mallet F. Direct involvement of HERV-W Env glycoprotein in human trophoblast cell fusion and differentiation. Mol Cell Biol 2003;23(10):3566—74.

[15] Fiddes JC, Goodman HM. The gene encoding the common alpha subunit of the four human glycoprotein hormones. J Mol Appl Genet 1981;1:3—18.

[16] Boorstein WR, Vamvakopoulos NC, Fiddes JC. Human chorionic gonadotropin beta-subunit is encoded by at least eight genes arranged in tandem and inverted pairs. Nature 1982;300:419—22.

[17] Rull K, Hallast P, Uuskula L, et al. Fine-scale quantification of hCG beta gene transcription in human trophoblastic and non-malignant non-trophoblastic tissues. Mol Hum Reprod 2008;14:23—31.

[18] Aldaz-Carroll L, Richon S, Dangles-Marie V, Cocquebert M, Fournier T, Troalen F, Stevens D, Guery B, Hersant AM, Guibourdenche J, Nordor A, Pecking A, Bellet D. Specific detection of type II human chorionic gonadotropin beta subunit produced by trophoblastic and neoplastic cells. Clin Chim Acta 2015;444:92—100.

[19] Cocquebert M, Berndt S, Segond N, Guibourdenche J, Murthi P, Aldaz-Carroll L, Evain-Brion D, Fournier T. Comparative expression of hCG β-genes in human trophoblast from early and late first-trimester placentas. Am J Physiol Endocrinol Metab 2012; 303:E950—8.

[20] Bo M, Boime I. Identification of the transcriptionally active genes of the chorionic gonadotropin beta gene cluster *in vivo*. J Biol Chem 1992;267. 3179e84.

[21] Miller-Lindholm AK, LaBenz CJ, Ramey J, Bedows E, Ruddon RW. Human chorionic gonadotropin-beta gene expression in first trimester placenta. Endocrinology 1997;138. 5459e65.

[22] Jameson JL, Lindell CM, Hsu DW, Habener JF, Ridgway EC. Expression of chorionic gonadotropin-beta-like messenger ribonucleic acid in an alpha subunit- secreting pituitary adenoma. J Clin Endocrinol Metab 1986;62. 1271e8.

[23] Rull K, Laan M. Expression of beta-subunit of hCG genes during normal and failed pregnancy. Hum Reprod 2005;20:3360—8.

[24] Buckberry S, Bianco-Miotto T, Bent SJ, Dekker GA, Roberts CT. Integrative transcriptome meta-analysis reveals widespread sex-biased gene expression at the human fetal-maternal interface. Mol Hum Reprod 2014;20:810—9.

[25] Knöfler M, Saleh L, Bauer S, Vasicek R, Griesinger G, Strohmer H, Helmer H, Husslein P. Promoter elements and transcription factors involved in differentiation-dependent human chorionic gonadotrophin-alpha messenger ribonucleic acid expression of term villous trophoblasts. Endocrinology 2000;141:3737—48.

[26] Knöfler M, Vasicek R, Schreiber M. Key regulatory transcription factors involved in placental trophoblast development—a review. Placenta 2001;22(Suppl. A). S83-92. Review.

[27] Knöfler M, Saleh L, Bauer S, Galos B, Rotheneder H, Husslein P, Helmer H. Transcriptional regulation of the human chorionic gonadotropin beta gene during villous trophoblast differentiation. Endocrinology 2004;145. 1685e94.

[28] Knöfler M. Regulation of hCG during normal gestation and in pregnancies affected by Down's syndrome. Mol Hum Reprod 1999;5. 895e7.

[29] Murthi P, Kalionis B, Cocquebert M, Rajaraman G, Chui A, Keogh RJ, Evain-Brion D, Fournier T. Homeobox genes and down-stream transcription factor PPARγ in normal and pathological human placental development. Placenta 2013;34. 299e309.

[30] Alsat E, Wyplosz P, Malassiné A, Guibourdenche J, Porquet D, Nessmann C, Evain-Brion D. Hypoxia impairs cell fusion and differentiation process in human cytotrophoblast, in vitro. J Cell Physiol 1996;168:346—53.

[31] Burton GJ, Jauniaux E, Watson AL. Maternal arterial connections to the placental intervillous space during the first trimester of human pregnancy: the Boyd collection revisited. Am J Obstet Gynecol 1999;181:718—24.

[32] Handschuh K, Guibourdenche J, Tsatsaris V, Guesnon M, Laurendeau I, Evain-Brion D, et al. Human chorionic gonadotropin produced by the invasive trophoblast but not the villous trophoblast promotes cell invasion and is down-regulated by peroxisome proliferator-activated receptor-gamma. Endocrinology 2007;148. 5011e9.

[33] Handschuh K, Guibourdenche J, Cocquebert M, Tsatsaris V, Vidaud M, Evain- Brion D, et al. Expression and regulation by PPARgamma of hCG alpha- and beta-subunits: comparison between villous and invasive extravillous trophoblastic cells. Placenta 2009;30. 1016e22.

[34] Barak Y, Nelson M, Ong ES, et al. PPARγ is required for placental, cardiac, and adipose tissue development. Mol Cell 1999;4:585—95.

[35] Kubota N, Terauchi Y, Miki H, et al. PPARgamma mediates highfat diet-induced adipocyte hypertrophy and insulin resistance. Mol Cell 1999;4:597—609.

[36] Nadra K, Quignodon L, Sardella C, Joye E, Mucciolo A, Chrast R, Desvergne B. PPARgamma in placental angiogenesis. Endocrinology 2010;151(10):4969—81.

[37] Schaiff WT, Barak Y, Sadovsky Y. The pleiotropic function of PPAR gamma in the placenta. Mol Cell Endocrinol 2006;249(1—2):10—5. Epub 2006 Mar 29. Review.

[38] Fournier T, Tsatsaris V, Handschuh K, Evain-Brion D. PPARs and the placenta. Placenta 2007;28:65—76.

[39] Fournier T, Guibourdenche J, Handschuh K, Tsatsaris V, Rauwel B, Davrinche C, Evain-Brion D. PPARγ and human trophoblast differentiation. J Reprod Immunol 2011;90(1):41—9.

[40] Tarrade A, Schoonjans K, Guibourdenche J, Bidart JM, Vidaud M, Auwerx J, et al. PPAR gamma/RXR alpha heterodimers are involved in human CG beta synthesis and human trophoblast differentiation. Endocrinology 2001;142. 4504e14.

[41] Schild RL, Schaiff WT, Carlson MG, Cronbach EJ, Nelson DM, Sadovsky Y. The activity of PPAR gamma in primary human trophoblasts is enhanced by oxidized lipids. J Clin Endocrinol Metab 2002;87. 1105e10.

[42] de Medeiros SF, Norman RJ. Human choriogonadotrophin protein core and sugar branches heterogeneity: basic and clinical insights. Hum Reprod Update 2009;15. 69e95.

[43] O'Connor J, Birken S, Lustbader J, Krichevsky A, Chen Y, Canfield R. Recent advances in the chemistry and immunochemistry of human chorionic gonadotropin: impact on clinical measurements. Endocr Rev 1994;15. 650e83.

[44] Kardana A, Elliott MM, Gawinowicz MA, Birken S, Cole LA. The heterogeneity of human chorionic gonadotropin (hCG). I. Characterization of peptide heterogeneity in 13 individual preparations of hCG. Endocrinology 1991;129:1541—50.

[45] Birken S, Krichevsky A, O'Connor J, Schlatterer J, Cole L, Kardana A, Canfield R. Development and characterization of antibodies to a nicked and hyperglycosylated form of hCG from a choriocarcinoma patient: generation of antibodies that differentiate between pregnancy hCG and choriocarcinoma hCG. Endocrine 1999;10:137—44.

[46] Cole LA. Hyperglycosylated hCG, a review. Placenta 2010;31:653—64.

[47] Loke Y, King A. Human implantation: cell biology and immunology. Cambridge: Cambridge University Press; 1993.

[48] Burton GJ, Jaunaiux E. Maternal vascularisation of the human placenta: does the embryo develop in a hypoxic environment? Gynecol Obstet Fertil 2001;29:503—8.

[49] Jauniaux E, Watson A, Burton G. Evaluation of respiratory gases and acid-base gradients in human fetal fluids and uteroplacental tissue between 7 and 16 weeks' gestation. Am J Obstet Gynecol 2001;184(5):998—1003.

[50] Zygmunt M, McKinnon T, Herr F, Lala PK, Han VK. hCG increases trophoblast migration in vitro via the insulin-like growth factor-II/mannose-6 phosphate receptor. Mol Hum Reprod 2005;11:261—7.

[51] Pavan L, Tarrade A, Hermouet A, Delouis C, Titeux M, Vidaud M, Thérond P, Evain-Brion D, Fournier T. Human invasive trophoblasts transformed with simian virus 40 provide a new tool to study the role of PPARgamma in cell invasion process. Carcinogenesis 2003;24:1325—36.

[52] Prast J, Saleh L, Husslein H, Sonderegger S, Helmer H, Knöfler M. Human chorionic gonadotropin stimulates trophoblast invasion through extracellularly regulated kinase and AKT signaling. Endocrinology 2008;149:979—87.

[53] Lee CL, Chiu PC, Hautala L, Salo T, Yeung WS, Stenman UH, Koistinen H. Human chorionic gonadotropin and its free β-subunit stimulate trophoblast invasion independent of LH/hCG receptor.

[54] Guibourdenche J, Handschuh K, Tsatsaris V, Gerbaud P, Leguy MC, Muller F, Brion DE, Fournier T. Hyperglycosylated hCG is a marker of early human trophoblast invasion. J Clin Endocrinol Metab 2010;95:E240—4.

[55] Berndt S, Perrier d'Hauterive S, Blacher S, Péqueux C, Lorquet S, Munaut C, Applanat M, Hervé MA, Lamandé N, Corvol P, van den Brûle F, Frankenne F,

Poutanen M, Huhtaniemi I, Geenen V, Noël A, Foidart JM. Angiogenic activity of human chorionic gonadotropin through LH receptor activation on endothelial and epithelial cells of the endometrium. FASEB J 2006;20:2630−2.

[56] Berndt S, Blacher S, Perrier d'Hauterive S, Thiry M, Tsampalas M, Cruz A, Péqueux C, Lorquet S, Munaut C, Noël A, Foidart JM. Chorionic gonadotropin stimulation of angiogenesis and pericyte recruitment. J Clin Endocrinol Metab 2009;94:4567−74.

[57] Berndt S, Blacher S, Munaut C, Detilleux J, Perrier d'Hauterive S, Huhtaniemi I, Evain-Brion D, Noël A, Fournier T, Foidart JM. Hyperglycosylated human chorionic gonadotropin stimulates angiogenesis through TGF-β receptor activation. FASEB J 2013;27: 1309−21.

[58] Sasaki Y, Ladner DG, Cole LA. Hyperglycosylated human chorionic gonadotropin and the source of pregnancy failures. Fertil Steril 2008;89. 1781e6.

[59] Cole LA. Hyperglycosylated hCG and pregnancy failures. J Reprod Immunol 2012;93. 119e22.

[60] Bersinger NA, Wunder DM, Nicolas M, Birkh€auser MH, Porquet D, Guibourdenche J. Serum hyperglycosylated human chorionic gonadotropin to predict the gestational outcome in vitro fertilization/intracytoplasmic sperm injection pregnancies. Fetal Diagn Ther 2008;24. 74e8.

[61] Chuan S, Homer M, Pandian R, Conway D, Garzo G, Yeo L, et al. Hyperglycosylated human chorionic gonadotropin as an early predictor of pregnancy outcomes after in vitro fertilization. Fertil Steril 2014;101. 392e8.

[62] Keikkala E, Vuorela P, Laivuori H, Romppanen J, Heinonen S, Stenman UH. First trimester hyperglycosylated human chorionic gonadotrophin in sérum - a marker of early-onset preeclampsia. Placenta 2013;34. 1059e65.

[63] Keikkala E, Ranta JK, Vuorela P, Leinonen R, Laivuori H, Vaisanen S, et al. Serum hyperglycosylated human chorionic gonadotrophin at 14-17 weeks of gestation does not predict preeclampsia. Prenat Diagn 2014;34. 699e705.

Molecular modeling of human chorionic gonadotropin glycosylation, nicking, and carboxyl terminal extension: influence on molecular folding and potential epitope recognition by common hCG antibodies

1.5

Stephen A. Butler, Nicholas Gibbons, Ray K. Iles

Introduction

The application of human chorionic gonadotropin (hCG) detection as a marker in pregnancy and oncology has been well described, and standardization of international reference preparations of hCG and hCG epitope mapping has been the focus of working groups for both the IFCC and ISOBM [1−5].

The heterodimeric α-β crystal structure of the hormone hCG was published over 20 years ago [6,7], and the triple loop structure stabilized by the central cystine knot has become quite familiar to hCG and glycoprotein biochemists (Fig. 1.5.1). The original primary sequences, relationships between α- and β-subunits, N-linked and O-linked glycosylations were first described in the 1970s and modified throughout the 1980s [8]. Briefly, the hCGα subunit consists of a 92-amino-acid peptide, including 10 cysteine residues that form five intramolecular disulfide bonds. The hCGβ subunit is a 145-amino-acid peptide, with 12 cysteine residues forming six intramolecular disulfide bonds, three of which form the central cystine knot

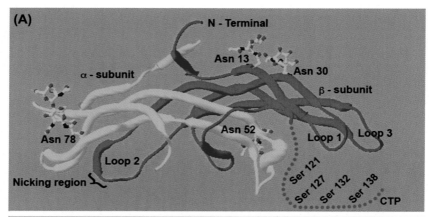

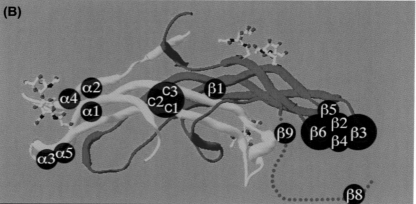

FIGURE 1.5.1 3D ribbon structure of hCG in familiar conformation as described by Lapthorn et al. [6] and produced from PDB accession code 1HRP shown here indicating key regions and epitope map.

(A) Top pane illustrates alpha (*cyan*) and beta (*red*) subunits their respective loop assignments, N-linked glycosylation points, nicking region, N-terminus and illustrative carboxyl terminal peptide (CTP) with 4 Serine residues which indicate the O-linked glycosylation points. (B) Bottom pane illustrates the same molecular conformation and view of hCG as seen in A but indicates major epitope locations as defined by the ISOBM TD-7 workshop on hCG and related molecules [4]. Images are redrawn from 1HRP and adapted to include regions of relevant interest.

[6,9] a structure which is highly conserved [10]. Peripheral disulfide bridges stabilize each subunit in a remarkably similar topological structure of two hairpin loops (loops 1 and 3) positioned opposite a third, much larger, long loop (the Keutman Loop/Loop 2) [6] (Fig. 1.5.1A).

The folding within hCG came after many attempts at crystallization were impeded by the extent of complex glycosylation [11,12]. Eventually, electron density maps produced tracings of the hCGα and hCGβ subunits; however, only amino acids 5 to 89 (of α) and amino acids 2 to 111 (of β) were ever resolved. The 34 amino acids of hCGβ's carboxyl terminal peptide (CTP) was also unresolved and was described as adopting a "random conformation" [6] although some efforts have been made to reveal the topography of this region subsequently [13]. In addition, this model was built not only missing key peptides but also missing key oligosaccharides; where all but the base sugars were cleaved from the molecule in order to obtain crystals. Despite being incomplete, this structure is still established as the model upon which extensive theoretical matching to antibody epitope binding has been mapped and studied [1−6,14,15], a version of which can be seen in Fig. 1.5.1B.

As a result, we currently rely on a molecular model that does not fully represent hCG in its native state and is observed as a deglycosylated variant lacking any representation of the carboxyl terminal peptide. If we go further, and factor in metabolic nicking of hCG in loop 2, which in some cases can represent 100% of the hCG determined by immunoassay [16] and the variability of CTP O-linked glycosylation, the overall effect of these modifications on molecular folding is unlikely to be inconsequential and hypothetical models have recently been offered to propose novel structures in the cases of hCGh and hCGβ [17,18].

Both the IFCC and ISOBM working groups on hCG have described the differences in hCG assay specificity for most of the commonly used antibodies [1−5]. The reports have extensively described inter-assay variability and between-method variation in the detection of hCG standards and QCs [19], in particular for the management of trophoblast diseases [20].

In light of these problems, we examined the structural variation of key hCG epitopes using bioinformatic molecular modeling tools to creating hCG models with the most common structural variants of N-linked and O-linked glycosylations, hCGβ Loop 2 nicking and CTP conformations.

Methods

In order to determine the structural changes in hCG affected by glycan and peptide structural permutations, we utilized a series of bioinformatics and molecular modeling packages to construct and manipulate the hCG model.

The crystal structure of hCG as determined by Lapthorn et al. [6] (accession code 1HRP) was obtained from the protein data bank. The effects of six oligosaccharides found linked to hCG were investigated and for simplicity are referred to herein by the "G, M, F" notation which describes the branched oligosaccharide by referring to the galactose, mannose, and fucose terminus of the oligosaccharide in a system employed previously for hCG as defined by Elliott et al. [16], and as shown in Fig. 1.5.2. The biantennary oligosaccharides GG and GGF which are found in high percentage concentrations on hCG molecules secreted under normal pregnancy

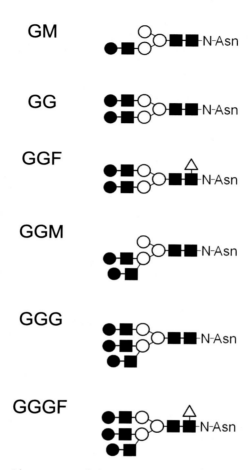

FIGURE 1.5.2 Common biantennary and triantennary glycan N-linked moieties found on hCG.

Figure indicates the six common glycan structures found on hCG using the standard structures and terminology for each monnosaccaride alongside terminal glycan abreviations as used by Elliott et al. [16] and here also for simplicity. ■ = GlcNAc, ○ = mannose, △ = Fucose, and ● = Galactose.

conditions and in the first IRP preparations of hCG, plus three triantennary oligosaccharides GGGF, GGG, GGM (Fig. 1.5.2) and a truncated biantennary oligosaccharide GM (Fig. 1.5.2) which are most prevalently found linked to variant forms of hCG in gestational trophoblastic diseases and other disorders of pregnancy but also in early pregnancy during implantation (these include variants such as hyperglycosylated hCG—hCGh).

N-linked oligosaccharides on asparagine residues were modeled as follows: The sugar-building module of HyperChem Professional (Hypercube Inc, Gainesville, FL, USA) was used to construct the various branches of the oligosaccharide GGGF, which were then linked to the peptide backbone to give the full oligosaccharides. Both asparagine glycosylation sites on hCG (Asn13 and Asn30) were glycosylated. For the other sugars, GGG and GM, monosaccharide units were removed sequentially from GGGF until the different required structures were reached.

To model the effects of nicking, the hCG backbone was broken in accordance with four previously reported nicking sites: Thr42-Arg43, Arg43-Val44, Val44-Leu45, and the most common Gly47-Val48 [16]. Artificial breaks were inserted into the HyperChem sequence 1HRP, and models were reminimized and allowed to form based on the nature of structure alone.

To examine the possible effects of the C-terminal peptide, this was modeled as a random coil structure using HyperChem Sequence Editor (Hypercube Inc.). In addition, O-linked oligosaccharides, both the trisaccharide and hexasaccharide forms were modeled and linked to appropriate serine residues to determine how normal and hyperglycosylated moieties might affect the overall structure of hCG, including the relative most likely position of the C-terminal peptide in each case.

Energy minimization was then carried out in these CTP modeling simulation experiments to give thermodynamically stable structures. Within HyperChem (Hypercube Inc.), the optimized potentials for liquid simulations all atom (OPLS A-A) force field method was used to determine minimum force field energy required for molecular interaction and therefore generated the most likely stable molecular conformation. The OPLS A-A force field was selected from other simulations as the most suited to both proteins and glycoproteins (oligosaccharides) in this study and is also a rapid approach which saves simulation time (it automatically groups hydrocarbons). The conditions used for minimization employed Polak-Ribeire conjugation gradient with termination conditions of 0.1 0 Kcal/($\mathring{A}$ mol). Deep View/Swiss PDB-viewer was used to analyze and present resulting structures, and Adobe Photoshop CC2014 was used to present and arrange figures and recolor where necessary to aid visualization and interpretation. No figures were manipulated in such a way to falsely present structures and are always shown as in Fig. 1.5.1A or as a mirror image of Fig. 1.5.1A. Therefore, any variability in structure shown is only due to the protein or oligosaccharide modifications reported.

Results and discussion

The achievable number of structural permutations for hCG is almost infinite, and most data generated in this study are therefore not shown or included in supplemental material. As such, a selection of only the most significant data has been presented to illustrate particular shifts in the molecular structure of hCG under certain conditions of glycosylation, nicking, and subsequent peptide folding; especially those which pertain to regions involving known epitopes. The results are presented as deviating, or not deviating, from the original model represented by 1HRP in the protein data bank (PDB) (Fig. 1.5.1A).

Generally, hCG is a very stable molecule primarily because of the cystine knot and subunit-subunit bonding. Overall, there is very little movement or refolding of peptide sequences in either the α-subunit or β-subunit, either after manually linking the different glycan moieties (GG, GM, GGF, GGM, GGG, GGGF) or after artificially breaking Loop 2 at the four known nicking sites (Thr42-Arg43, Arg43-Val44, Val44-Leu45, and Gly47-Val48). The exceptions to this are the effects seen in Loop 1 and Loop 3 and on the CTP of hCGβ where regions involving epitopes β2, β3, β4, β5, β6, β8, and β9 are found (see Fig. 1.5.1B). The epitopes β2—β6 are found on the first and third loops formed from two clusters of amino acids (β20—25 and β68—77). Loop 3 is potentially more important as all (β2—β6) epitopes involve significant amino acids contained in this loop (see Fig. 1.5.1).

α-/β-subunit glycosylation versus β-subunit glycosylation alone

Surprisingly, α-subunit glycosylation does not appear to have any effect over the folding of hCG, and very few structural modifications can be seen. In contrast, the glycosylation of hCGβ on Asn13 and Asn30 gives rise to multiple shifts, some of which occur in key epitope regions of the molecule. A comparison of five hCG glycoforms, where both subunits are glycosylated, in comparison to five where only the β-subunit is glycosylated alone, shows that in most glycoforms there does not seem to be any great difference in peptide structure or folding (GGGF, GGF GGM, GG). However, in the triantennary hyperglycosylated form GGG, there are clear changes when heterodimer subunits are both hyperglycosylated compared with glycosylation of β-subunit alone. Triantennary glycosylation (GGG) appears to exert very strong forces over the shape of the molecule particularly in terminal loop regions (Fig. 1.5.2) and appears to be the only hCGα glycovariant which does this; this is of little interest in clinical chemistry as hCGα—GGG is a particularly rare form [16]. It is immediately apparent that the majority of influence exerted by variation in glycosylation (and nicking) pertains to structural shifts in the hCGβ peptide affecting only β-epitopes. Ironically, it is these epitopes which have been selected specifically to identify, and quantify, hCG in order to solve specificity relating to cross-reactivity with LHβ.

Peptide folding and positioning of loops 1 and 3 for different hCG glycoforms: implication on the position of amino acids involved in epitopes β2—β6

The addition of glycans GG, GGF, GGM, and GGGF appears to exert only a minimal effect giving rise to subtle deviations in peptide structure and amino acid repositioning with respect to Loop 1 (Fig. 1.5.3) and Loop 3 (Fig. 1.5.4); a moderate effect can perhaps be seen in Loop 3 with the addition of GGF (Fig. 1.5.4D). In contrast, addition of the glycans GM, and more notably GGG, appears to distinctly affect the

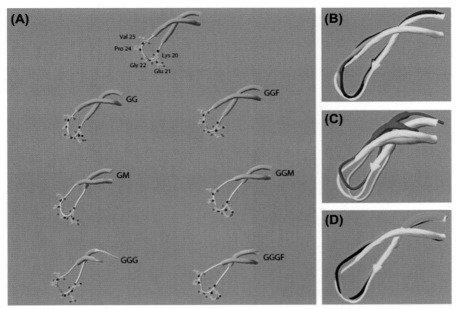

FIGURE 1.5.3 Structural effects on the peptide of hCG following the addition of six different glycans on hCGβ loop 1: impact on hCG epitopes β3 and β6.

The effects of six different oligosaccharides were modeled for the glycosylation on Asn13 & Asn30 and are shown here for loop 1 (A). GG and GGF, which are the glycoforms most prevalent in normal pregnancy and GM, GGM, GGG and GGGF are the glycoforms prevalent in either diabetic pregnancy, choriocarcinoma or very early pregnancy. Amino acids known to be important in contributing to affinity of epitopes in loop 1 are shown: Lys20, Glu21, Gly22, Pro24 and Val25. Key antigenic amino acids are seen to be displaced significantly in GM and GGG in addition to the extent of beta-pleated regions. Pro24 and Val25, (in conjunction with Arg68, Gly71 & Gly 75 from loop 3) are key amino acids in epitope β3. Lys20, Glu21 & Gln22, (in conjunction with Gly75 & Asn77 from loop 3) are key amino acids in epitope β6. The form of loop 1 in hCGβ from the crystal structure model as solved by Lapthorn et al is shown as a comparison (A - *top centre*). (B), (C) and (D) show a differently affected loop 1, overlaid on Lapthorn model (*yellow*). Specifically, (B) indicates the minimal effect seen as a result of the addition of GG (*blue*) and GGF (*orange*) glycans when compared to Lapthorn non-glycosylated model (*yellow*).
(C) indicates the divergence from the non-glycosylated model (*yellow*) seen after the addition of GGG (*red*) and GM (*pale blue*), and (D) shows the minimal effect of GGM (green) and GGGF (*purple*) glycans on loop 1 when compared to the Lapthorn model loop 1 (*yellow*).

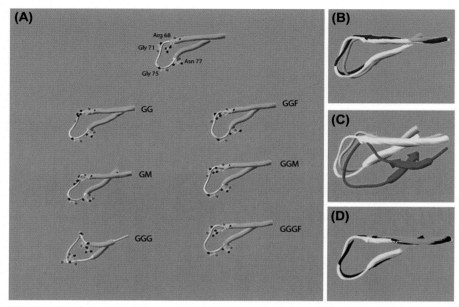

FIGURE 1.5.4 Structural effects on the peptide of hCG following the addition of six different glycans on hCGβ loop 3: impact on hCG epitopes β2, β4, β5, β6 and possibly β3.

The effects of six different oligosaccharides were modeled for the glycosylation of Asn13 & Asn30 and are shown for loop 4 (A). GG and GGF, which are the glycoforms most prevalent in normal pregnancy and GM, GGM, GGG and GGGF are the glycoforms prevalent in either diabetic pregnancy or choriocarcinoma or very early pregnancy. Amino acids know to be important in contributing to epitopes in loop 3 are shown: Arg68, Gly71, Gly75 and Asn77. Key antigenic amino acids which are seen to be significantly displaced include Arg68, Gly71 & Gly 75 (in conjunction with Pro24 & Val25 from loop 1) and are key amino acids in epitope β3. Gly75 & Asn77 (in conjunction with Lys20, Glu21 & Gln22, from loop 1) are key amino acids in epitope β6. Arg 68 is critical for antibodies which bind hCG eptiopes β2, β4 & β5. The form of loop 3 in hCGβ from the crystal structure model as solved by Lapthorn et al is shown as a comparison (A - top centre). (B), (C) and (D) show a differently affected loop 3, overlaid on Lapthorn model (yellow). Specifically, (B) and (D) indicates the minimal effect seen as a result of the addition of GG (blue), GGF (orange), GGM (green) and GGGF (purple) glycans when compared to Lapthorn non-glycosylated model (yellow). (C) indicates the divergence from the non-glycosylated model (yellow) seen after the addition of GGG (red) and GM (pale blue), and (D) shows the minimal effect of GGM and GGGF glycans on loop 3 when compared to the Lapthorn model loop 3 (yellow).

positions of Loop 1 and Loop 3 and result in significantly altered structures (Figs. 1.5.3C and 1.5.4C). Importantly, these alterations are so considerable as to affect the position of key amino acids involved in binding antibodies to epitopes β2–β6 (Figs. 1.5.1 and 1.5.5). It is worth mentioning that GGG is most common

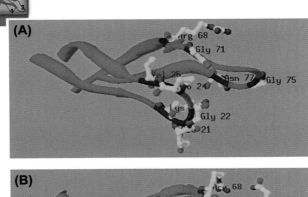

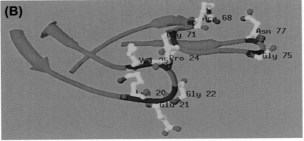

FIGURE 1.5.5 Structural comparison of key amino acid positions in loop 1 and loop 3 with and without hyperglycosylation.

The positions of loop 1 and loop 3 (labeled 1 and 3 in insert) are shown in the Lapthorn model (A) and when compared to the same region with hyperglycosylation (GGG) modeled on Asn13 and Asn30 on the beta subunit in hCG (B). Key amino acids required for binding mapped epitopes β2-β6 are shown in full as ball and stick structures protruding from the ribbon peptide backbone (*red*). Pro 24 and Val 25 move only slightly between A and B but their involvement in eptitope β3 is in conjunction with Arg 68, Gly 71 and Gly 75 all three of which shift position quite considerably. Lys 20, Glu 21 and Gly 22 on loop 1 together with Asn 77 and Gly 75 on loop 3 are key amino acids for antibody binding to epitope β6 and are all displaced between the two models, especially with regard to loop-to-loop associations. Most significant is the shift in position of Arg 68 which is critical for the affinity of antibodies binding epitopes β2, β4 and β5.

in hCGh which is prevalent in very early pregnancy and in trophoblastic diseases as are GM forms [21], both instances where quantification of hCG variants is particularly problematic [19,20].

As seen in Fig. 1.5.5, amino acids Pro24 and Val25 on Loop 1 appear to move only slightly between the two molecular variants of 1HRP and GGG. However, Arg68, Gly71, and Gly75 on Loop 3 are all seen to shift position quite considerably and these are key amino acids in epitope β3 in conjunction with Pro24 and Val25. In addition, Lys20, Glu21, and Gly22 on Loop 1 and Asn77 and Gly75 on Loop 3 are all also displaced, especially with regard to inter-loop associations, and are all implicated in the epitope β6. Perhaps the most significant single shift is in the position of Arg68, which has been described as critical for antibody affinity to epitopes β2, β4, and β5 [4,5].

Peptide folding and positioning of loops 1 and 3 for different hCG glycoforms: implication of enzymatic nicking of loop 2

Subunit nicking enzymes are known to cleave hCGβ at different positions in Loop 2 of hCGβ which is also called the Keutman loop. The most common nick site is at Gly47-Val48 and occurs in both normal and abnormal pregnancies. hCGβ is also cleaved at several less common positions, most notably in choriocarcinoma, and these can occur between Val44-Leu45, Arg43-Val44, and Thr42-Arg43 [16,22]. Nicking of any kind has been shown to variably affect the ability of antibodies to detect hCG [22] and as a consequence affect immunoassay quantification.

We examined the effects of nicking at all four sites in Loop 2 on the relative positions of Loop 1 (epitopes β3 and β6) and on Loop 3 (epitopes β2−β6). The overall effect of nicking alone is quite limited, especially with nicking at 47−48 and shows very little change to the overall structure when compared with 1HRP. Loop 1 appears to be affected the most, and these shifts are more significant with the less common nicking sites. However, when considered in combination with glycosylation, nicking has a more profound effect altering the relative positions of these antigenic amino acids in both Loop 1 and Loop 3 (Figs. 1.5.5 and 1.5.6). These peptide shifts are most significant in hyperglycosylated variants than in hCG with biantennary oligosaccharides which again highlights the problems associated with detecting hCG present in early pregnancy and gestational trophoblastic diseases.

Peptide folding and positioning of loops 1 and 3 for different hCG glycoforms and nicking: implication of fucosylation

It is evident that the presence of hyperglycosylation in the form of GGG has a profound effect on position of the amino acids in loops 1 and 3 and that nicking appears to exacerbate these changes. However, perhaps the most interesting finding from this study is that hCG with fucosylated oligosaccharides GGF and GGGF is quite unchanged and ribbon structures are almost perfectly overlaid on 1HRP (as seen in Fig. 1.5.7A).

Fucosylation at the base N-acetylglucosamine residue of the sugar moiety seems to provide structural stability to hCG folding and exerts a correcting force over that of the larger triantennary branched portion of the oligosaccharide. Fucosylation, over nicking and hyperglycosylation, appears to make the ribbon "snap" back into place as seen clearly in Fig. 1.5.7A. Importantly, this also means that fucosylation stabilizes the positions of the antigenic epitopes found on loops 1 and 3, even

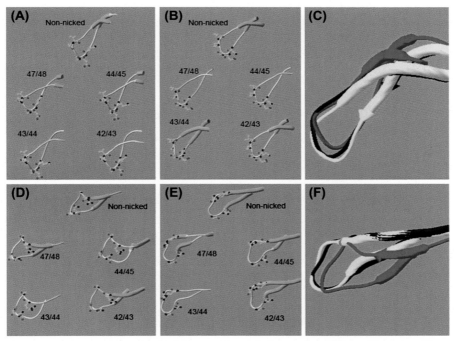

FIGURE 1.5.6 The effect of Loop 2 nicking and fucosylation on the positions of Loop 1 and Loop 3 in the β-subunit of hCG: potential impact on hCG epitopes β2-β6.

The effects of four different nicking sites Gly47-Val48, Val44-Leu45, Arg43-Val44 and Thr42-Arg43 were modeled and the effect on Loop 1 (A), (B) & (C) and Loop 3 (D), (E) & (F) are shown for two glycoforms GGG (A) & (D) and GGGF (B) & (E). Amino acids known to be important in contributing to epitopes in Loops 1 and 3 are shown as in Figs. 1.5.3 and 1.5.4 and can be clearly seen to shift position with the loops. Nicking alone appears to have very little effect on the overall structure of hCG and only in combination with certain glycoforms do we see shifts in Loops 1 and 3 which are ablated when the same structures a modeled to include a fucose residue (for structures with fucose residues see Fig. 1.5.2). The effects of nicking on two particular glycoforms, hCG-GGG and hCG-GGGF are shown here to illustrate the effects of hyperglycosylation and also of fucosylation, which seems to stabilise hCG structure.

when the proteins are nicked, in both biantennary and triantennary glycoforms. The stabilizing effect might be explained through the electrostatic interactions (hydrogen bonds) between fucose and the adjacent amino acids in the ascending and descending peptide of the loop. In particular, in nonfucosylated GG or GGG, the N-linked oligosaccharides protrude freely from the peptide which then adopts a more loosely associated loop. In the presence of fucose, however, the fucosylated oligosaccharide

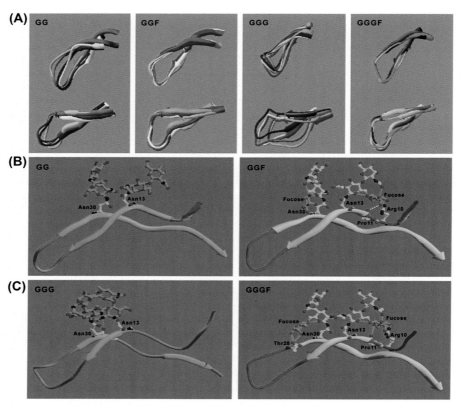

FIGURE 1.5.7 The effect of Nicking and Fucosylation on the stability of Loops 1 and 3 in hCGβ with biantennary and triantennary glycosylation.

(A) displays Loop 1 (*above*) and Loop 3 (*below*) displaying the loop as it would appear with and without fucosylated oligosaccharides. Each loop is overlaid on the others to show variability as a result of all four kinds of nicking (Gly47-Val48, Val44-Leu45, Arg43-Val44 and Thr42- Arg43) in loop 2 of hCGβ. Panel illustrates the effect of nicking and glycosylation on loops 1 and 3 that become variable with GG (*blue*) and GGG (*pink*), however, this effect is nullified with the addition of fucose on the biantennary oligosaccarides GGF (*orange*) and triantennary oligosaccharides GGGF (*green*). Refer to Fig. 1.5.2 for structures, both Asn 13 and 30 have been glycosylated to the same extent in each case. (B) and (C) display examples of the nullifying effect of fucose on N-linked glycosylation moieties. The re-stabilising of loop 1 may be explained through the electrostatic interactions (hydrogen bonds) between fucose and adjacent amino acids in the peptide of hCGβ. Hydrogen bonds are shown as dotted lines in green for strong interactions and white for weaker interactions. (B) GG and GGF. In the first pane Loop 1 is shown with non fucosylated biantennary oligosaccharides attached at Asn13 and Asn 30; the oligosaccharides float freely and the loop appears to be distorted. In the second pane native hCG with fucose belonging to the Asn13 linked oligosaccharide GGF forms attached to Asn13 appears to associate with Pro11 and the fucosylated oligosaccharide attached to Asn30 appears to associate with Thr28 (Fig. 1.5.7B and 1.5.7C).

The ability of fucose to interact with surface amino acids in and around the glycosylated asparagine residues suggest that fucosylated glycoforms are the default glycoforms found in hCG. Fucose also appears to have this role when the β-subunit has been subjected to nicking although different amino acids may be recruited into the interaction and stability as seen in Table 1.5.1. There may also be an implication in subunit to subunit interaction where fucosylated oligosaccharides on Asn52 and Asn78 of the α-subunit interact similarly with amino acids on the β chain.

The critical involvement of fucose suggests that α-(1,6)-fucosyltransferase plays an important part in the biochemistry of hCG synthesis. Furthermore, any deficiency in α-(1,6)-fucosyltransferase activity is likely to produce hCG deficient in fucosylated oligosaccharides and therefore a form of hCG with altered loops 1 and 3 of the β-subunit and poor α-β subunit interaction. In either case, these significantly altered loops which can be seen in Fig. 1.5.5 surely result in poorly defined epitopes and reduced antibody recognition of hCG molecules especially such as those seen in early pregnancy and in GTD.

Peptide folding and positioning of the carboxyl terminal peptide: implication on the positions of epitopes β8 and β9

Unglycosylated hCG gives rise to a CTP which adopts a "random conformation" [6], but being random does not mean the terminal peptide is linear and does not mean there are no interactions with the core molecule. This is especially true of a glycosylated peptide when this, as we have seen above, introduces opportunity for interactions between the sugar moieties and amino acids to stabilize the tertiary structure. Indeed, single amino acid substitutions have been shown to secure the conformation of the CTP and radically affect immunopotency in other studies [23]. Here a "random coil" model of the CTP was built on 1HRP with existing biantennary N-linked glycosylations. These models were allowed to form in the most thermodynamically stable conformation, the four most natural of these are shown in

---

hydrogen bonds with Pro11 of the b -subunit, while the fucose belonging to the oligosaccharide GGF attached to Asn30 forms hydrogen bonds with the adjacent amino acid Thr28; the oligosaccharides are constrained and the loop is apparently stabilised. (C) GGG and GGGF. In the first pane Loop 1 is shown with non fucosylated biantennary oligosaccharides attached at Asn13 and Asn 30, the oligosaccharides float freely and the loop appears distorted. In the second pane, fucose of the Asn13 linked GGGF appears to form hydrogen bonds with Arg10, Pro11 and Asn13 and the fucose of the oligosaccharide attached to Asn30 belonging to GGGF interacts with Thr28; the oligosaccharides are constrained and the loop is apparently stabilised.

Table 1.5.1 Amino acid residues that potentially interact with a 1–6 linked fucose residue of the N-linked glycosylation moieties attached to the beta-subunit of hCG.

hCG Glycoform and Loop 2 Nicking Position	Amino Acid forming hydrogen bonds with Fucose residue on Oligosaccharide bound to Asn[13]	Amino Acid forming hydrogen bonds with Fucose residue on Oligosaccharide bound to Asn[30]
hCG-GGF non nicked	Arg[10], Pro[11]	Asn[30]
hCG-GGF 47-48	Arg[10], Pro[11]	Val[29]
hCG-GGF 44-45	Pro[11], Asn[13]	–
hCG-GGF 43-44	Pro[11], Ala[14]	Thr[28]
hCG-GGF 42-43	Arg[10], Pro[11]	Thr[28]
hCG-GGGF non nicked	Arg[10], Pro[11]	Thr[28]
hCG-GGGF 47-48	Arg[10], Pro[11], Thr[15]	Thr[28]
hCG-GGGF 44-45	Arg[10], Thr[15]	Thr[28]
hCG-GGGF 43-44	Arg[10]	Thr[28], Val[29]
hCG-GGGF 42-43	Arg[10]	Thr[28]

Fig. 1.5.6 along with their energy readings in kcal/mol, where lower energy readings indicate higher stability and more likely natural positions.

Three of four conformations are very similar and provide further evidence for the most likely configuration and position of the CTP in unglycosylated hCG. It has also been possible to demonstrate the effect of normal (trisaccharide) and hyperglycosylated (hexasaccharide) O-linked sugars on the position of the CTP by adding the oligosaccharides and then reapplying minimization to display the most thermodynamically stable orientation. Peptide configuration energy tables for four most likely CTPs with trisaccharide glycosylation and with hexasaccharide glycosylation (along with no glycosylation) are shown in Fig. 1.5.8. Data indicate that CTP 1 (Fig. 1.5.8A1) is the most unlikely and is not rendered any more favorable by glycosylation which does not fit with our understanding of side chain interaction (-9995.98, -9744.03, and -9990.28 kcal/mol, respectively). CTP 2, while possible in an unglycosylated hCG, becomes less likely with glycosylation (-11097.11 verses -10480.10 and -10289.41) (Fig. 1.5.8A2). However, CTP 3 (-9429.76 verses -11332.66 and -11872.21 kcal/mol) (Fig. 1.5.8A3) and CTP 4 (-9550.01 verses -11471.09 and -11819.24 kcal/mol) (Fig. 1.5.8A4) stabilize with glycosylation and appear to adopt a less likely random position further highlighting the necessity of glycosylation on the natural position of the CTP in hCG.

Upon nicking at the four recognized sites described previously, classic trisaccharide glycosylation in CTP 3 and hyperglycosylated (hexasaccharide) hCG in CTP 4

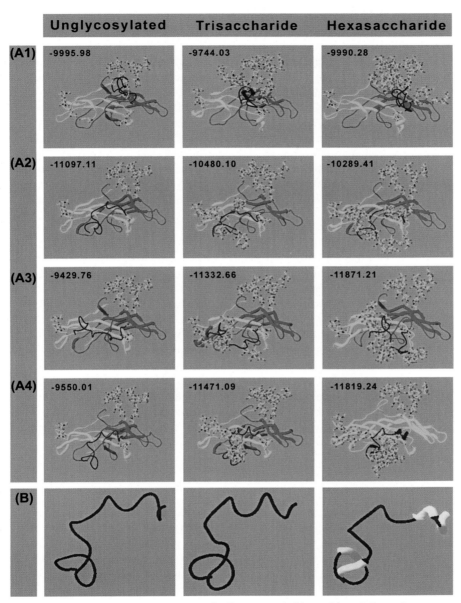

FIGURE 1.5.8 Modelling the thermodynamically most probable position of the carboxy terminal peptide of the beta-subunit of human chorionic gonadotropin in the intact hetrodimeric form of hCG — effect of glycosylation and CTP folding on eptitopes β8 and β9.

did not change significantly and maintained thermodynamically stable positions and hence epitopes. However, if the CTP is not in a confirmation which is thermodynamically optimal when nicking occurs, there is likely to be a major refolding of the CTP. This highlights again the importance of glycosylation on the position of this peptide and supports the case that 1HRP is not necessarily a natural structure for hCG and that the CTP in this structure could well be considered random.

Thus, glycosylated hCG likely favors a particular and stable CTP conformation, with or without nicking, and as a result presents two clear epitopes (β8 and β9, see Fig. 5.1) which are immunopotent and against which many high-affinity antibodies have been generated. However, of particular interest, when hyperglycosylated the CTP forms two distinct β pleated sheet regions which correspond exactly with these epitopes (Fig. 5.8B). It is highly likely that hyperglycosylation of the CTP affects the ability of CTP antibodies to recognize and bind sufficiently epitopes β8 and β9.

Implication

The suggestion that certain glycovariants of hCG, particularly in combination with nicking, bring about significant topological shifts in key epitope regions goes someway to explaining why there is such wide variation in assay and antibody specificity [19,20,24,25]. This is especially important when quantifying variant hCG glycoforms in early pregnancy, gestational trophoblastic diseases, and cancer where these glycoforms are particularly prevalent and sensitivity and specificity are critical [26–30]. These observations are not only important in the design and application of hCG immunoassays but also in the ongoing studies to develop anti-hCG vaccines for contraception and as adjuvant cancer therapies [31–33]. The ability to specifically detect hCG has now moved beyond immunoassay, and perhaps one solution may lie in the detection of hCG using mass spectrometry where not only sensitivity increases but the ability to qualitatively assess the hCG is now also possible [34–38].

Plates (A1)–(A4) illustrate hCG (As shown in Fig. 1.5.1) with the four most thermodynamically stable CTP conformations found in this study. In each case the relative CTP (Asp112-Gln145 in *dark blue*) position is shown in an unglycosylated form and also when Ser residues at Ser121, Ser127, Ser132 and Ser131 were glycosylated with trisaccharides and also hexasaccharides. Total energy readings for hCG were taken with the CTP attached in different random coil conformations and are indicated in the *top left* hand corner of each plate; Energy readings are in kcal/mol where lower numbers indicate higher stability and more likely natural positions. Figure plates in (B) show the detail of the CTP positions alone and enlarged from that seen above in (A4). The beta pleated sheet regions which occur as a result of hexasacchartide glycosylation correspond to regions associated with epitopes β8 and β9 (as seen in Fig. 1.5.1B).

Conclusion

The N-linked and O-linked sugars associated with the most common glycoforms of hCG do not appear to cause any significant movement in the common antigenic epitopes other than limited local movement of amino acid residue side chains, and if anything, these structures are more sound than any nonnative deglycosylated hCG. However, in the glycoforms associated with abnormal pregnancy, early pregnancy, and trophoblastic diseases, there are significant changes in the positioning of the peptides, including the CTP, and large displacements of side chain residues, protein folding, and epitopes occur. Hydroxyl groups on the fucose residues have the potential to interact and form H-bonds with proximal amino acids which appears to restabilize the peptide and the positions of amino acids in key epitopes. O-linked hyperglycosylation is likely to affect key epitopes β8 and β9 in the CTP where thermodynamically stable conformations include regions of β pleated sheets which are absent in native CTPs. These findings suggest that the detection and quantification of hCG by immunoassay in pregnancy and cancer not be entirely fit for purpose and antibodies may not be seeing the entire picture. Alternative or supplementary diagnostic tools, such as mass spectrometry which take a more qualitative approach, may be a useful addition in certain cases.

References

[1] Sturgeon CM, Berger P, Bidart JM, Birken S, Burns C, Norman RJ, et al. Differences in recognition of the 1st WHO international reference reagents for hCG-related isoforms by diagnostic immunoassays for human chorionic gonadotropin. Clin Chem 2009;55: 1484–91.

[2] Bristow A, Berger P, Bidart JM, Birken S, Norman R, Stenman UH, et al. Establishment, value assignment, and characterization of new WHO reference reagents for six molecular forms of human chorionic gonadotropin. Clin Chem 2005;51:177–82.

[3] Birken S, Berger P, Bidart JM, Weber M, Bristow A, Norman R, et al. Preparation and characterization of new who reference reagents for human chorionic gonadotropin and metabolites. Clin Chem 2003;49:144–54.

[4] Berger P, Sturgeon C, Bidart JM, Paus E, Gerth R, Niang M, et al. The ISOBM TD-7 Workshop on hCG and related molecules. Towards user-oriented standardization of pregnancy and tumor diagnosis: assignment of epitopes to the three-dimensional structure of diagnostically and commercially relevant monoclonal antibodies directed against human chorionic gonadotropin and derivatives. Tumour Biol 2002;23:1–38. Available from: http://www.ncbi.nlm.nih.gov/pubmed/11893904.

[5] Berger P, Paus E, Hemken PM, Sturgeon C, Stewart WW, Skinner JP, et al. Candidate epitopes for measurement of hCG and related molecules: the second ISOBM TD-7 workshop. Tumor Biol 2013;34:4033–57.

[6] Lapthorn AJ, Harris DC, Littlejohn A, Lustbader JW, Canfield RE, Machin KJ, et al. Crystal structure of human chorionic gonadotropin. Nature 1994;369:455–61. Available from: http://www.ncbi.nlm.nih.gov/pubmed/8202136.

[7] Wu H, Lustbader JW, Liu Y, Canfield RE, Hendrickson WA. Structure of human chorionic gonadotropin at 2.6 A resolution from MAD analysis of the selenomethionyl protein. Structure 1994;2:545—58. Available from: http://www.ncbi.nlm.nih.gov/pubmed/7922031.

[8] Cole LA, Butler SA. Structure, synthesis, secretion, and function of hCG. Elsevier Hum Chorionic Gonadotropin 2010:49—62. Available from: https://linkinghub.elsevier.com/retrieve/pii/B9780123849076000050.

[9] Murray-Rust J, McDonald NQ, Blundell TL, Hosang M, Oefner C, Winkler F, et al. Topological similarities in TGF-beta 2, PDGF-BB and NGF define a superfamily of polypeptide growth factors. Structure 1993;1:153—9. Available from: http://www.ncbi.nlm.nih.gov/pubmed/8069627.

[10] Vitt UA, Hsu SY, Hsueh AJ. Evolution and classification of cystine knot-containing hormones and related extracellular signaling molecules. Mol Endocrinol 2001;15:681—94. Available from: http://www.ncbi.nlm.nih.gov/pubmed/11328851.

[11] Harris DC, Machin KJ, Evin GM, Morgan FJ, Isaacs NW. Preliminary X-ray diffraction analysis of human chorionic gonadotropin. J Biol Chem 1989;264:6705—6.

[12] Lustbader JW, Birken S, Pileggi NF, Kolks MA, Pollak S, Cuff ME, et al. Crystallization and characterization of human chorionic gonadotropin in chemically deglycosylated and enzymatically desialylated states. Biochemistry 1989;28:9239—43. Available from: http://www.ncbi.nlm.nih.gov/pubmed/2611225.

[13] Venkatesh N, Krishnaswamy S, Meuris S, Murthy GS. Epitope analysis and molecular modeling reveal the topography of the C-terminal peptide of the β-subunit of human chorionic gonadotropin. Eur J Biochem 1999;265:1061—6. Available from: https://doi.org/10.1046/j.1432-1327.1999.00828.x.

[14] Lapthorn AJ, Berger P. Standardization of epitopes for human chorionic gonadotropin (hCG) immunoassays. Curr Med Chem 2016:3481—94. Available from: http://www.eurekaselect.com/node/142655/article.

[15] Berger P, Lapthorn AJ. The molecular relationship between antigenic domains and epitopes on hCG. Mol Immunol 2016;76:134—45. Available from: http://www.ncbi.nlm.nih.gov/pubmed/27450517.

[16] Elliott MM, Kardana A, Lustbader JW, Cole LA. Carbohydrate and peptide structure of the α- and β-subunits of human chorionic gonadotropin from normal and aberrant pregnancy and choriocarcinoma. Endocrine 1997;7:15—32. Available from: http://link.springer.com/10.1007/BF02778058.

[17] Cole LA. hCG structure: a logical perspective. Hainan Medical College Asian Pac J Reprod 2012;1:287—92. Available from: https://doi.org/10.1016/S2305-0500(13)60094-9.

[18] Cole LA. Three-dimensional structures of hCG and hyperglycosylated hCG. Elsevier Hum Chorionic Gonadotropin 2015:45—50. Available from: https://linkinghub.elsevier.com/retrieve/pii/B9780128007495000055.

[19] Cole LA, Sutton JM, Higgins TN, Cembrowski GS. Between-method variation in human chorionic gonadotropin test results. Clin Chem 2004;50:874—82.

[20] Cole LA, Shahabi S, Butler SA, Mitchell H, Newlands ES, Behrman HR, et al. Utility of commonly used commercial human chorionic gonadotropin immunoassays in the diagnosis and management of trophoblastic diseases. Clin Chem 2001;47:308—15.

[21] Butler SA, Khanlian SA, Cole LA. Detection of early pregnancy forms of human chorionic gonadotropin by home pregnancy test devices. Clin Chem 2001;47:2131—6.

[22] Cole LA, Kardana A, Ying FC, Birken S. The biological and clinical significance of nicks in human chorionic gonadotropin and its free β-subunit. Yale J Biol Med 1991; 64:627—37.

[23] Charrel-Dennis M, Terrazzini N, McBride JD, Kaye P, Martensen PM, Justesen J, et al. The human chorionic gonadotropin-β arginine 68 to glutamic acid substitution fixes the conformation of the C-terminal peptide. Mol Endocrinol 2005;19:1803—11. Available from: https://academic.oup.com/mend/article-lookup/doi/10.1210/me.2004-0109.

[24] Grenache DG, Greene DN, Dighe AS, Fantz CR, Hoefner D, McCudden C, et al. Falsely decreased human chorionic gonadotropin (hCG) results due to increased concentrations of the free ?? subunit and the ?? core fragment in quantitative hCG assays. Clin Chem 2010;56:1839—44.

[25] Gregor CR, Cerasoli E, Schouten J, Ravi J, Slootstra J, Horgan A, et al. Antibody recognition of a human chorionic gonadotropin epitope (hCGβ66-80) depends on local structure retained in the free peptide. J Biol Chem 2011;286:25016—26.

[26] Cole LA, Butler SA. Hyperglycosylated human chorionic gonadotropin and human chorionic gonadotropin free beta-subunit: tumor markers and tumor promoters. J Reprod Med 2008;53:499—512. Available from: http://www.ncbi.nlm.nih.gov/pubmed/18720925.

[27] Cole LA, Khanlian SA, Riley JM, Butler SA. Hyperglycosylated hCG in gestational implantation and in choriocarcinoma and testicular germ cell malignancy tumorigenesis. J Reprod Med 2006;51:919—29. Available from: http://www.ncbi.nlm.nih.gov/pubmed/17165440.

[28] Cole LA, Butler SA, Khanlian SA, Giddings A, Muller CY, Seckl MJ, et al. Gestational trophoblastic diseases: 2. Hyperglycosylated hCG as a reliable marker of active neoplasia. Gynecol Oncol 2006;102:151—9. Available from: http://www.ncbi.nlm.nih.gov/pubmed/16631241.

[29] Butler SA, Cole LA, Chard T, Iles RK. Dissociation of human chorionic gonadotropin into its free subunits is dependent on naturally occurring molecular structural variation, sample matrix and storage conditions. Ann Clin Biochem 1998;35(Pt 6):754—60. Available from: http://www.ncbi.nlm.nih.gov/pubmed/9838989.

[30] Lempiäinen A, Hotakainen K, Blomqvist C, Alfthan H, Stenman UH. Hyperglycosylated human chorionic gonadotropin in serum of testicular cancer patients. Clin Chem 2012;58:1123—9.

[31] Talwar GP, Gupta JC, Rulli SB, Sharma RS, Nand KN, Bandivdekar AH, et al. Advances in development of a contraceptive vaccine against human chorionic gonadotropin. Expert Opin Biol Ther 2015;15:1183—90. Available from: http://www.ncbi.nlm.nih.gov/pubmed/26160491.

[32] Morse MA, Chapman R, Powderly J, Blackwell K, Keler T, Green J, et al. Phase I study utilizing a novel antigen-presenting cell-targeted vaccine with toll-like receptor stimulation to induce immunity to self-antigens in cancer patients. Clin Cancer Res 2011;17:4844—53.

[33] Kvirkvelia N, Chikadze N, Makinde J, McBride JD, Porakishvili N, Hills FA, et al. Investigation of factors influencing the immunogenicity of hCG as a potential cancer vaccine. Clin Exp Immunol 2018;193:73—83. Available from: http://www.ncbi.nlm.nih.gov/pubmed/29601077.

[34] Lund H, Snilsberg AH, Halvorsen TG, Hemmersbach P, Reubsaet L. Comparison of newly developed immuno-MS method with existing DELFIA(®) immunoassay for

human chorionic gonadotropin determination in doping analysis. Bioanalysis 2013;5: 623—30. Available from: http://www.ncbi.nlm.nih.gov/pubmed/23425277.

[35] Butler SA, Luttoo J, Freire MOT, Abban TK, Borrelli PTA, Iles RK. Human chorionic gonadotropin (hCG) in the secretome of cultured embryos: hyperglycosylated hCG and hCG-free beta subunit are potential markers for infertility management and treatment. Reprod Sci 2013;20.

[36] Lund H, Paus E, Berger P, Stenman U-H, Torcellini T, Halvorsen TG, et al. Epitope analysis and detection of human chorionic gonadotropin (hCG) variants by monoclonal antibodies and mass spectrometry. Tumour Biol 2014;35:1013—22. Available from: http://www.ncbi.nlm.nih.gov/pubmed/24014048.

[37] Iles RK, Cole LA, Butler SA. Direct analysis of hCGβcf glycosylation in normal and aberrant pregnancy by matrix-assisted laser desorption/ionization time-of-flight mass spectrometry. Int J Mol Sci 2014;15:10067—82.

[38] Woldemariam GA, Butch AW. Immunoextraction-tandem mass spectrometry method for measuring intact human chorionic gonadotropin, free β-subunit, and β-subunit core fragment in urine. Clin Chem 2014;60:1089—97. Available from: http://www. ncbi.nlm.nih.gov/pubmed/24899693.

Why hCG is glycosylated

1.6

Laurence A. Cole

Human chorionic gonadotropin (hCG) subunit genes code for two independent molecules, the hormone hCG which acts on a luteinizing hormone (LH)/hCG joint hormone receptor and the autocrine hyperglycosylated hCG which acts on a transforming growth factor-β (TGF-β) receptor [1−4].

The hCG family of molecule is the most glycosylated glycoproteins in the human genome (Table 1.6.1), sugar accounting for 29% (hormone hCG) and 37% (extravillous cytotrophoblast hCG) of molecular weight [5,6]. Here I discuss why hCG is glycosylated, why hCG contains such a high proportion of sugar side chains, and what the sugar side chains do.

Oligosaccharides and acidity of hCG

Chorionic gonadotropin (CG), both the hormone hCG and the autocrine hyperglycosylated hCG drove the evolution of humans starting with early primates Aotus and Callicebus [7−9]. First came the evolution of CG from LH by deletion mutation of LH β-subunit in Aotus and Callicebus. The introduction of CG advanced these species by starting hemochorial placentation.

The first CG was isoelectric point (pI) 6.9 or a neutral form of CG with just three N-linked and two O-linked sugar side chains. The introduction of CG and hemochorial placentation improved fetal feeding efficiency which started brain expansion enzymes increasing the size of the primitive brain. Slowly, as primate species evolved to hominid species and as hominid species evolved to humans, the CG became more and more acidic, as did the efficiency and circulating half-life of CG and the effectiveness of hemochorial placentation. With this, the brain grew and grew leading to the increasing effectiveness of brain expansion enzymes and the evolution of humans. In the predecessor species of Aotus and Callicebus, the lemur and tarsier, the brain was 0.07% of total body weight. In Aotus and Callicebus, the brain was 0.17% of body weight. In the baboon, the brain size was 0.47% of body weight, in orangutan the brain size was 0.74% of body weight. In *Homo habilis*, the brain size was 1.2% of body weight, and in humans, the brain size was 2.4% of body weight (Table 1.6.2). Parallel to increasing brain size, evolved CG. In lemur and tarsier, LH had a pI of 8.0 with just three N-linked oligosaccharides, Aotus and Callicebus had a pI of 6.9 with three N-linked and two O-linked sugars, orangutan had a pI of 4.9 with three N-linked

100 Years of Human Chorionic Gonadotropin. https://doi.org/10.1016/B978-0-12-820050-6.00006-0

Table 1.6.1 The six primary variants of chorionic gonadotropin (CG).

Parameter	Placental hormone hCG	Hyperglycosylated hCG	Pituitary sulfated hCG	Cancer hCG	Cancer-free β-subunit	Fetal hCG
Source cells	Syncytiotrophoblast cells	Cytotrophoblast cells	Pituitary gonadotrope cells	Trophoblastic malignancy cells	Nontrophoblastic malignancy cells	Fetal kidney and liver cells
Mode of action	Endocrine	Autocrine	Endocrine	Autocrine	Autocrine	NonEndocrine
Total MW	36,525	39,149	35,943	40,461	26,271	Variable
Site of action	LH/hCG receptor	TGFβ antagonism	LH/hCG receptor	TGFβ antagonism	TGFβ antagonism	Fetal organ
Amino acids α-subunit	92	92	92	92	-	Variable
Amino acids β-subunit	145	145	145	145	145	Variable
Peptide MW	25,813	25,813	25,813	25,813	15,543	Variable
O-linked sugar units	4	4	4	4	4	Not determined
Type O-linked sugars	Type 1	Type 2	Type 1 + SO$_4$	Type 2	Type 2	Not determined
N-linked sugar units	4	4	4	4	2	Not determined
Type N-linked sugars	Biantennary	Biantennary	Biantennary + SO$_4$	Triantennary β	Triantennary	Not determined
Sugar side chain MW	10,712	13,336	10,130	14,648	10,728	Not determined
Percentage sugars	29%	34%	28%	36%	41%	Not determined

MW, molecular weight; SO$_4$, sulfated sugars.

Table 1.6.2 The acidity of luteinizing hormone (LH) and chorionic gonadotropin (CG).

Molecule	Species	Isoelectric point (pI)	Circulating half-life	Biological potency	Brain size % Body Weight	No. of oligosaccharides
LH	Lemur	8.0	0.33 h	1X	0.07%	3 N-linked, 0 O-linked
CG	Aotus/Callicebus	6.9	2.4 h	7.3X	0.17%	3 N-linked, 2 O-linked
CG	Baboon				0.47%	3 N-linked, 3 O-linked
CG	Orangutan	4.9	6.0 h	18.2X	0.74%	3 N-linked, 3 O-linked
CG	*Homo habilis*				1.2%	3 N-linked, 4 O-linked
CG	Human	3.5	36 h	109X	2.4%	4 N-linked, 4 O-linked

and three O-linked oligosaccharides, and humans had a pI of 3.5 with four N-linked and four O-linked sugar side chains [1−3] (Table 1.6.2).

In conclusion, the increasing acidity of CG drove the evolution of humans. The hormone CG drove the evolution of hemochorial placentation, and the autocrine hyperglycosylated hCG drove the growth of the villus tissue of hemochorial placentation and the essential implantation of hemochorial placentation.

Super acidic, pI = 3.5, hCG is needed by the human fetus to develop a large human brain and to promote efficient hemochorial placentation to promote brain enhancement genes and to develop the species that we call humans.

Oligosaccharides and function of hCG

There are two forms of hCG, the hormone hCG as secreted by syncytiotrophoblast cells, and the autocrine hyperglycosylated hCG as secreted by cytotrophoblast cells and the autocrine extravillous cytotrophoblast hCG as secreted by extravillous cytotrophoblast cells. Structurally, the only difference between the hormone and the autocrines is the four O-linked oligosaccharides on the C-terminal peptide of the β-subunit and the triantennary N-linked oligosaccharides. There are type 1 O-linked oligosaccharides on the hormone hCG and type 2 O-linked oligosaccharide on the autocrine hyperglycosylated hCG and extravillous cytotrophoblast hCG, and biantennary N-linked oligosaccharides on the hormone hCG and hyperglycosylated hCG, and triantennary N-linked oligosaccharides on the β-subunit of extravillous cytotrophoblast hCG.

The presence of type 1 and type 2 oligosaccharides on the β-subunit C-terminal peptide very much affects the folding of the hCG molecule [10] (Fig. 1.6.1), and whether or not the molecule can be cleaved by a nicking enzyme. The hormone hCG with its type 1 O-lined oligosaccharides has a C-terminal peptide that folds into the β30-β59 loop blocking nicking. This generally prevents nicking, keeping the molecule intact. The advantage is that the hCG/LH receptor only responds to nonnicked and nondissociated hCG molecules. In this respect, this protects hCG. The autocrine hyperglycosylated hCG, in contrast, has type 2 O-linked oligosaccharides. Its β-subunit C-terminal peptide does not fold into the β30-β59 loop and does not block nicking [10] (Fig. 1.6.1). The autocrine hyperglycosylated hCG is rapidly nicked upon secretion, and after nicking rapidly dissociates into an hCG α-subunit and a nicked hCG β-subunit. The advantage is that nicked hCG β-subunit is the substrate for the TGF-β receptor [10].

Why oligosaccharides were added to hCG

N-linked oligosaccharides are semiautomatically added at sites with the amino acid sequence Asn-Xxx-Ser/Thr. O-linked oligosaccharides are formed at Pro/Ser-Ser

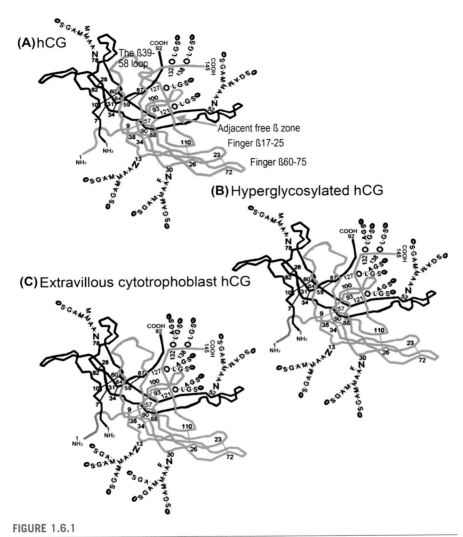

FIGURE 1.6.1

The three-dimensional structure of the hormone hCG, the autocrine hyperglycosylated hCG, and the autocrine extravillous cytotrophoblast hCG as shown by the computer modeling of Stephen Butler [10] seen in Chapter 1.5.

sites that can optimally sterically fit an oligosaccharide. CG first came about in Aotus and Callicebus primates, and oligosaccharides were fitted when amino acid sequence accommodated glycosylation.

As discussed in the lay book "God Mastered Human Evolution, Bringing Cancer To an End: The Life Story of Laurence A. Cole," published in 2019, author Laurence

A. Cole, Ph.D., God must have been involved in the story of human evolution, both in the design of the CG molecule, and how it through so many changes in evolution leading through the stepwise increase in acidity in over 50 + species from Aotus/Callicebus to humans. Somehow, God seemed to design a molecule to facilitate the evolution of humans, a very idealistic molecule to accommodate such extreme hyperglycosylation, 30%−37% sugar.

I state no further information on how hCG was created to fulfill both promotion of hemochorial placentation and implantation here or how glycosylation facilitated the optimal nicking/nonnicking and processing of the hormone hCG and the autocrine hyperglycosylated hCG. You must now research it and make up your own mind as to whether God was involved. Simply accept that a very ideal molecule, hCG, was somehow created, somehow fulfilled the seemingly never-ending acidity evolution of humans, and how one set of genes somehow met the two needed molecules to fulfill hemochorial placentation and its needed implantation.

The fact is that excessive carbohydrate side chains were added to hCG to make the ideal hormone and the ideal TGF-β autocrine. This is what happened.

References

[1] Butler SA, Ikram MS, Mathieu S, Iles RK. The increase in bladder carcinoma cell population induced by the free beta subunit of hCG is a result of an anti-apoptosis effect and not cell proliferation. Br J Cancer 2000;82:1553−6.

[2] Berndt S, Blacher S, Munuat C, Detilleux J, Evain-Brion D, Noel A, Fournier T, Foidart JM. Hyperglycosylated human chorionic gonadotropin stimulates angiogenesis through TGF-ß receptor activation. FASEB J 2013;12:1309−21.

[3] Cole LA, Dai D, Butler SA, Leslie KK, Kohorn EI. Gestational trophoblastic diseases: 1. Pathophysiology of hyperglycosylated hCG-regulated neoplasia. Gynecol Oncol 2006;102:144−9.

[4] Dufau ML. The luteinizing hormone receptor. Annu Rev Physiol 1998;60:461−96.

[5] Elliott MM, Kardana A, Lustbader JW, Cole LA. Carbohydrate and Peptide structure of the α- and ß- subunits of human chorionic gonadotropin from normal and aberrant pregnancy and choriocarcinoma. Endocrine 1997;7:15−32.

[6] Valmu L, Alfthan H, Hotakainen K, Birken S, Stenman UH. Site-specific glycan analysis of human chorionic gonadotropin beta-subunit from malignancies and pregnancy by liquid chromatography - electrospray mass spectrometry. Glycobiology 2006;16:1207−18.

[7] Cole LA. hCG and hyperglycosylated hCG in the establishment and evolution of hemochorial placentation. J Reprod Immunol 2009;82:112−8.

[8] Cole LA. Chapter 36: evolution of hCG, evolution of humans, evolution of human pregnancy disorders and cancer. In: Cole LA, Butler SA, editors. Human chorionic gonadotropin (hCG). Burlington MA: Elsevier; 2010. p. 363−76.

[9] Cole LA. The evolution of the primate, hominid and human brain. Primatology 2015;4: 100124.

[10] Cole LA. The minute structural difference between the hormone hCG and the identical amino acid sequence TGFß autocrine hyperglycosylated hCG. Am J Obstet Gynecol 2018 (in press).

Detection and quantitation

Detecting hCG that is not there—Anecdote

2.1

Stephen A. Butler

My research with hCG started 25 years ago as an undergraduate on placement in the Department of Reproductive Medicine at St Bartholomew's Hospital in London. Prof. Timothy Chard was the Chair. I was working in a basement laboratory deep under Bart's East wing which specialized in the study of oncofetal antigens and was run by Dr. Ray Iles. I cut my teeth on RIAs, IRMAs, and some early RT PCR to detect the ectopic expression of hCGβ by carcinoma of the bladder, among other cancers. At the time, I did not realize that this early exposure to the problems of working with "old school" immunoassays would provide the perfect insight into the subtleties of antibody-based sandwich assays which I would need to draw on later in my career.

I completed my placement, my degree dissertation, and then my Ph.D. all at the Williamson Laboratory with Ray, all the time focused on the ectopic expression of hCG and its subunits in cancer. In 1999, I started my Postdoc Fellowship at Yale University School of Medicine in the laboratory of Prof. Laurence (Larry) Cole. Larry had contacted me several months before, inviting me to work with him in the United States once I finished my Ph.D. in London, and I had jumped at the chance. My 2-year project would be to isolate and identify hCG from pregnancy urine to determine structural variation in different trimesters and any structure-function associations with disorders of pregnancy and gestational trophoblastic diseases.

Once I arrived at Yale, I was immediately introduced to the immunoassays, microtiter plate ELISAs now (no more radioisotopes), we used seven or eight of them in total. Each assay cleverly used a different antibody pair to detect a different hCG variant, and by combining data from all of the assays, it was possible to profile the hCG in the sample. This became the basis for the USA hCG Reference Service which received samples from all across the United States, and abroad, to "profile" hCG properties which were not immediately evident from the single assay available to the investigating physician. It was during one such investigation that we first received a sample from Washington from a woman who had persistent serum hCG and by the end of her treatment had had numerous surgeries including a hysterectomy and partial lung lobectomy.

At the reference service we received many cases like this one, and they were becoming more and more common. Rather than risk any more needless therapy we chose to publish our methods and the stepwise checks and assays that any biochemistry laboratory could perform to quickly identify false positive hCG [1]. We publicized the phenomenon in leading clinical chemistry and OB/GYN journals [2,3] and documented and published all the cases we had seen [4]. This was not addressing the problem though, and the assay manufacturer still refused to look into the cause of the recurrent false positives, claiming it would cost millions of dollars to identify and modify a validated clinical assay.

Over the course of just 2 days, with hardly any sleep, I deconstructed the validated clinical platform assay, reducing it to the component reagents and rebuilt it, so it could be run using a microtiter plate. Systematically, I replaced each component reagent with alternatives to identify the step of the assay which could be responsible for the false positives. At around 4 a.m. on the second night, I ran a permutation which gave me the answer, goat serum. Under the normal operation of the platform assay, undiluted samples were incubated in buffers which did not contain any animal serum, this provided the opportunity for heterophilic antibodies to cross-link capture and tracer antibodies to produce a false-positive signal. Because these samples always gave rise to apparent, low, persistent levels of hCG, the samples were never diluted. Infuriatingly, if any of the false-positive samples had been diluted just 1:1 in the preparatory assay dilution buffer, the false-positive signal would have disappeared. The dilution buffer in the assay contained goat serum and, as I had learned from running all those old school IRMAs, animal serum contains masses of nonspecific antibodies and proteins that effectively "mop up" the heterophilic antibodies in the sample and reduce nonspecific signals. It did not take a year of research, and it did not take millions of dollars and revalidation, the assay manufacturer just needed to add a note on the system to say that all samples must be diluted in assay buffer.

References

[1] Butler SA, Cole LA. Use of heterophilic antibody blocking agent (HBT) in reducing false-positive hCG results. Clin Chem 2001;47(7):1332—3.

[2] Butler SA, Cole LA. False positive hCG. Obstet Gynecol 2002;99(3):516—7.

[3] Cole LA, Butler SA. False positive or phantom hCG result: a serious problem. Clin Lab Int 2001;25:9—14.

[4] Cole LA, Butler S. Detection of hCG in trophoblastic disease. The USA hCG reference service experience. J Reprod Med 2002;47(6):433—44.

robust, cost-effective, and straight forward detection of hCG, including hCGβ, hCGβcf, hCGα, hCGh, and other forms is now possible with the use of MALDI-ToF mass spectrometry.

MALDI for detection of hCG family molecules

The concept of MALDI was introduced in 1985 [27] and later Karas and Hillenkam [28] have introduced the use of organic matrix in mass spectrometry, thus enabling an analysis of molecules larger than 10,000 Da. With this groundbreaking technology, the analysis of proteins, including hCG, has improved and expanded. Also, the detection of hCG in the biological fluids, especially urine, has improved as the matrix used in the acquisition process, sinapinic acid (3,5-dimethoxy-4-hydroxycinnamic acid), is insensitive to the ionic contaminants such as urea, even in relatively high concentrations (1 M) [29]. MALDI offers the ability to measure hCG in a variety of biofluids without the necessity of specialist preparation such as the requirement of specific, expensive antibodies. It is also a method of soft ionization; therefore, the molecules can be observed in their original proteoforms and any qualitative changes such as between hCG and hCGh are easily identified due to observed mass shift as shown previously [20,30]. Besides these advantages, MALDI offers a high-throughput and sensitive method, reaching detection limits of 0.25 fmol for pure protein preparations and only requiring 1 μL of a sample [31].

MALDI-ToF mass spectrometry as a quantitative tool for hCG detection

MALDI-ToF has already been described as a quantitative tool [32], yet in general, it is not considered a quantitative method. Nevertheless, it was used for the detection and extent of albuminuria [33], quantification of glycated hemoglobin [34], and cardiac α- and β-Myosin heavy chain proteins extracted from human heart right atrium [35].

Given that hCG has several variants that vary in size and thus the occurring mass shift can be readily recognized in mass spectrometry, we have explored the possibility of MALDI as a tool to provide a relative quantification for hCG variants. Fig. 2.2.2 shows six species of hCG (hCGβcf [H++], hCGβcf, hCGα, hCGβ, hCG, and hCGββ dimers in panel A to F) obtained from SkyBio hCG preparation and for the hCGβcf preparations as described later.

Relative quantification of hCGβcf and hCG

The hCGβcf used in this study was extracted from pooled 80 L of urine of 22 pregnant women from the laboratory of Prof. L.A. Cole. The hCG and hCGβ were

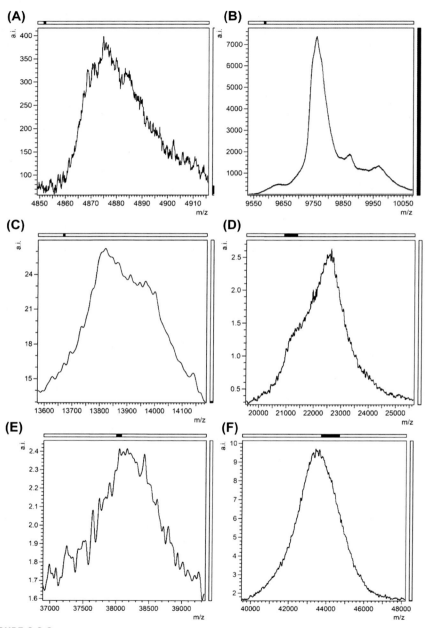

FIGURE 2.2.2

Variants of hCG as analyzed by MALDI-ToF MS. In the panels A to F are hCGβcf [H++], hCGβcf, hCGα, hCGβ, hCG, and hCGββ dimers. Axis represents relative peak intensity (y) and mass to charge ratio (m/z) (x). Gaussian smoothing was applied for visualization purposes.

separated, and smaller molecules including 50% hCGβcf and hCG α subunit. The crude protein was freeze-dried and stored in −20°C. One milligram of the powder was weighted and reconstituted in 100 μL of mass spectrometry grade water (Romil, UK). For the hCG, SkyBio preparation was used (120 U/l) and reconstituted as per requirements.

The analysis was done using sinapinic acid matrix (SA) (Sigma, Aldrich) on a benchtop MALDI 8020 (Shimadzu, UK) in a positive linear mode. Starting with a stock solution, further doubling dilutions were prepared to up to 1 in 16,384 for both molecules. All samples were run in duplicates in case of crystallization problems. Reproducibility was ensured by averaging 8500 shots in total per each sample well.

An automated computational method was developed in R [36], using MALDI-quantForeign and MALDIquant packages to import and preprocess the data [37,38]. Data were imported and baseline removed using Statistics—sensitive nonlinear iterative peak clipping (SNIP) algorithm [39]. We have previously identified that hCGβcf is detectable in a region of 9750 m/z, thus peak maximum intensity was extracted from a range of 9700 m/z to 9820 m/z. For hCG, hCGβ, and its dimer, the range was 35,000 m/z to 39,000 m/z, 20,000 m/z to 24,000 m/z, and 40,000 m/z to 46,000 m/z, respectively, providing a wide range to avoid missing the peak due to potential mass shift. Identified maximum peak intensity values with corresponding dilution coefficient were exported to a data frame for the construction of the calibration curve.

However, the actual protein concentration is not known for the hCGβcf molecule, the detection limit exceeding signal-to-noise ratio of 3 (SNR = 3) was at a 1 in 256 dilution. In Fig. 2.2.3, top left is the standard curve of intensity over the dilution coefficient, where $R^2 = 0.98$, showing a strong negative correlation with dropping in signal intensity with increasing dilution coefficient. Diluting further, the signal intensity was lost and thus the reference curve was not appropriate for quantification for samples of unknown mass.

For the intact hCG molecule, the intensity of the signal was suppressed due to oversaturation starting with stock and dilution of one in two, four, and eight. However, 1 in 16 and 1 in 32 and 1 in 64 have shown an optimal quality signal, based on intensity strength and with further dilution the signal was lost. In this range, the correlation of a natural log of the intensity signal was perfect, with $R^2 = 1$ (Fig. 2.2.3). Nevertheless, the standard used in the study was stored for prolonged time and thus free subunits where observed at the higher intensity compared with the intact molecule. For example, hCGβ signal was seen in the range of 1 in 8 to 1 in 2048 and lost in a following doubling dilution of 1 in 4096, where it was optimal based on the strength of intensity at 1 in 16. The dilution range for hCGα was from 1 in 32 to 1 in 2048. The optimal dilution, based on the highest intensity of the spectra was 1 in 256, where the point with highest residual error is observed. Both hCGα and hCGβ were positively correlated with R^2 of 0.81 and 0.95.

We have observed high correlation, where the correlation coefficient ranged from $R^2 = 0.81$ to 1 for the intact hCG molecule. There is a lack of quantitative methods

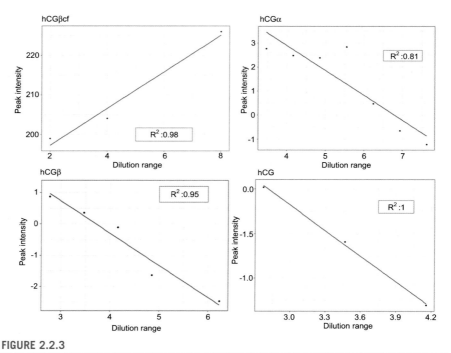

FIGURE 2.2.3

Calibration curves of hCGβcf, hCGα, hCGβ, and hCG. Plotted here the peak intensity over the dilution range value, showing a strong correlation, $R^2 = 0.98$, 0.81, 0.95, and 1 for all molecules, respectively. All data had a natural log transformation applied before visualization.

for the determination of low hCG levels [40], thus this is a very important finding, showing that MALDI-ToF can play a role not only in the identification of various qualitative changes of hCG but also as a quantitative tool detecting hCG in a very low concentration. Since some pathologies, such as early pregnancy loss, are defined by inherently very low hCG levels, this method of hCG quantitative and qualitative analysis would add additional benefits to the accurate measure. Furthermore, the required sample size is miniature (1 μL), thus for those patients that require continuous invasive testing, it can be a great advantage.

In this chapter, we have briefly overviewed the detection of hCG molecule and its variants over the years of development, in particular, what challenges were associated with accurate and precise detection. Furthermore, the most recent technology, benchtop MALDI has been shown to be able to produce a standard reference curve of hCGβcf, hCGα, hCGβ, and hCG in a particular dilution range providing the evidence of quantification of hCG in MALDI. Most importantly, no additional sample preparation or reagents is required in order to detect different isoforms, glycoforms, and biodegradation products of hCG, as was shown with hCG analyzed in this chapter. To conclude, MALDI-ToF technology is a suitable tool for the analysis and relative quantification of hCG molecule and its variant and will play a major role in the clinical pathology and early pregnancy monitoring in the future.

References

[1] Curry SL, et al. Hydatidiform mole: diagnosis, management, and long-term followup of 347 patients. Obstet Gynecol 1975;45(1):1−8.

[2] Saller B, et al. 'Testicular cancer secretes intact human choriogonadotropin (hCG) and its free beta-subunit: evidence that hCG (+ hCG-beta) assays are the most reliable in diagnosis and follow-up. Clin Chem 1990;36(2):234−9.

[3] Barnhart K, et al. Prompt diagnosis of ectopic pregnancy in an emergency department setting. Obstet Gynecol 1994;84(6):1010−5.

[4] Brizot ML, et al. Maternal serum hCG and fetal nuchal translucency thickness for the prediction of fetal trisomies in the first trimester of pregnancy. Br Int J Obstet Gynaecol 1995;102(2):127−32. Wiley Online Library.

[5] Ferreira HP. The relative merits of the various biological tests for pregnancy. Postgrad Med J 1954;30(345):355. BMJ Publishing Group.

[6] Aschheim S, Zondek B. Hypophysenvorderlappenhormon und Ovarialhormon im Harn von Schwangeren. J Mol Med 1927;6(28):1322. Springer.

[7] Friedman MH, Lapham ME. A simple, rapid procedure for the laboratory diagnosis of early pregnancies. Am J Obstet Gynecol 1931;21(3):405−10. Elsevier.

[8] Shapiro HA, Zwarenstein H. A rapid test for pregnancy on *Xenopus laevis*. Nature 1934;133(3368):762. Nature Publishing Group.

[9] Stone B. Clinical value of the Aschheim-Zondek test for pregnancy. South Med J 1930;23(8):747−9.

[10] Hurry E. A laboratorians view of pregnancy testing. Am J Med Technol 1982;48(12):971.

[11] Brody S, Carlström G. Estimation of human chorionic gonadotrophin in biological fluids by complement fixation. Lancet 1960;276(7141):99. Elsevier.

[12] Wide L, Gemzell CA. An immunological pregnancy test. Eur J Endocrinol 1960;35(II):261−7.

[13] Shimizu SY, et al. Chorigonadotropin measured by use of monoclonal antibodies in a two-site immunoradiometric assay. Clin Chem 1982;28(3):546−7.

[14] Köhler G, Milstein C. Continuous cultures of fused cells secreting antibody of predefined specificity. Nature 1975;256(5517):495. Nature Publishing Group.

[15] Van Weemen BK, Schuurs A. Immunoassay using antigen—enzyme conjugates. FEBS Lett 1971;15(3):232−6. Wiley Online Library.

[16] Wada HG, et al. Enzyme immunoassay of the glycoprotein tropic hormones. Clin Chem 1982;28:1862−6.

[17] Leavitt SA. A private little revolution: the home pregnancy test in American culture. Bull Hist Med 2006;80(2):317−45. Johns Hopkins University Press.

[18] Cole LA. Human chorionic gonadotropin (hCG) and hyperglycosylated hCG, seven semi-independent critical molecules: a review. J Mol Oncol Res 2017;1(1):22−4.

[19] Elliott MM. Carbohydrate and peptide structure of the alpha and beta subunits of chorionic gonadotropin (hCG): characteristics and variants in 32 subunit preparations from normal and aberrant pregnancy and choriocarcinoma. Endocrine 1997;7:15−32.

[20] Butler SA, et al. Human chorionic gonadotropin (hCG) in the secretome of cultured embryos: hyperglycosylated hCG and hCG-free beta subunit are potential markers for infertility management and treatment. Reprod Sci 2013;20(9):1038−45. Sage Publications Sage CA: Los Angeles, CA.

[21] Cole LA. Hyperglycosylated hCG, a review. Placenta 2010;31(8):653−64. Elsevier.

[22] Iles RK, et al. Direct and rapid mass spectral fingerprinting of maternal urine for the detection of Down syndrome pregnancy. Clini Proteomics BioMed Central 2015; 12(1):9. https://doi.org/10.1186/s12014-015-9082-9.

[23] Gronowski AM, et al. False-negative results in point-of-care qualitative human chorionic gonadotropin (hCG) devices due to excess hCGβ core fragment. Clin Chem 2009;55(7):1389−94.

[24] Nerenz RD, Song H, Gronowski AM. Screening method to evaluate point-of-care human chorionic gonadotropin (hCG) devices for susceptibility to the hook effect by hCG β core fragment: evaluation of 11 devices. Clin Chem 2014;60(4):667−74.

[25] Cole LA, et al. Between-method variation in human chorionic gonadotropin test results. Clin Chem 2004;50(5):874−82.

[26] Bock JL. HCG assays: a plea for uniformity. Am J Clin Pathol 1990;93(3):432−3. Oxford University Press Oxford, UK.

[27] Karas M, Bachmann D, Hillenkamp F. Influence of the wavelength in high-irradiance ultraviolet laser desorption mass spectrometry of organic molecules. Anal Chem 1985;57(14):2935−9. ACS Publications.

[28] Karas M, Hillenkamp F. Laser desorption ionization of proteins with molecular masses exceeding 10,000 daltons. Anal Chem 1988;60(20):2299−301. ACS Publications.

[29] Beavis RC, Chait BT. High-accuracy molecular mass determination of proteins using matrix-assisted laser desorption mass spectrometry. Anal Chem 1990;62(17): 1836−40. https://doi.org/10.1021/ac00216a020. American Chemical Society.

[30] Lund H, et al. Exploring the complementary selectivity of immunocapture and MS detection for the differentiation between hCG isoforms in clinically relevant samples. J Proteome Res 2009;8(11):5241−52. ACS Publications.

[31] Ng EWY, Wong MYM, Poon TCW. Advances in MALDI mass spectrometry in clinical diagnostic applications. In: Chemical diagnostics. Springer; 2013. p. 139−75.

[32] Bucknall M, Fung KYC, Duncan MW. Practical quantitative biomedical applications of MALDI-TOF mass spectrometry. J Am Soc Mass Spectrom 2002;13(9):1015−27. https://doi.org/10.1016/S1044-0305(02)00426-9.

[33] Cho YT, et al. The study of interferences for diagnosing albuminuria by matrix-assisted laser desorption ionization/time-of-flight mass spectrometry. Clin Chim Acta 2012; 413(9−10):875−82. https://doi.org/10.1016/j.cca.2012.01.029. Elsevier B.V.

[34] Biroccio A, et al. A quantitative method for the analysis of glycated and glutathionylated hemoglobin by matrix-assisted laser desorption ionization-time of flight mass spectrometry. Anal Biochem 2005;336(2):279−88. Elsevier.

[35] Helmke SM, et al. 'Simultaneous quantification of human cardiac α-and β-myosin heavy chain proteins by MALDI-TOF mass spectrometry. Anal Chem 2004;76(6): 1683−9. ACS Publications.

[36] Team RC. A language and environment for statistical computing. Vienna, Austria2014': R Foundation for Statistical Computing; 2014. URL, https://www.R-project.org.

[37] Gibb S, Strimmer K. Maldiquant: A versatile R package for the analysis of mass spectrometry data. Bioinformatics 2012;28(17):2270−1. https://doi.org/10.1093/bioinformatics/bts447.

[38] Gibb S. MALDIquantForeign: import/Export routines for MALDIquant. R package version 0.7. 2014.

[39] Ryan CG, et al. SNIP, a statistics-sensitive background treatment for the quantitative analysis of PIXE spectra in geoscience applications. Nucl Instrum Methods Phys Res Sect B Beam Interact Mater Atoms 1988;34(3):396−402. Elsevier.

[40] Reis MF, et al. Quantification of urinary chorionic gonadotropin in spontaneous abortion of pre-clinically recognized pregnancy: method development and analytical validation. Int J Hyg Environ Health 2007;210(3−4):419−27. Elsevier.

[41] MIDGLEY JR AR. Radioimmunoassay: a method for human chorionic gonadotropin and human luteinizing hormone. Endocrinology 1966;79(1):10−8. Oxford University Press.

[42] Vaitukaitis JL, Braunstein GD, Ross GT. A radioimmunoassay which specifically measures human chorionic gonadotropin in the presence of human luteinizing hormone. Am J Obstet Gynecol 1972;113(6):751−8. Elsevier.

Pregnancy failures and false-positive hCG tests

2.3

Laurence A. Cole

Introduction

The USA hCG Reference Service is a specialty consulting service specializing in false-positive hCG assay cases and gestational trophoblastic disease cases. Here we present the latest findings with false-positive hCG cases. The USA hCG Reference Service discovered the cause of problems for the 2001 outbreak, a clear defect in the Abbott AxSym assay [1], and disclosed methods to determine false-positive hCG [2,3], quiescent pregnancy, aftereffect of a recently aborted or terminated pregnancy in 2001 [4], the most common cause of a false-positive hCG test, and discovered familial hCG, the genetic false-positive hCG syndrome in 2012 [5]. These cases and pituitary sulfated hCG cases, heterophilic antibodies cases, and cancer cases appear to be all of the causes of false-positive hCG pregnancy tests.

The USA hCG Reference Service started at Yale University in 1998, when I was constantly bugged by 12 US physicians to investigate why their patients were false-positive in a commercial hCG test. Physicians tested for hCG, and once a patient was shown to be positive, pregnancy was confirmed one or two or 3 weeks later by ultrasound. When repeated ultrasound showed no pregnancy, a false-positive hCG test was considered. In early days, 1998—2005, chemotherapy and surgery were commonly used to treat false-positive cases.

The USA hCG Reference Service charged cases $974. Of this, approximately $100 was paid to Tricore Laboratories Inc. and Quest Diagnostics to run a follicle-stimulating hormone (FSH), total hCG, total urine hCG, and hyperglycosylated hCG assay, and $120 was paid to send serum samples on dry ice by federal express to University of Alberta Hospital in Edmonton, Canada, the only laboratory in America willing to run an hCG free β-subunit test. In the fall 2017, the USA hCG Reference Service was partly closed, only examining urgent or specialty cases. In 2018 and 2019, the USA hCG Reference Service examined five cases with familial hCG syndrome, two cases with quiescent pregnancy hCG, and one case with cancer. These cases were not included in this study. The USA hCG Reference Service was closed in 2017 because of the repetitiveness of the service and problem with health insurance services.

100 Years of Human Chorionic Gonadotropin. https://doi.org/10.1016/B978-0-12-820050-6.00009-6

Material and methods

As a commercial consulting service, the USA hCG Reference Service ordered the following tests.

The serum total hCG was run by the service (1998–2009) by Tricore Laboratories Inc. (2010–14) and Quest Diagnostics Inc. (2015–17). The service measured total hCG on a Siemens Immulite 1000 automated analyzer using the manufacturer's WHO fourth I.S. internal hCG standard. Tests were run exactly according to manufacturer's guidelines. Tricore Diagnostics Inc. measured total hCG on the Siemens Immulite 2000 automated analyzer, and Quest Inc. measured total hCG using the Siemens Centaur test.

The serum FSH test was run by the service (1998–2009) by Tricore Laboratories Inc. (2010–14) and Quest Diagnostics Inc. (2015–17). The service measured FSH on a Siemens Immulite 1000 automated analyzer using the manufacturer's second I.S. internal FSH standard. Tests were run exactly according to manufacturer's guidelines. Tricore Diagnostics Inc. measured total hCG on the Siemens Immulite 2000 automated analyzer, and Quest Inc. measured total hCG using the Siemens Centaur test.

Urine hCG was a problem; a quantitative hCG was needed and only a qualitative hCG was permitted by the federal drug administration in the United States. The urine test was run by the service (1998–2009). Urine was run on the Siemens Immulite 1000 total hCG test together with urine standards (recombinant hCG). I used the Tricore Laboratories serum total hCG (2010–15) and the Quest Diagnostics serum total hCG (2015–17). In each cases, I took urine and diluted it 1:1 with normal male serum and then submitted it for serum total hCG tests. I then multiplied the results by two.

Hyperglycosylated hCG and extravillous cytotrophoblast hCG were measured by the service (1998–2009) using the B152 immunoassay and C5 hCG standards. The test was run as described previously [4]. In 2002, I set up the identical B152 test at Quest Diagnostics Inc. They have run the test as described ever since. Quest Diagnostics ran the test (2010–17).

The free β-subunit was another problem. The free β-subunit test was run by the service (1998–2009). The service used the FBT11 assay as previously described [4]. The test used CR129 β-subunit standard calibrated in nanograms per milliliter. The only free β-subunit test ran in the United States is the Perkin-Elmer DELFIA test. They have told all laboratories that the test can only be used for Down syndrome screening and have banned all other applications. I send serum samples on dry ice to University of Alberta Hospital in Edmonton, Alberta, Canada, the only laboratory willing to run test for us. They ran all serum free β-subunit tests 2010–17.

Results and discussion

Table 2.3.1 shows the overall experience of the USA hCG Reference Service with 307 cases. The principal cause of false-positive hCG pregnancy tests was by far quiescent pregnancy. It causes 48% of false-positive hCG pregnancy tests. Quiescent

Table 2.3.1 The overall experience of the USA hCG Reference Service.

Quiescent pregnancy	147 cases	48%
Pituitary sulfated hCG	32 cases	10%
Heterophilic antibody	73 cases	24%
Familial hCG syndrome	14 cases	4.6%
Cancer	41 cases	13%
Total	307 cases	

pregnancy occurs when a biochemical pregnancy or spontaneous abortion leaves residual tissue that persistently, for approximately 1 year, produces hCG and causes false-positive pregnancy tests. Heterophilic antibodies are the second most common cause of false-positive pregnancy test. Heterophilic antibodies or cross-species antibodies in the maternal blood can cross-link the capture and tracer antibody used in not properly protected hCG assays, causing false-positive hCG pregnancy results. Cancer is the third most common cause of false-positive results in a hCG assay. Cancer naturally produces extravillous cytotrophoblast hCG and its free β-subunit [6]. As such it can lead to a false-positive hCG pregnancy test. Patient needs to see an oncologist or gynecological oncologist to have cancer identified. Pituitary sulfated hCG is the fourth most common cause of false-positive hCG in pregnancy tests. Detectable pituitary sulfated hCG is produced naturally by menopausal and perimenopausal women. Familial hCG syndrome is the fifth most common cause of false-positive hCG pregnancy tests. Familial hCG syndrome is a genetic defect leading to men and women producing hCG outside of pregnancy, and one of their parents and possibly their children producing hCG [5,7]. It is thought that familial hCG syndrome evolves from fetal hCG produced during pregnancy, with the fetus not stopping production of hCG, leading to hCG production during life.

Table 2.3.2 shows the USA hCG Reference Service experience with 307 cases. Pituitary sulfated hCG was found in 32 cases. As shown, it was found with symptoms of perimenopause or oligomenorrhea, with symptoms of menopause or amenorrhea, or in those with history of oophorectomy and amenorrhea. Pituitary sulfated hCG production was marked by the presence of a high concentration of FSH (FSH >30 IU/L). This can be used to identify pituitary sulfated hCG cases (Table 2.3.2).

Quiescent pregnancy was diagnosed in 147 cases (Table 2.3.2). Hyperglycosylated hCG and extravillous cytotrophoblast hCG are essential for proper blastocyst implantation [8,9]. The absence or near absence of production of these markers causes failure of implantation [8,9], biochemical pregnancy, and spontaneous abortions and leads to quiescent false-positive pregnancies. The absence of significant hyperglycosylated hCG (<5% of total hCG) is a potent indicator of quiescent pregnancies and should be used in their diagnosis (Table 2.3.2).

Heterophilic antibodies were diagnosed with 73 cases (Table 2.3.2). Heterophilic antibodies are large glycoproteins and never cross the kidney or get into the urine.

Table 2.3.2 The USA hCG Reference Service experience, 1998–2017.

Symptoms and history	Age	Total hCG, IU/L	Hyperglycosylated hCG, IU/L hCG	FSH IU/L	Diagnosis
Perimenopause/oligomenorrhea	35	2.3	<0.50	93	Pituitary sulfated hCG
Perimenopause/oligomenorrhea	48	3.9	<0.50	15	Pituitary sulfated hCG
Perimenopause/oligomenorrhea	39	4.8	<0.50	82	Pituitary sulfated hCG
Perimenopause/oligomenorrhea	46	5.0	<0.50	82	Pituitary sulfated hCG
Perimenopause/oligomenorrhea	49	6.8	<0.50	142	Pituitary sulfated hCG
Perimenopause/oligomenorrhea	69	6.9	<0.50	117	Pituitary sulfated hCG
Perimenopause/oligomenorrhea	49	8.0	<0.50	137	Pituitary sulfated hCG
Perimenopause/oligomenorrhea	43	9.1	<0.50	108	Pituitary sulfated hCG
Perimenopause/oligomenorrhea	39	9.2	<0.50	144	Pituitary sulfated hCG
Perimenopause/oligomenorrhea	34	45	<0.50	111	Pituitary sulfated hCG
Menopause/amenorrhea	54	4.0	<0.50	65	Pituitary sulfated hCG
Menopause/amenorrhea	65	4.5	<0.50	103	Pituitary sulfated hCG
Menopause/amenorrhea	55	4.6	<0.50	39	Pituitary sulfated hCG
Menopause/amenorrhea	52	4.8	<0.50	82	Pituitary sulfated hCG
Menopause/amenorrhea	46	5.0	<0.50	77	Pituitary sulfated hCG
Menopause/amenorrhea	54	6.0	<0.50	37	Pituitary sulfated hCG
Menopause/amenorrhea	69	6.9	<0.50	151	Pituitary sulfated hCG
Menopause/amenorrhea	58	7.3	<0.50	63	Pituitary sulfated hCG
Menopause/amenorrhea	58	7.3	<0.50	63	Pituitary sulfated hCG
Menopause/amenorrhea	58	7.4	<0.50	61	Pituitary sulfated hCG
Menopause/amenorrhea	53	7.5	<0.50	51	Pituitary sulfated hCG
Menopause/amenorrhea	48	7.7	<0.50	60	Pituitary sulfated hCG
Menopause/amenorrhea	54	8.5	<0.50	88	Pituitary sulfated hCG
Menopause/amenorrhea	52	10	<0.50	144	Pituitary sulfated hCG

Menopause/amenorrhea	66	10	<0.50	54	Pituitary sulfated hCG
Menopause/amenorrhea	53	11	<0.50	76	Pituitary sulfated hCG
Menopause/amenorrhea	50	12	<0.50	92	Pituitary sulfated hCG
Menopause/amenorrhea	53	12	<0.50	72	Pituitary sulfated hCG
Menopause/amenorrhea	50	13	<0.50	133	Pituitary sulfated hCG
Menopause/amenorrhea	54	13	<0.50	131	Pituitary sulfated hCG
Oophorectomy/amenorrhea	28	13	<0.50	134	Pituitary sulfated hCG
Oophorectomy/amenorrhea	34	13	<0.50	63	Pituitary sulfated hCG
No symptoms, history of failure	19	<1.0	<0.50		Quiescent pregnancy
No symptoms, history of failure	29	2.4	<0.50		Quiescent pregnancy
No symptoms, history of failure	22	3.1	<0.50		Quiescent pregnancy
No symptoms, history of failure	43	3.3	<0.50		Quiescent pregnancy
No symptoms, history of failure	43	3.3	<0.50		Quiescent pregnancy
No symptoms, history of failure	42	3.4	<0.50		Quiescent pregnancy
No symptoms, history of failure	42	3.4	<0.50		Quiescent pregnancy
No symptoms, history of failure	33	3.7	<0.50		Quiescent pregnancy
No symptoms, history of failure	34	5.0	<0.50		Quiescent pregnancy
No symptoms, history of failure	33	5.5	<0.50		Quiescent pregnancy
No symptoms, history of failure	33	5.5	<0.50		Quiescent pregnancy
No symptoms, history of failure	31	5.7	<0.50		Quiescent pregnancy
No symptoms, history of failure	28	5.9	<0.50		Quiescent pregnancy
No symptoms, history of failure	40	6.0	<0.50		Quiescent pregnancy
No symptoms, history of failure	39	6.0	<0.50		Quiescent pregnancy
No symptoms, history of failure	37	6.4	<0.50		Quiescent pregnancy
No symptoms, history of failure	34	6.6	<0.50		Quiescent pregnancy
No symptoms, history of failure	23	6.6	<0.50		Quiescent pregnancy
No symptoms, history of failure	24	7.3	<0.50		Quiescent pregnancy

Continued

Table 2.3.2 The USA hCG Reference Service experience, 1998–2017.—cont'd

Symptoms and history	Age	Total hCG, IU/L	Hyperglycosylated hCG, IU/L hCG	FSH IU/L	Diagnosis
No symptoms, history of failure	27	7.5	<0.50		Quiescent pregnancy
No symptoms, history of failure	31	8.0	<0.50		Quiescent pregnancy
No symptoms, history of failure	25	8.2	<0.50		Quiescent pregnancy
No symptoms, history of failure	34	8.6	<0.50		Quiescent pregnancy
No symptoms, history of failure	36	11	<0.50		Quiescent pregnancy
No symptoms, history of failure	26	11	<0.50		Quiescent pregnancy
No symptoms, history of failure	30	12	<0.50		Quiescent pregnancy
No symptoms, history of failure	30	12.7	<0.50		Quiescent pregnancy
No symptoms, history of failure	19	12.9	0.77		Quiescent pregnancy
No symptoms, history of failure	35	13	<0.50		Quiescent pregnancy
No symptoms, history of failure	39	13	<0.50		Quiescent pregnancy
No symptoms, history of failure	32	14	<0.50		Quiescent pregnancy
No symptoms, history of failure	33	14	<0.50		Quiescent pregnancy
No symptoms, history of failure	19	15	<0.50		Quiescent pregnancy
No symptoms, history of failure	28	15	<0.50		Quiescent pregnancy
No symptoms, history of failure	21	16	<0.50		Quiescent pregnancy
No symptoms, history of failure	24	17	<0.50		Quiescent pregnancy
No symptoms, history of failure	20	17	<0.50		Quiescent pregnancy
No symptoms, history of failure	20	17	<1.0		Quiescent pregnancy
No symptoms, history of failure	28	18.7	<0.44		Quiescent pregnancy
No symptoms, history of failure	41	23	<0.50		Quiescent pregnancy
No symptoms, history of failure	25	23	<0.50		Quiescent pregnancy
No symptoms, history of failure	36	23	<0.50		Quiescent pregnancy
No symptoms, history of failure	33	23	<0.50		Quiescent pregnancy

No symptoms, history of failure	17	24	<0.50	Quiescent pregnancy
No symptoms, history of failure	22	24	<0.50	Quiescent pregnancy
No symptoms, history of failure	21	24	<0.50	Quiescent pregnancy
No symptoms, history of failure	53	27	<0.50	Quiescent pregnancy
No symptoms, history of failure	31	27	<0.50	Quiescent pregnancy
No symptoms, history of failure	23	29	<0.50	Quiescent pregnancy
No symptoms, history of failure	29	35	<0.50	Quiescent pregnancy
No symptoms, history of failure	35	35	<0.50	Quiescent pregnancy
No symptoms, history of failure	29	35	<0.50	Quiescent pregnancy
No symptoms, history of failure	28	37	<0.50	Quiescent pregnancy
No symptoms, history of failure	27	37	<0.50	Quiescent pregnancy
No symptoms, history of failure	31	38	<0.50	Quiescent pregnancy
No symptoms, history of failure	27	41	<0.50	Quiescent pregnancy
No symptoms, history of failure	33	44	<0.50	Quiescent pregnancy
No symptoms, history of failure	30	46	<0.50	Quiescent pregnancy
No symptoms, history of failure	35	46	<0.50	Quiescent pregnancy
No symptoms, history of failure	44	49	<0.50	Quiescent pregnancy
No symptoms, history of failure	34	52	<0.50	Quiescent pregnancy
No symptoms, history of failure	34	52	<0.50	Quiescent pregnancy
No symptoms, history of failure	31	55	<0.50	Quiescent pregnancy
No symptoms, history of failure	32	55	<0.50	Quiescent pregnancy
No symptoms, history of failure	36	59	<0.50	Quiescent pregnancy
No symptoms, history of failure	40	62	<0.50	Quiescent pregnancy
No symptoms, history of failure	38	70	<0.50	Quiescent pregnancy
No symptoms, history of failure	35	79	<0.50	Quiescent pregnancy
No symptoms, history of failure;	25	81	<0.50	Quiescent pregnancy

Continued

Table 2.3.2 The USA hCG Reference Service experience, 1998–2017.—cont'd

Symptoms and history	Age	Total hCG, IU/L	Hyperglycosylated hCG, IU/L hCG	FSH IU/L	Diagnosis
No symptoms, history of failure	47	94	<0.50		Quiescent pregnancy
No symptoms, history of failure	43	100	<0.50		Quiescent pregnancy
No symptoms, history of failure	28	106	<0.50		Quiescent pregnancy
No symptoms, history of failure	30	127	<0.50		Quiescent pregnancy
No symptoms, history of failure	43	139	<0.50		Quiescent pregnancy
No symptoms, history of failure	24	212	<0.50		Quiescent pregnancy
No symptoms, history of failure	22	245	<0.50		Quiescent pregnancy
No symptoms, history of failure	24	5.0	<0.50		Quiescent pregnancy
No symptoms, history of failure	20	12	<0.50		Quiescent pregnancy
No symptoms, history of failure	21	3.0	<0.50		Quiescent pregnancy
No symptoms, history of failure	48	13	<0.50		Quiescent pregnancy
History of mole, treated for choriocarcinoma	18	2.9	<0.50		Quiescent pregnancy
History of mole, treated for choriocarcinoma	7.7	3.1	<0.50		Quiescent pregnancy
History of mole, treated for choriocarcinoma	34	3.5	<0.50		Quiescent pregnancy
History of mole, treated for choriocarcinoma	27	3.6	<0.50		Quiescent pregnancy
History of mole, treated for choriocarcinoma	31	4.9	<0.50		Quiescent pregnancy
History of mole, treated for choriocarcinoma	35	5	<0.50		Quiescent pregnancy
History of mole, treated for choriocarcinoma	22	6.6	<0.50		Quiescent pregnancy
History of mole, treated for choriocarcinoma	26	7.1	<0.50		Quiescent pregnancy
History of mole, treated for choriocarcinoma	30	7.2	<0.50		Quiescent pregnancy
History of mole, treated for choriocarcinoma	47	8.2	<0.66		Quiescent pregnancy
History of mole, treated for choriocarcinoma	28	8.3	<1.0		Quiescent pregnancy
History of mole, treated for choriocarcinoma	15	9.6	<0.50		Quiescent pregnancy
History of mole, treated for choriocarcinoma	51	9.8	<0.50		Quiescent pregnancy

History of mole, treated for choriocarcinoma	37	11	<0.50	Quiescent pregnancy
History of mole, treated for choriocarcinoma	35	11	<0.50	Quiescent pregnancy
History of mole, treated for choriocarcinoma	20	13	<0.50	Quiescent pregnancy
History of mole, treated for choriocarcinoma	35	13	<0.50	Quiescent pregnancy
History of mole, treated for choriocarcinoma	43	13	<0.50	Quiescent pregnancy
History of mole, treated for choriocarcinoma	38	15	<0.50	Quiescent pregnancy
History of mole, treated for choriocarcinoma	32	16	<0.50	Quiescent pregnancy
History of mole, treated for choriocarcinoma	43	16	<0.50	Quiescent pregnancy
History of mole, treated for choriocarcinoma	27	16	<0.50	Quiescent pregnancy
History of mole, treated for choriocarcinoma	26	17	<0.50	Quiescent pregnancy
History of mole, treated for choriocarcinoma	45	19	<0.50	Quiescent pregnancy
History of mole, treated for choriocarcinoma	37	20	2.8	Quiescent pregnancy
History of mole, treated for choriocarcinoma	19	21	<0.50	Quiescent pregnancy
History of mole, treated for choriocarcinoma	18	22	<0.50	Quiescent pregnancy
History of mole, treated for choriocarcinoma	34	23	<0.50	Quiescent pregnancy
History of mole, treated for choriocarcinoma	28	23	<0.50	Quiescent pregnancy
History of mole, treated for choriocarcinoma	20	26	<0.50	Quiescent pregnancy
History of mole, treated for choriocarcinoma	34	27	<0.50	Quiescent pregnancy
History of mole, treated for choriocarcinoma	34	29	<0.50	Quiescent pregnancy
History of mole, treated for choriocarcinoma	31	29	<0.50	Quiescent pregnancy
History of mole, treated for choriocarcinoma	31	31	<0.50	Quiescent pregnancy
History of mole, treated for choriocarcinoma	39	39	<0.50	Quiescent pregnancy
History of mole, treated for choriocarcinoma	39	42	<0.50	Quiescent pregnancy
History of mole, treated for choriocarcinoma	20	43	<0.50	Quiescent pregnancy
History of mole, treated for choriocarcinoma	39	51	<0.50	Quiescent pregnancy
History of mole, treated for choriocarcinoma	39	53	<0.50	Quiescent pregnancy
History of mole, treated for choriocarcinoma	29	57	<0.50	Quiescent pregnancy
History of mole, treated for choriocarcinoma	30	61	<0.33	Quiescent pregnancy
History of mole, treated for choriocarcinoma	26	61	<0.50	Quiescent pregnancy

Continued

Table 2.3.2 The USA hCG Reference Service experience, 1998–2017.—cont'd

Symptoms and history	Age	Total hCG, IU/L	Hyperglycosylated hCG, IU/L hCG	FSH IU/L	Diagnosis
History of mole, treated for choriocarcinoma	36	75	<0.50		Quiescent pregnancy
History of mole, treated for choriocarcinoma	27	79.4	<0.44		Quiescent pregnancy
History of mole, treated for choriocarcinoma	33	93	<0.50		Quiescent pregnancy
History of mole, treated for choriocarcinoma	30	117	21		Quiescent pregnancy
History of mole, treated for choriocarcinoma	38	2.0	<0.50		Quiescent pregnancy
History of mole, treated for choriocarcinoma	31	7.6	<0.50		Quiescent pregnancy
History of mole, treated for choriocarcinoma	31	9.9	<0.50		Quiescent pregnancy
History of mole, treated for choriocarcinoma	20	12	<0.50		Quiescent pregnancy
History of mole, treated for choriocarcinoma	28	15	<0.50		Quiescent pregnancy
History of mole, treated for choriocarcinoma	36	37	<0.50		Quiescent pregnancy
History of mole, treated for choriocarcinoma	32	38	<0.66		Quiescent pregnancy
History of mole, treated for choriocarcinoma	30	43	<0.50		Quiescent pregnancy
History of mole, treated for choriocarcinoma	29	48	<0.50		Quiescent pregnancy
History of mole, treated for choriocarcinoma	39	2.0	<0.50		Quiescent pregnancy
History of mole, treated for choriocarcinoma	33	2.1	<0.50		Quiescent pregnancy
History of mole, treated for choriocarcinoma	44	3.2	<0.50		Quiescent pregnancy
History of mole, treated for choriocarcinoma	35	5.8	<0.50		Quiescent pregnancy
History of mole, treated for choriocarcinoma	40	10	<0.50		Quiescent pregnancy
History of mole, treated for choriocarcinoma	28	11	<0.50		Quiescent pregnancy
History of mole, treated for choriocarcinoma	39	13	<0.50		Quiescent pregnancy
History of mole, treated for choriocarcinoma	29	20	<0.66		Quiescent pregnancy
History of mole, treated for choriocarcinoma	34	30	<0.50		Quiescent pregnancy
History of mole, treated for choriocarcinoma	37	99	<0.50		Quiescent pregnancy
History of mole, treated for choriocarcinoma	44	107	<0.50		Quiescent pregnancy

	Serum hCG IU/L	Urine hCG IU/L	Assay	Result	False-positive hCG test
No symptoms, no history	12	<1.0	Abbott AxSym	6.0	Heterophilic antibody
No symptoms, no history	15	<1.0	Abbott AxSym	8.4	Heterophilic antibody
No symptoms, no history	<1.0	<1.0	Abbott AxSym	12	Heterophilic antibody
No symptoms, no history	<1.0	<1.0	Abbott AxSym	16	Heterophilic antibody
No symptoms, no history	17	<1.0	Abbott AxSym	17	Heterophilic antibody
No symptoms, no history	<1.0	<1.0	Abbott AxSym	20	Heterophilic antibody
No symptoms, no history	<1.0	<1.0	Abbott AxSym	21	Heterophilic antibody
No symptoms, no history	<1.0	<1.0	Abbott AxSym	24	Heterophilic antibody
No symptoms, no history	<1.0	<1.0	Abbott AxSym	33	Heterophilic antibody
No symptoms, no history	<1.0	<1.0	Abbott AxSym	38	Heterophilic antibody
No symptoms, no history	15	<1.0	Abbott AxSym	41	Heterophilic antibody
No symptoms, no history	6.3	<1.0	Abbott AxSym	50	Heterophilic antibody
No symptoms, no history	5.4	<1.0	Abbott AxSym	50	Heterophilic antibody
No symptoms, no history	23	<1.0	Abbott AxSym	57	Heterophilic antibody
No symptoms, no history	<1.0	<1.0	Abbott AxSym	60	Heterophilic antibody
No symptoms, no history	<1.0	10.5	Abbott AxSym	79	Heterophilic antibody
No symptoms, no history	110	<1.0	Abbott AxSym	80	Heterophilic antibody
No symptoms, no history	<1.0	<1.0	Abbott AxSym	81	Heterophilic antibody
No symptoms, no history	15	<1.0	Abbott AxSym	82	Heterophilic antibody
No symptoms, no history	18	<1.0	Abbott AxSym	97	Heterophilic antibody
No symptoms, no history	13	<1.0	Abbott AxSym	120	Heterophilic antibody
No symptoms, no history	<1.0	<1.0	Abbott AxSym	122	Heterophilic antibody
No symptoms, no history	10	<1.0	Abbott AxSym	139	Heterophilic antibody
No symptoms, no history	9.9	<1.0	Abbott AxSym	151	Heterophilic antibody
No symptoms, no history	3.6	<1.0	Abbott AxSym	160	Heterophilic antibody

Continued

Table 2.3.2 The USA hCG Reference Service experience, 1998–2017.—cont'd

	Serum	Urine	False-positive hCG test		
	hCG IU/L	hCG IU/L	Assay	Result	
No symptoms, no history	<1.0	<1.0	Abbott AxSym	168	Heterophilic antibody
No symptoms, no history	<1.0	<1.0	Abbott AxSym	190	Heterophilic antibody
No symptoms, no history	<1.0	<1.0	Abbott AxSym	200	Heterophilic antibody
No symptoms, no history	<1.0	<1.0	Abbott AxSym	212	Heterophilic antibody
No symptoms, no history	42	<1.0	Abbott AxSym	275	Heterophilic antibody
No symptoms, no history	<1.0	<1.0	Abbott AxSym	284	Heterophilic antibody
No symptoms, no history	6.1	<1.0	Abbott AxSym	300	Heterophilic antibody
No symptoms, no history	<1.0	<1.0	Abbott AxSym	300	Heterophilic antibody
No symptoms, no history	179	<1.0	Abbott AxSym	350	Heterophilic antibody
No symptoms, no history	<1.0	<1.0	Abbott AxSym	350	Heterophilic antibody
No symptoms, no history	21	<1.0	Abbott AxSym	351	Heterophilic antibody
No symptoms, no history	13	<1.0	Abbott AxSym	385	Heterophilic antibody
No symptoms, no history	<1.0	<1.0	Abbott AxSym	400	Heterophilic antibody
No symptoms, no history	<1.0	<1.0	Abbott AxSym	402	Heterophilic antibody
No symptoms, no history	3.3	<1.0	Abbott AxSym	1010	Heterophilic antibody
No symptoms, no history	<1.0	<1.0	Beckman Access	25	Heterophilic antibody
No symptoms, no history	<1.0	<1.0	Beckman Access	40	Heterophilic antibody
No symptoms, no history	<1.0	<1.0	Beckman Access	84	Heterophilic antibody
No symptoms, no history	<1.0	<1.0	Beckman Access	95	Heterophilic antibody
No symptoms, no history	31	26	Beckman DXI	36	Heterophilic antibody
No symptoms, no history	<1.0	<1.0	Beckman DXI	50	Heterophilic antibody
No symptoms, no history	<1.0	<1.0	Ortho Vitros Eci	80	Heterophilic antibody
No symptoms, no history	<1.0	<1.0	Ortho Vitros Eci	41	Heterophilic antibody
No symptoms, no history	<1.0	<1.0	Ortho Vitros Eci	100	Heterophilic antibody
No symptoms, no history	<1.0	<1.0	Ortho Vitros Eci	9.1	Heterophilic antibody

Case details	Sex	Age	Total hCG IU/L	Free β IU/L	
No symptoms, no history	1.6	<1.0	Roche Elecsys	13.2	Heterophillic antibody
No symptoms, no history	<1.0	<1.0	Siemens ACS180	20	Heterophillic antibody
No symptoms, no history	<1.0	<1.0	Siemens Centaur	23	Heterophillic antibody
No symptoms, no history	13	<1.0	Siemens Centaur	27	Heterophillic antibody
No symptoms, no history	<1.0	<1.0	Siemens Centaur	37	Heterophillic antibody
No symptoms, no history	<1.0	<1.0	Siemens Centaur	40	Heterophillic antibody
No symptoms, no history	<1.0	<1.0	Siemens Centaur	6.1	Heterophillic antibody
No symptoms, no history	<1.0	<1.0	Siemens Centaur	404	Heterophillic antibody
No symptoms, no history	<1.0	<1.0	Siemens Centaur	15	Heterophillic antibody
No symptoms, no history	5.9	<1.0	Siemens Centaur	30	Heterophillic antibody
No symptoms, no history	<1.0	<1.0	Siemens Centaur	11	Heterophillic antibody
No symptoms, no history	4.4	<1.0	Siemens Centaur	11	Heterophillic antibody
No symptoms, no history	<1.0	<1.0	Siemens Centaur	16	Heterophillic antibody
No symptoms, no history	<1.0	<1.0	Siemens Centaur	80	Heterophillic antibody
No symptoms, no history	<1.0	<1.0	Siemens Centaur	25	Heterophillic antibody
No symptoms, no history	<1.0	<1.0	Siemens Centaur	23	Heterophillic antibody
No symptoms, no history	<1.0	<1.0	Siemens Dimension	23	Heterophillic antibody
No symptoms, no history	<1.0	<1.0	Siemens Dimension	14	Heterophillic antibody
No symptoms, no history	<1.0	<1.0	Siemens Dimension	20	Heterophillic antibody
No symptoms, no history	<1.0	<1.0	Siemens Dimension	19	Heterophillic antibody
No symptoms, no history	4.2	<1.0	Siemens Immulite	11	Heterophillic antibody
No symptoms, no history	4.8	<1.0	Siemens Immulite	14.3	Heterophillic antibody
No symptoms, no history	5.7	<1.0	Siemens Immulite	11	Heterophillic antibody
Case details	**Sex**	**Age**	**Total hCG IU/L**	**Free β IU/L**	
Case 1	F	32	43	34	Familial hCG syndrome
Case 1 Sister	F	34	34		Familial hCG syndrome
Case 1 Mother	F	54	54		Familial hCG syndrome
Case 2	M	32	2.0	1.3 (65%)	Familial hCG syndrome

Continued

Table 2.3.2 The USA hCG Reference Service experience, 1998–2017.—cont'd

Case details	Sex	Age	Total hCG IU/L	Free β IU/L	
Case 2 Brother	M	28	1.1		Familial hCG syndrome
Case 2 Father	M	50	1.3		Familial hCG syndrome
Case 3	M	22	2.8	1.7 (61%)	Familial hCG syndrome
Case 3 Father	M	45	3.3		Familial hCG syndrome
Case 4	F	28	201	113 (56%)	Familial hCG syndrome
Case 4 Sister	F	27	153		Familial hCG syndrome
Case 4 Father	M	53	142		Familial hCG syndrome
Case 5	M	22	1.8	1.0 (55%)	Familial hCG syndrome
Case 5 Mother	F	55	2.5		Familial hCG syndrome
Case 6	F	33	216	121 (56%)	Familial hCG syndrome
Case 6 Father	M	56	201		Familial hCG syndrome
Case 7	F	28	32	17 (53%)	Familial hCG syndrome
Case 7 Son	M	3	24		Familial hCG syndrome
Case 8	F	58	9.4	7.6 (81%)	Familial hCG syndrome
Case 8 Daughter	F	22	Only urine tested 2.5		Familial hCG syndrome
Case 9	M	20	25	1.2 (60%)	Familial hCG syndrome
Case 9 Father	M	46	Only urine tested 1.6		Familial hCG syndrome
Case 9 Brother	M	16	Only urine tested 4.0		Familial hCG syndrome
Case 10	M	28	<1.0	<0.03 6.8	Familial hCG syndrome
Case 10 Father	M	52	<1.0	10	Familial hCG syndrome
Case 11	M	24	<1	27	Familial hCG syndrome
Father	M	55	2.2	85	Familial hCG syndrome
Brother	M	18	0.59	55	Familial hCG syndrome
Case 12	F	21	<1	26	Familial hCG syndrome
Case 12 Sister	F	19	<1	19	Familial hCG syndrome

	Sex	Age	Total hCG IU/L	Hyperglycosylated hCG	Free β IU/L	final diagnosis
Case 12 Mother	F	51		<1	22	Familial hCG syndrome
Case 13	M	29		<1	2.1 (100%) 4.2	Familial hCG syndrome
Case 13 Father	F	55		<1	3.2	Familial hCG syndrome
Case 14	F	26		17	13 (76%) 15	Familial hCG syndrome
Case 14 Mother	F	51		12	10	Familial hCG syndrome
No symptoms		31	305	310	59	Choriocarcinoma
No symptoms		39	1929	1991	273	Choriocarcinoma
No symptoms		19	1208	720	76	Choriocarcinoma
No symptoms		15	214	162	29	Choriocarcinoma
No symptoms		32	22	74	<0.5	Choriocarcinoma
No symptoms		40	99	112	1.0	Choriocarcinoma
No symptoms		39	80,400	88,550	216	Choriocarcinoma
No symptoms		26	206	58	145	Cervical cancer
No symptoms		31	6.6	2.6	6.6	Cervical cancer
No symptoms		52	274	79	198	Renal carcinoma
No symptoms		22	6.4	4.1	10	Ductal breast cancer
No symptoms		40	27.9	8.6	22	Ductal breast cancer
No symptoms		17	1.0	0.21	0.54	Endometrial cancer
No symptoms		21	1.5	3.3	8.3	Endometrial cancer
No symptoms		34	160	68	172	Endometrial cancer
No symptoms		33	19	5.9	15	Hepatocellular cancer
No symptoms		27	209	54	136	Lobular breast cancer
No symptoms		20	235	73	183	Lobular breast cancer
No symptoms		37	3.1	2.0	5	Small cell lung cancer

Continued

Table 2.3.2 The USA hCG Reference Service experience, 1998–2017.—cont'd

	Age	Total hCG hCG IU/L	Hyperglycosylated hCG	Free β final diagnosis IU/L	
No symptoms	21	46	13	34	Ovarian cancer
No symptoms	14	4.9	1.2	3.0	Ovarian cancer
No symptoms	21	320	132	329	Ovarian cancer
No symptoms	17	110	29	72	Ovarian cancer
No symptoms	26	12	4.4	11	Ovarian cancer
No symptoms	19	21	10	25	Ovarian cancer
No symptoms	21	150	61	153	Ovarian cancer
No symptoms	18	10	2.1	5.2	Ovarian cancer
No symptoms	25	16.5	4.7	12	Ovarian cancer
No symptoms	50	41	16	41	Ovarian cancer
No symptoms	37	2.3	1.4	3.4	Ovarian cancer
No symptoms	31	3.5	7.8	19	Ovarian cancer
No symptoms	45	43	20	49	Renal carcinoma
No symptoms	34	1.9	8	20	Small cell lung cancer
No symptoms	46	11	4.4	11	Hepatic cancer
No symptoms	26	24.4	6.8	17	Vulvar cancer
No symptoms	39	119	43	108	Bladder cancer
No symptoms	50	129	202	504	Bladder cancer
No symptoms	40	223	67	167	Bladder cancer
No symptoms	26	249	79	198	Bladder cancer
No symptoms	54	564	171	428	Bladder cancer
No symptoms	25	683	112	281	Bladder cancer
No symptoms	29	48	14	35	Uterine cancer

The presence of heterophilic antibodies is best diagnosed by showing the absence of any hCG cross-reactivity in urine. This is the standard test for detecting these pregnancy failures (Table 2.3.2).

Familial hCG syndrome was detected in 14 cases. This is best demonstrated by showing that the majority of hCG immunoreactivity is coming from free β-subunit. It is confirmed by demonstration that either the father or the mother is producing false-positive hCG (Table 2.3.3).

Cancer is another cause of false-positive pregnancy hCGs (Table 2.3.4). You can only rule out quiescent pregnancy, pituitary sulfated hCG, heterophilic antibodies, and familial hCG syndrome and refer patient to an oncologist or gynecology oncologist.

Table 2.3.3 False-positive hCG results due to familial hCG syndrome.

Case	Sex	Age	Serum hCG IU/L	Serum hCG Free β IU/L	Total Urine hCG IU/L
Case 1	F	32	43	34 (79%)	3.0
Case 1 Sister	F	34	34		2.0
Case 1 Mother	F	54	54		2.0
Case 2	M	32	2.0	1.3 (65%)	26
Case 2 Brother	M	28	1.1		4.0
Case 2 Father	M	50	1.3		1.6
Case 3	M	22	2.8	1.7 (61%)	54
Case 3 Father	M	45	3.3		27
Case 4	F	28	201	113 (56%)	83
Case 4 Sister	F	27	153		100
Case 4 Father	M	53	142		670
Case 5	M	22	1.8	1.0 (55%)	2.9
Case 5 Mother	F	55	2.5		2.8
Case 6	F	33	216	121 (56%)	24
Case 6 Father	M	56	201		178
Case 7	F	28	32	17 (53%)	27
Case 7 Son	M	3	24		12
Case 8	F	58	9.4	7.6 (81%)	1.5
Case 8 Daughter	F	22	Only urine tested		2.5
Case 9	M	20	2.0	1.2 (60%)	25
Case 9 Father	M	46	Only urine tested		1.6
Case 9 Brother	M	16	Only urine tested		4.0
Case 10	M	28	<1.0	<0.03	6.8
Case 10 Father	M	52	<1.0		10
Case 11	M	24	<1		27
Father	M	55	2.2		85

Continued

Table 2.3.3 False-positive hCG results due to familial hCG syndrome.—*cont'd*

Case	Sex	Age	Serum hCG IU/L	Serum hCG Free β IU/L	Total Urine hCG IU/L
Brother	M	18	0.59		55
Case 12	F	21	<1		26
Case 12 Sister	F	19	<1		19
Case 12 Mother	F	51	<1		22
Case 13	M	29	<1	2.1(100%)	4.2
Case 13 Father	F	55	<1		3.2
Case 14	F	26	17	13(76%)	15
Case 14 Mother	F	51	12		10

Table 2.3.4 Cancer as a cause of false-positive hCG result, 49 cases.

Age	Total hCG Serum IU/L	Hyperglycosylated hCG serum IU/L	Free β IU/L	Final Histology
31	305	310	59	Choriocarcinoma
39	1929	1991	273	Choriocarcinoma
19	1208	720	76	Choriocarcinoma
15	214	162	29	Choriocarcinoma
32	22	74	<0.5	Choriocarcinoma
40	99	112	1.0	Choriocarcinoma
39	80,400	88,550	216	Choriocarcinoma
53	3.1	0.17	1.9	Placental site trophoblastic
37	224	<0.36	70	Placental site trophoblastic
26	116	46	3.4	Testicular germ cell
31	673,000	880,000	445	Testicular germ cell
26	206	58	145	Cervical cancer
31	6.6	2.6	6.6	Cervical cancer
52	274	79	198	Clear cell renal carcinoma
22	6.4	4.1	10	Ductal breast cancer
40	27.9	8.6	22	Ductal breast cancer
17	1.0	0.21	0.54	Endometrial adenocarcinoma
21	1.5	3.3	8.3	Endometrial adenocarcinoma
34	160	68	172	Endometrial adenocarcinoma
33	19	5.9	15	Hepatocellular carcinoma
27	209	54	136	Lobular breast cancer
20	235	73	183	Lobular breast cancer
37	3.1	2.0	5	Non—small cell lung cancer
21	46	13	34	Ovarian dysgerminoma
14	4.9	1.2	3.0	Ovarian dysgerminoma

Table 2.3.4 Cancer as a cause of false-positive hCG result, 49 cases.—*cont'd*

Age	Total hCG Serum IU/L	Hyperglycosylated hCG serum IU/L	Free β IU/ L	Final Histology
21	320	132	329	Ovarian dysgerminoma
17	110	29	72	Ovarian dysgerminoma
26	12	4.4	11	Ovarian dysgerminoma
19	21	10	25	Ovarian dysgerminoma
21	150	61	153	Ovarian dysgerminoma
18	10	2.1	5.2	Ovarian dysgerminoma
25	16.5	4.7	12	Ovarian dysgerminoma
50	41	16	41	Ovarian serous
37	2.3	1.4	3.4	Ovarian serous
31	3.5	7.8	19	Ovarian serous
45	43	20	49	Papillary renal carcinoma
29	6.8	2.7	6.8	Prostate adenocarcinoma
37	13.3	5.2	13	Prostate adenocarcinoma
51	31.1	10	25	Prostate adenocarcinoma
34	1.9	8	20	Small cell lung cancer
46	11	4.4	11	Squamous cell hepatic cancer
26	24.4	6.8	17	Squamous vulvar cancer
39	119	43	108	Urothelial bladder
50	129	202	504	Urothelial bladder
40	223	67	167	Urothelial bladder
26	249	79	198	Urothelial bladder
54	564	171	428	Urothelial bladder
25	683	112	281	Urothelial bladder
29	48	14	35	Uterine mixed Mullerian

All told diagnosis of a case of false-positive pregnancy tests is simple, you just have to order a serum total hCG, a serum FSH, a serum hyperglycosylated hCG (B152), and a urine total hCG test.

References

[1] Cole LA, Khanlian SA. Easy fix for clinical laboratories for the false positive defect with the Abbott AxSym total ß-hCG test. Clin Biochem 2004;37:344−9.

[2] Butler SA, Cole LA. Use of heterophilic antibody blocking agent (HBT) in reducing false-positive hCG results. Clin Chem 2001;47(7):1332−3.

[3] Butler SA, Cole LA. False positive hCG. Obstet Gynecol 2002;99(3):516−7.

[4] Cole LA, Butler SA. False positive or phantom hCG result: a serious problem. Clin Lab Intl 2001;25:9−14.

[5] Cole LA. Familial hCG. J Reprod Immunol 2012;93:52–7.

[6] Cole LA. Hyperglycosylated hCG drives malignancy in most or all human cancers: tying all research together. J Analyt Oncol 2018;7:14–21.

[7] Cole LA, Butler SA. Familial hCG syndrome: production of variable, degraded or mutant form of hCG. J Reprod Med 2014;59:435–42.

[8] Sasaki Y, Ladner DG. Cole LA hyperglycosylated hCG the source of pregnancy failures. Fertil Steril 2008;89. 1871-1786.

[9] Cole LA. Hyperglycosylated hCG and pregnancy failures. J Reprod Immunol 2012;93:119–22.

The home pregnancy test 2.4

Sarah Johnson

One of the most important questions a woman may have in her life is "Am I Pregnant?" Today's home pregnancy test is able to provide her with this answer in a convenient, discrete, and reliable way. Over 65 million packs of pregnancy tests are sold across Europe per annum, illustrating the tremendous importance of these products to women. But the home pregnancy test in its current form was only possible due to innovative work by scientists at Unipath[1] who pioneered the development of the lateral flow test.

Lateral flow technology: complex immunochemistry made user-friendly

Laboratory-based immunoassays require skilled personnel, laboratory equipment, a controlled environment, and several hours to achieve a reliable result. So, they are definitely not suitable for use by untrained women at a time of stress in their own home. A new technology was needed to convert a complex laboratory method to something very simple to use and which could still work after being stocked on the shelves of a pharmacy or supermarket for years; this led to the development of the lateral flow test.

Like standard immunoassay tests, lateral flow assays rely on the specific binding of the target, in this case, human chorionic gonadotropin (hCG), by labeled antibodies and the subsequent removal of any unbound antibodies from the test zone. In lateral flow tests, this is accomplished simply by fluid flow through porous membranes. The technology has been widely exploited in other applications where quick results are needed in nonlaboratory environments. Examples include home fertility testing, drugs of abuse and infectious disease testing in both humans and animals. The technology's versatility means that different sample fluids can be used including urine, blood, saliva or even solid materials broken down in buffer, an example being allergen testing in foods [1].

---

[1] Unipath products are now made by SPD Swiss Precision Diagnostics GmbH.

100 Years of Human Chorionic Gonadotropin. https://doi.org/10.1016/B978-0-12-820050-6.00010-2

Principles of a pregnancy test

Pregnancy tests employ a sandwich immunoassay using two antibodies that recognized different epitopes of hCG [35]. One of the antibodies is immobilized as a test line on a nitrocellulose test strip, while the second antibody is labeled with a colored marker and is located upstream of the result zone but remains freely mobile, so is often referred to as the mobile phase. The mobile phase consists of colored latex particles or gold sol coated with one of the antibodies that are dried down on glass fiber or other suitable substrate, often in the presence of sugars, which assist resolution.

When urine is applied to the test, it tracks through the test via capillary flow. First, the sample encounters reagents to normalize the urine, such as buffers and detergents, ensuring that the conditions for the antibody reaction are optimized. The reagent mixes tend to be proprietary to the test and are crafted to maintain test performance throughout its shelf life. When the sample encounters the mobile phase, the particles move with the fluid and track up the strip. If hCG is present in the urine, it is bound by the antibodies on the particles forming the first half of the sandwich immunoassay.

On reaching the test line, if hCG is present it is bound at the line and with it, the associated particle bound antibody also becomes immobilized, forming a visible line. If no hCG is present, the particles move across the test line to the end of the strip, so no line is formed. The principles of the lateral flow immunoassay are shown in Fig. 2.4.1.

Visually read home pregnancy tests, also known as line tests, also employ a control test so that the user can check that they have conducted the test correctly and that the test is still working. This typically consists of a separate immunoassay on the same lateral flow strip. A separate control line is plotted on the nitrocellulose strip, with an antibody that should always enable particle binding if sample is applied correctly and the test has not been denatured. Examples of antibody used on the test line include anti-species antibodies such as anti-mouse. In this case, if the particle-bound hCG antibody is a mouse monoclonal antibody, any particles that make it past the test line can be bound by the control line. This system has drawbacks

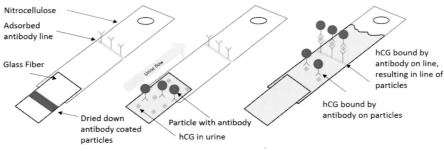

FIGURE 2.4.1

Principles of a lateral flow test.

though, as when hCG levels are very high, there may not be enough particles that make it past the test line to form a visible control line. Therefore, most tests use a separate population of antibody-coated control particles that do not participate in the hCG immunoassay to ensure a test line is always formed, for example, using a mouse monoclonal antibody to a different protein such as CEA.

Digital tests

Many women struggle with the ambiguity of reading a faint line and want a test that provides an unequivocal result. This led to the development of digital tests, which provide the user a clear Pregnant or Not Pregnant result. The underlying principles of digital tests are the same as visual tests, except they incorporate electronic components which measure either light reflectance or light transmission at the test line and signal processing algorithms to determine the result which is displayed on an LCD screen.

The reader and optical electronics within Clearblue digital tests measure light which is emitted from a red LED onto the nitrocellulose strip. The amount of light which is either transmitted through or reflected back from the strip is then detected by a photodiode. When a test line is present, the blue latex absorbs the light so that less can be detected. The amount of light absorbed by the latex line is proportional to the strength of the line on the strip and results in a reduction in signal attenuation. Embedded software processes this electrical signal according to various thresholds and rule-sets. The optical geometry of the digital reader and electronics is arranged such that light can be emitted and detected at various points on the strip including the test and control zones as well as regions on either side of these lines which can be used as a reference to set a baseline value. Rule-sets regarding rate of fluid flow mean that test errors due to improper movement of reagents can be identified and displayed to the user, negating the need for the immunoassay-based control system that is used in visual tests.

hCG as a biomarker for pregnancy

Home pregnancy tests detect the presence of urinary levels of hCG which is a clinically accurate marker of pregnancy. Levels of hCG rise rapidly and predictably in the earliest days of pregnancy [2,3], and it usually first appears in urine 9—10 days following the estimated day of conception [4]. This makes hCG an ideal urinary marker for quickly and accurately assessing whether a woman is pregnant or not.

The reported range in hCG concentration by day of pregnancy is highly dependent on the reference method used to date the pregnancy. When a highly accurate method such as determining the day of ovulation (and hence conception as the life span of the unfertilized egg is less than 1 day) is applied, urinary intact hCG levels are remarkably consistent for the first 3 weeks following conception. However, if a less precise reference method is used, such as ultrasound crown rump length measurement or last menstrual period, then variation is more pronounced [5,6].

Different forms of hCG show different profiles of hCG rise. Free β-hCG tends to appear in urine at one-tenth the concentration of intact hCG, whereas β-core hCG is initially not present in urine at the earliest stages of pregnancy but can become the predominant form at 6 weeks following conception [7].

Home pregnancy test accuracy

Home pregnancy tests can be very accurate, with some tests having robust data to show they are >99% accurate in detecting pregnancy from the day the period is due. But, some currently marketed tests have shown lower accuracy in studies. A recent study examining the analytical sensitivity and women's interpretation of eight home pregnancy tests found varying degrees of accuracy between products. The best performing test (Clearblue Digital) returned >99% correct results when tested at the device sensitivity and read by users, in comparison with the worst performing test which only 33% of users correctly interpreted [36]. An important factor in pregnancy test performance is usability.

Usability

Home pregnancy tests come in different formats (as shown in Fig. 2.4.2), some more easy to use than others. Midstream tests (line tests or digital tests) are designed to enable the user to sample directly onto the test, via a wick. Users can also choose to dip these tests into a collected sample if they prefer. Cassettes were originally created for point-of-care and laboratory testing but are now available for consumers to buy. They require the user to collect a sample, then use a pipette to apply the sample to the testing well. Strip tests were developed as an economical product for healthcare professionals to use and, like cassettes tests, are also now available for consumers to buy directly. A study comparing consumer use of the various device formats found not only did consumers find strip and cassette tests to be harder to

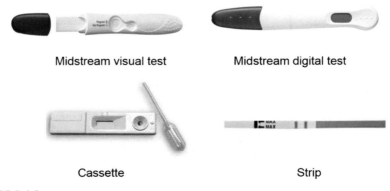

Midstream visual test   Midstream digital test

Cassette   Strip

FIGURE 2.4.2

Pregnancy Test formats.

use, but they were less accurate than midstream tests in consumers hands [8]. There was <3% discrepancy between technician and lay-user results for midstream tests, which rose to 30% for cassettes and 40% for strips, when testing at device sensitivity. This indicates that test usability is extremely important for accurate results.

Home pregnancy test instructions are also critical to usability and in some cases have been found to be lacking [9], using technical language that is not accessible to those with low literacy. Given nearly 30% of reproductive aged women have literacy skills that are basic or less [10,11], poor instructions can lead to test errors or misinterpretation of results.

However, even the best tests are not 100% accurate. Some of the more common reasons for erroneous results are described below.

Testing too early?

A home pregnancy test provides a pregnant result when hCG has been detected in urine. However, if a woman conducts a test too early, then she will receive a negative result even though she has conceived because hCG is either not present yet or too low to detect. Confirming pregnancy as soon as possible has important benefits, so many tests are sensitive enough to provide results 5 or 6 days before the missed period.

For women either desiring or avoiding pregnancy, knowing early allows them to make appropriate medical and lifestyle decisions as early as possible. For example, prompting pregnant women to modify their diet; begin taking pregnancy supplements; and avoiding risks to the developing fetus through the use of pharmaceuticals, alcohol, and occupational exposure to mutagens/teratogens. A recent study by Prior et al. [12] examined the alcohol consumption of 5036 pregnant women and found that over half of women reported some use of alcohol while trying to conceive, but the majority stopped drinking, or at least reduced their alcohol consumption, on obtaining a positive pregnancy test. They concluded that promoting early awareness of pregnancy status was more effective than promoting abstinence from alcohol among all who could conceive, and this is likely to apply to other important health messages relating to behavior in pregnancy. During 2016, an independent study on home pregnancy testing was commissioned by SPD. Of 336 American women who had used a home pregnancy test in the last 12 months, 29% reported they had tested before they missed their period.

The conundrum for many women though is knowing when their period is due. If the woman has been using home ovulation tests, then this is relatively simple as the luteal phase is very consistent [13], so testing 15 days after ovulation would provide reliable results. If only the last menstrual period is known, prediction is much trickier because over 50% of women have cycles that vary in length by 5 or more days across a 6-month period [3]. In addition, many women have poor perception of the cycle characteristics [14]. The effect of unpredictability of cycle length on likelihood of receiving a positive pregnancy test is shown in Fig. 2.4.3. Examination of first appearance of hCG in urine in relation to day of LH surge demonstrates a 4-day timeframe. Using LMP, results in first appearance of hCG occurring across a 21-day timeframe.

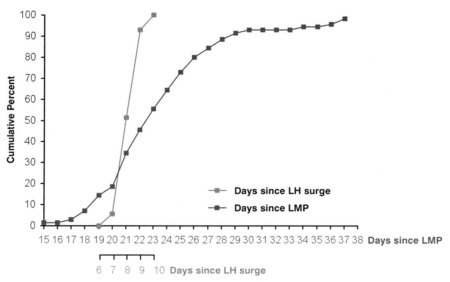

FIGURE 2.4.3

First appearance of hCG when referenced from LH surge or from LMP.

Data taken from SPD study on daily urine samples from women trying to conceive, where LH surge and first appearance of hCG were measured by AutoDELFIA. Data from 86 women who conceived.

To put this into context, if a woman believes she normally has a 24-day cycle, but ovulates on day 18 in her conception cycle, the day she would expect her period to occur on would be only 6 days after ovulation; far too early to get a positive result. Most home pregnancy tests advise women who receive a Not Pregnant result, but who have not yet had their period to test again in 2—3 days time.

False positive results

Testing during later reproductive life

hCG is a heterodimeric glycoprotein hormone which is structurally similar to the other gonadotropins (FSH, LH, and TSH). These hormones all share a common α subunit and have a unique β subunit. Small quantities of hCG may be produced by the pituitary gland in conjunction with synthesis of these structurally similar hormones.

In menopause, the production of pituitary hCG has been shown to increase [15,16]. As women approach menopause and the number of ovarian follicles available for recruitment each cycle falls, more FSH is required in order to stimulate the remaining follicles and as a consequence FSH levels rise. Elevated FSH levels may also persist in menopause for some women. This increase in FSH production in peri- and postmenopausal women can result in coproduction of small amounts of hCG in the pituitary gland.

Elevated levels of hCG in perimenopause have been reported, with Snyder et al. [17] finding 1.3% of the population they examined having serum hCG levels greater than 5 mIU/mL. In a recent urine collection study done by SPD, urine samples from 100 perimenopausal women (classified as age 41−55) were collected and analyzed. The range of urinary hCG was found to be 0−8.4 mIU/mL with 3% of the volunteers having a concentration of 5 mIU/mL hCG or higher.

The production of hCG can also occur in some postmenopausal women [17,18]. Serum levels as high as 13mIU/mL have been reported, with 6.7% of women having a hCG concentration greater than 5mIU/mL [17]. SPD have also collected urine samples from postmenopausal women (classified as age 56−65), and in a collection from 100 women a urinary hCG concentration range of 0−8.9 mIU/mL was observed, with 3% of volunteers having a concentration of 5mIU/mL or higher.

In the United States and across much of the developed world, women are waiting longer to start a family. Between 2000 and 2014, the mean age of first-time mothers in the United States increased by 1.4 years from 24.9 to 26.3 [19] and between 2000 and 2012 first birth rates for women aged 35−39 and 40−44 years increased by 24% and 35%, respectively [20]. More recently, data from the US Department of Health and Human Services for the year 2017 [21] show birth rates have declined for nearly all age groups of women under 40 years, but rose for women in their early 40s. The provisional birth rate for women aged 40−44 years in 2017 was 11.6 births per 1000 women, up 2% from 2016. The rate for this age group has generally risen since 1982.

Perimenopause, which may last up to 10 years can begin in a woman's 30s (ACOG FAQ047, 2015) [34], causes shifts in hormone levels, and may affect ovulation causing irregular menstrual cycles. Menopause, which on average occurs at age 51, but before the age of 40 in 1% of women [22], can occur suddenly and without warning. Many women have poor understanding of their fertility and will be unaware that they are experiencing peri-/postmenopause. The disruption to a woman's menstrual cycle in perimenopause, or their absence in menopause, could be mistaken for a missed period and prompt her to take a pregnancy test.

The increasing population of older women seeking to conceive will inevitably result in more peri- and postmenopausal women using home pregnancy tests, potentially leading to an increase in false positive results, should that woman use a high sensitivity test that does not discriminate between pituitary hCG and hCG from pregnancy.

If a woman with pituitary-derived hCG in her urine due to peri-/postmenopause takes a high-sensitivity (10 mIU/mL) pregnancy test, it is possible that she may get a positive result leading her to believe, incorrectly, that she is pregnant.

Pituitary hCG is produced in conjunction with high levels of FSH, hence their concentrations are highly correlated [17], whereas in pregnancy FSH concentrations are very low. Fig. 2.4.4A illustrates the correlation of FSH and hCG concentrations in urine samples collected from pre-, peri-, and postmenopausal woman. This contrasts with the hormone profile observed in pregnancy where hCG concentration rapidly increases and FSH concentration remains low (Fig. 2.4.4B).

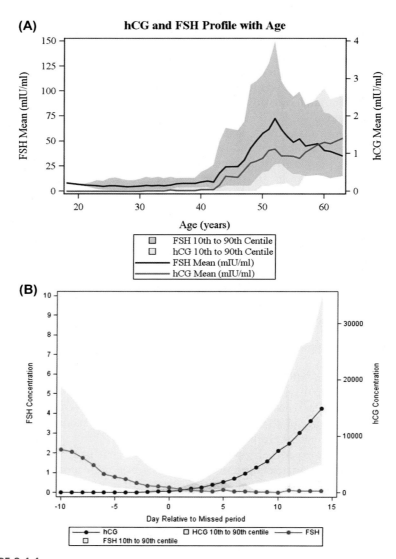

FIGURE 2.4.4

(A) Mean, 10th, and 90th centiles of urinary FSH and hCG concentrations in pre-, peri-, and postmenopausal women (FSH and hCG in mIU/mL). 397 urine samples (97 pre- (age 18–40), 150 peri (age 41–55)-, and 150 postmenopausal (age 56–65)) were collected from volunteers who participated in a urine collection study SPD conducted. (B) Median, 10th, and 90th centiles urinary FSH and hCG concentrations in early pregnancy (FSH and hCG in mIU/mL). 5778 urine samples were collected from 243 volunteers who participated in a urine collection study SPD conducted.

Pituitary hCG can therefore be distinguished from hCG derived from pregnancy due to the differences in urinary FSH concentrations (and correlation between hCG and FSH), between the peri- and postmenopausal cohort and the pregnant cohort. A low level of FSH indicates pregnancy and a high level of FSH indicates pituitary hCG. This has been described previously in the literature [17,23].

Exogenous hCG

hCG-containing medications such as Pregnyl, Profasi, Novarel, and Ovidrel may be used to stimulate ovulation. Serum hCG falls to undetectable levels within 72 hours of administration. All currently marketed pregnancy tests would be affected by the administration of a hCG-containing medication and contain information about this limitation for use in their instruction leaflet.

Familial hCG syndrome

This is a very rare disorder in which persistently elevated hCG levels are found in otherwise healthy men and nonpregnant women and can result in false positive pregnancy test results [24] and appears to be inherited. Twenty-five cases have been reported worldwide [25].

Gestational trophoblastic disease, e.g., hydatidiform mole and choriocarcinoma

Positive pregnancy tests are often returned for a group of rare tumors that involve abnormal growth of cells inside a woman's uterus. These tumors are usually accompanied by elevated hCG levels, often with levels far exceeding those seen in a normal pregnancy. Incidence is estimated at 1 in every 1000 pregnancies in the United States [26].

Other cancers

Elevated concentrations of β-hCG have been reported in the serum of patients with nontrophoblastic malignancies such as lung, breast, ovarian, and gastrointestinal cancers. This is a rare finding and usually a sign of aggressive disease as elevated serum levels of β-hCG are strongly associated with poor prognosis [27]. It is likely that urinary levels would be high and provide a positive result with a home pregnancy test.

End-stage renal disease

Since hCG is largely excreted by the kidneys, its level in serum can be elevated in dialysis patients even if not pregnant [28] and can result in false positive pregnancy test results, for example [29]. End-stage renal disease is rare, and such women are under clinical management and therefore do not represent the intended user of a home pregnancy test.

False negative results

High-dose hook

When very high levels of hCG are present and all antibody binding sites in the test have been saturated, the strength of signal reaches a plateau. When levels of hCG rise beyond this point, the sandwich assay suffers from what is known as the high-dose hook affect. At this point, the signal begins to decline because binding sites in the result zone are occupied with analyte before the analyte bound to the label has time to reach it. Again, the rate of decline is proportional to the amount of analyte present in the sample. There are very effective technical remedies to prevent high-dose hook from delivering false negative results at high hCG concentrations, for example, appropriate antibody selection and titration of reagent concentrations. All modern home pregnancy tests should demonstrate that they do not suffer from high-dose hook before being made available to consumers.

β-Core hCG

β-Core hCG is a small, truncated form that is only found in urine and can become the predominant form in later pregnancy [30–32]. We have found very high ratios of β-core hCG in comparison with intact hCG at the end of the first trimester. In SPD studies, the urine sample with the highest amount of β-core hCG relative to intact hCG was from a woman at 9 weeks' postconception and contained 11,693 pmol/mL intact hCG and 785,924 pmol/mL βcf-hCG (ratio 67.2) [7].

High levels of β-core hCG can produce false negative results in some home pregnancy tests via a mechanism similar to high-dose hook. It can be problematic for sandwich immunoassay that employs one antibody that recognizes β-core hCG, but the second antibody does not. At high β-core levels, this truncated form is able to saturate all the antibody binding sites on the antibody that recognizes it, but it will not form a sandwich because the second antibody fails to recognize it. Therefore, the binding of intact (or free beta, dependent on assay) will essentially be blocked, so insufficient signal is formed to give a positive result. As with the high-dose hook effect, appropriate assay design should minimize likelihood of β-core hCG interference, and validation work should demonstrate negligible effect prior to making the product available to consumers.

Miscarriage

Many women, after receiving a positive home pregnancy test, will obtain a subsequent negative result when testing again at a later date. Some women are told by healthcare professionals that this is a "false positive" result because it is thought to be a more palatable message than the often true meaning of these results; that the woman has suffered from a miscarriage. This message is doing women an injustice as although very distressing for some women, disguising the truth ultimately does no favor as it hides how common miscarriage is and perpetuates the idea that miscarriage is shameful and something that should not be talked about. Early

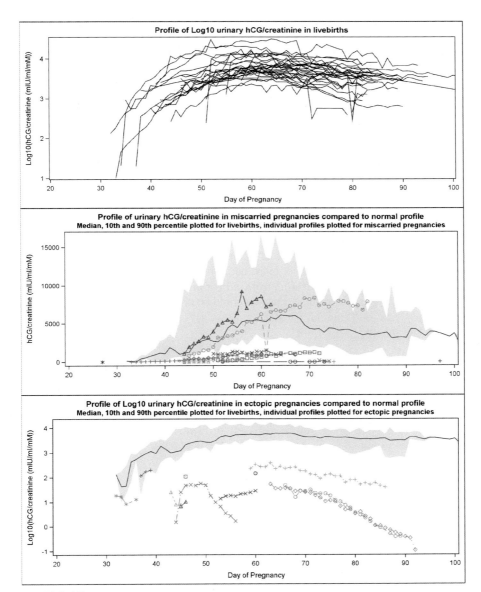

FIGURE 2.4.5

Daily urinary hCG profiles (AutoDELFIA) from women who attended an early pregnancy unit due to high-risk pregnancy or early pregnancy symptoms. Profiles are for from 49 viable pregnancies, 17 miscarriages and 11 ectopic pregnancies. For miscarriage and ectopic pregnancy graphs, each color represents a different volunteer. The median and 10th-90th centile ranges of hCG in the viable pregnancies are overlain.

loss is very common; our estimates from our conception studies are that one in four conceptions will result in a miscarriage.

We have extensively studied the trajectory of hCG in early pregnancy loss and found that in many cases it differs from a viable pregnancy from the very earliest stages. Fig. 2.4.5 shows the daily urinary hCG levels for viable pregnancies, and miscarriage and ectopic pregnancies from a cohort of women who attended an early pregnancy unit either due to high-risk pregnancy or symptoms of early loss [33]. It can be seen that the daily, urinary hCG profile differs substantially between the groups, such that it is possible to derive mathematical models to predict loss based on hCG tracking [35,37].

Ectopic pregnancy

Ectopic pregnancy is where the embryo implants at a site outside of the uterus. This can be life-threatening, for example, if implanted in the fallopian tube, a progressive ectopic pregnancy can cause rupture. The urinary hCG levels of some ectopic pregnancies can be below the threshold of a home pregnancy test, so give a "false negative" result. Therefore, special consideration should be given to any woman suspecting pregnancy and suffering from pain or bleeding, even if a home pregnancy test produces a negative result because it could be an ectopic pregnancy. Most home pregnancy test will include a statement to say ectopic pregnancies can give misleading results.

Decline in hCG levels following miscarriage

Following an early loss, many women are instructed to take home pregnancy tests in the weeks following the loss to check hCG levels return to normal. Although the half-life of hCG is estimated to be 24—36 h, there is very little data on how long it takes for urinary levels to return to baseline following early loss. SPD collected daily urine samples from 348 women who become pregnant. Samples were collected preconception until the month following their expected period. There were 54 losses reported before 12 weeks, but only 40 of these volunteers recorded bleeding during the study period. Peak hCG concentration was reached a median of 3 days after the expected period (range 4 to 25 days) at 29.3 mIU/mL (range 4—7557mIU/mL). On average, onset of bleeding occurred 3 days after hCG peak level but ranged widely from 14 days before hCG peak to 10 days afterward. Median time for hCG levels to decline to <1 mIU/mL (baseline) from peak was 5.5 days (range 2—23 days). The time to decline was highly correlated with peak hCG concentration ($P=<0.0001$). Time for hCG to decline to baseline from onset of bleeding was also variable; median was 2 days after bleeding started, but hCG levels could return to baseline as early as 25 days before onset of bleeding and up to 13 days after onset. The median days of bleeding was 5 days (range 1—14 days) and correlated with peak hCG concentration ($P = .0148$) and day of peak hCG concentration ($P = .0054$). Given the wide heterogeneity in hCG decline following early loss, some women are likely to need multiple measurements to

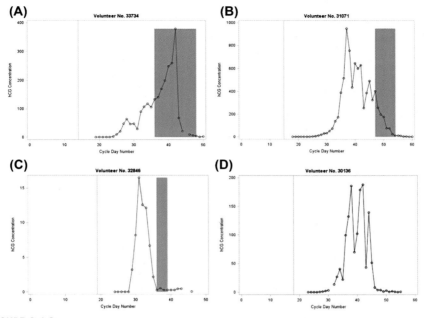

FIGURE 2.4.6

Examples of urinary hCG trajectories in early pregnancy loss. Blue bars indicate days on which the volunteer reported bleeding, with day of ovulation marked by a line. (A) Bleeding before hCG reaches peak levels, (B) bleeding during hCG decline, (C) bleeding after hCG returned to baseline, (D) no bleeding reported.

track the decline back to baseline. Examples of individual hCG profiles in early loss are shown in Fig. 2.4.6.

Conclusions

The principle of lateral flow technology has significant advantages over other more complicated forms of sample analyses. It is this fact along with its relative low cost and versatility which has enabled it to become the platform for home pregnancy tests. When well designed, with good usability features, clear instructions and a robust assay, home pregnancy tests provide highly accurate results to women at one of the most important times of their life.

Declaration of Interest

S. Johnson is an employee of SPD Development Company Ltd, a fully owned subsidiary of SPD Swiss Precision Diagnostics GmbH; the manufacturer of Clearblue pregnancy tests.

References

[1] Ehrenkranz JRL. Home and point-of-care pregnancy tests: a review of the technology. Epidemiology 2002;13(3S):S15—8.

[2] Nepomnaschy PA, Weinberg CR, Wilcox AJ, Baird DD. Urinary hCG patterns during the week following implantation. Hum Reprod 2008;23(2):271—7.

[3] Johnson SR, Miro F, Barrett S, Ellis JE. Levels of urinary human chorionic gonadotropin (hCG) following conception and variability of menstrual cycle length in a cohort of women attempting to conceive. Curr Med Res Opin 2009;25(3):741—8.

[4] Wilcox AJ, Baird DD, Weinberg CR. Time of implantation of the conceptus and loss of pregnancy. N Engl J Med 1999;340(23):1796—9.

[5] Larsen J, Buchanan P, Johnson S, Godbert S, Zinaman M. Human chorionic gonadotropin as a measure of pregnancy duration. Int J Gynecol Obstet 2013;123:189—95.

[6] Mahendru A, Wilhem-Benartizi S, Wilkinson I, McEniery C, Johnson S, Lees C. Gestational length assignment based on last menstrual period, first trimester crown-rump length, ovulation, and implantation timing. Arch Gynecol Obstet 2016;294(4):867—76.

[7] Johnson S, Eapen S, Smith P, Warren G, Zinaman M. Significance of pregnancy test false negative results due to elevated levels of β-core fragment hCG. J Immunoass. Immunochem 2017;38(4):449—55.

[8] Pike J, Godbert S, Johnson S. Comparison of volunteers' experience of using, and accuracy of reading, different types of home pregnancy test formats. Expert Opin Med Diagn 2013;7:435—41.

[9] Wallace L, Zite N, Homewood V. Making sense of home pregnancy test instructions. J Women's Health 2009;18:363—8.

[10] National Center for Educational Statistics. National assessment of adult literacy: a first look at the literacy of America's adults in the 21st century. NCES Publication No: 2006470. 2005.

[11] Rutherford J, Homan R, MacDonald J. Low literacy: a hidden problem in family planning clinics. J Fam Plan Reprod Health Care 2006;32:235—40.

[12] Prior J, Patrick SW, Sundermann AC, Wu P, Hartmann KE. Pregnancy intention and maternal alcohol consumption. Obstet Gynaecol 2017;129(4):727—33.

[13] Johnson S, Marriott L, Zinaman M. Can apps and calendar methods predict ovulation with accuracy? Curr Med Res Opin 2018;34(9):1587—94.

[14] Zinaman M, Johnson S, Ellis J, Ledger W. Accuracy of perception of ovulation day in women trying to conceive. Curr Med Res Opin 2012;28:749—54.

[15] Odell WD, Griffin J. Pulsatile secretion of human chorionic gonadotropin in normal adults. N Engl J Med 1987;317:1688—91.

[16] Stenman UH, Alfthan H, Ranta T, Vartiainen E, Jalkanen J, Seppala M. Serum levels of human chorionic gonadotropin in nonpregnant women and men are modulated by gonadotropin-releasing hormone and sex steroids. J Clin Endocrinol Metab 1987;64:730—6.

[17] Snyder JA, Haymond S, Parvin CA, Gronowski AM, Grenache DG. Diagnostic considerations in the measurement of human chorionic gonadotropin in aging women. Clin Chem 2005;51:1830—5.

[18] Alfthan H, Haglund C, Dabek J, Stenman UH. Concentrations of human choriogonadotropin, its beta-subunit, and the core fragment of the beta-subunit in serum and urine of men and non-pregnant women. Clin Chem 1992;38:1981—7.

[19] Mathews TJ, Hamilton BE. Mean age of mothers is on the rise: United States 2000 — 2014. NCHS Data Brief 2016;232.

[20] Mathews TJ, Hamilton BE. First births to older mothers continue to rise. NCHS Data Brief 2014;152.

[21] Hamilton BE, Martin JA, Osterman MJK, Driscoll AK, Rossen LM. Division of vital statistics. National Center for Health Statistics; 2018. Report No 004.

[22] Haller-Kikkatalo K, Uibo R, Kurg A, Salumets A. The prevalence and phenotypic characteristics of spontaneous premature ovarian failure: a general population registry-based study. Hum Reprod 2015;30(5):1229−38.

[23] Gronowski AM, Fantz CR, Parvin CA, Sokoll LJ, Wiley CL, Wener MH, Grenache DG. Use of serum FSH to identify perimenopausal women with pituitary hCG. Clin Chem 2008;54(4):652−6.

[24] Cole LA, Bulter S. Familial hCG syndrome: production of variable, degraded or mutant forms of hCG. J Reprod Med 2014;59(9−10):435−42.

[25] Tan A, Van der Merwe A, Low X, Chrystal K. Familial hCG syndrome: a diagnostic challenge. Gynecol Oncol Rep 2014;10:47−8.

[26] American Cancer Society. What are the key statistics about gestational trophoblastic disease?. 2016. Available at: http//www.cancer.org/cancer/gestational-trophoblastic-disease/about/key-statistics.html.

[27] Stenman U, Alfthan H, Hotakainen K. Human chorionin gonadotropin in cancer. Clin Biochem 2004;37(7):549−61.

[28] Schwarz A, Post KG, Keller F, Molzahn M. Value of human chorionic gonadotropin measurements in blood as a pregnancy test in women on maintenance hemodialysis. Nephron 1985;39:341−3.

[29] Soni S, Menon MC, Bhaskaran M, Jhaveri KD, Molmenti E, Muoio V. Elevated human chorionic gonadotropin levels in patients with chronic kidney disease: case series and review of literature. Indian J Nephrol 2013;23(6):424−7.

[30] Gronowski AM, Cervinski M, Stenman UH, Woodworth A, Ashby L, Scott MG. False-negative results in point-of-care qualitative human chorionic gonadotropin (hCG) devices due to excess hCGbeta core fragment. Clin Chem 2009;55:1389−94.

[31] Grenache DG, Greene DN, Dighe AS, Fantz CR, Hoefner D, McCudden C, Sokoll L, Wiley CL, Gronowski AM. Falsely decreased human chorionic gonadotropin (hCG) results due to increased concentrations of the free beta subunit and the beta core fragment in quantitative hCG assays. Clin Chem 2010;56(12):1839−44.

[32] Nerenz RD, Butch AW, Woldemariam GA, Yarbrough ML, Grenache DG, Gronowski AM. Estimating the hCGβcf in urine during pregnancy. Clin Biochem 2016;49(3):282−6.

[33] Walker J, Shillito J, Johnson S. Daily urinary hCG levels in viable, miscarriage and ectopic pregnancy from women attending an early pregnancy unit. [Unpublished].

[34] The American College of Obstetricians and Gynocologists. The menopause years. Women's health: frequently asked questions. 047. 2015.

[35] Gnoth C, Johnson S. Strips of hope: accuracy of home pregnancy tests and new developments. Geburtshilfe Frauenheilkd 2014;74:661−9.

[36] Johnson S, Cushion M, Bond S, Godbert S, Pike J. Comparison of analytical sensitivity and women's interpretation of home pregnancy tests. Clin Chem Lab Med 2015;53:391−402.

[37] Marriott L, Zinaman M, Abrams KR, Crowther MJ. Johnson S Analysis of urinary human chorionic gonadotrophin concentrations in normal and failing pregnancies using longitudinal, cox proportional hazards and two-stage modelling. Ann Clin Biochem 2017;54(5):548−57.

Human chorionic gonadotropin determination using mass spectrometry

Trine Grønhaug Halvorsen, Léon Reubsaet

Introduction

Human chorionic gonadotropin (hCG) exists as a heterodimer which consists of an α-subunit and a β-subunit. Only the β-subunit is specific for hCG as the α-subunit also is present in other proteins [1]. Determination of hCG in serum and urine has been carried out for a very long time for diagnostic purposes (e.g., in pregnancy, ovarium cancer, and testicular cancer). Initially, the amount or presence of *total* hCG was used for this purpose. Later on, the determination of various hCG glycoforms and isovariants made it possible to get a more differentiated diagnostic profile [2]. For the purpose of this overview, glycoforms are defined as variations in glycosylation pattern on hCG, while isovariants are variations in the protein backbone. The structure of these isovariants will be discussed in detail later. As hCG appears on the WADA list of prohibited substances, it is also being investigated in relation to doping [3,4]. At the present moment, immunometric assays are the gold standard for the determination of hCG and its glycoforms and isovariants in biological matrixes [5]. Since the first report in 1995 [6] on the use of mass spectrometry for the determination of hCG, its added value has been proven over time. The ability of the mass spectrometry to determine glycoforms and isovariants certainly addressed some of the common challenges and disadvantages occurring in immunometric assays like cross-reactivity [7]. Several reviews have been published where hCG, among other proteins, has been mentioned as an example of how mass spectrometry can be used to perform the analysis [4,7−11]. In these cases, the focus was broader, e.g., on structural qualitative analysis of endogenous occurring gonadotropins and on proteins in drug formulations, in targeted quantitative analysis of biomarkers using immunoextractions or more general, in biopharmaceutical analyses. This overview is the first to show use of mass spectrometry in the determination of hCG which only focuses on hCG itself. We have chosen to focus this overview on the protein backbone of hCG. Here we will not discuss the mass spectrometry of the O- and N-glycans of hCG, neither will we discuss all the hCG glycoforms based on the heterogeneity caused by variation in the glycan composition. It will, however, discuss the consequences of glycosylation on the determination of the protein backbone. This overview will give insight in the efforts to determine hCG using both the top-down and bottom-up approaches. It will discuss the need and use of enzymes in the analytical workflow, especially if the protein backbone of hCG and its isovariants are investigated. Also, the need and use of monoclonal antibodies in the sample pretreatment is elaborated on, as this is been an essential element to be able to do mass spectrometric determination of hCG and its isovariants at the required low detection levels.

Intact hCG determination: the top-down MS approach

Mass spectrometric determination of hCG using a top-down approach is susceptible to large variations in the measured m/z values. Due to the microheterogeneous nature of hCG, primarily caused by variation in glycosylation, it is challenging to get an accurate mass determination. Laidler et al. were the first to describe the MALDI-TOF analysis of intact hCG giving masses for the α-subunit (m/z 13 408), β–subunit (m/z 21 446), and the intact heterodimer (m/z 35 140)[6]. MALDI-TOF has been the most reported combination of ionization and mass spectrometer for the top-down determination of intact hCG, the α-subunit, and the β-subunit [6,12–14] (see Figs. 2.5.1 and 2.5.2) as well as the determination of the β-core fragment of hCG [15,16]. The advantage of combining MALDI with TOF mass spectrometry is that it is able to detect singly charged species.

In 2006, the first chromatographic separation of intact species followed by electrospray ion-trap mass spectrometry was described [17]. This approach results in

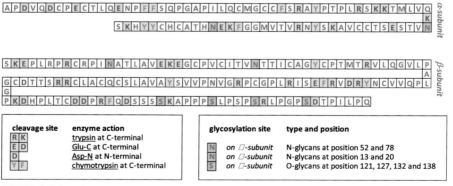

FIGURE 2.5.1

Amino acid sequence of hCG subunits (top: α, bottom: β), cleavage sites of various enzymes and glycosylation sites.

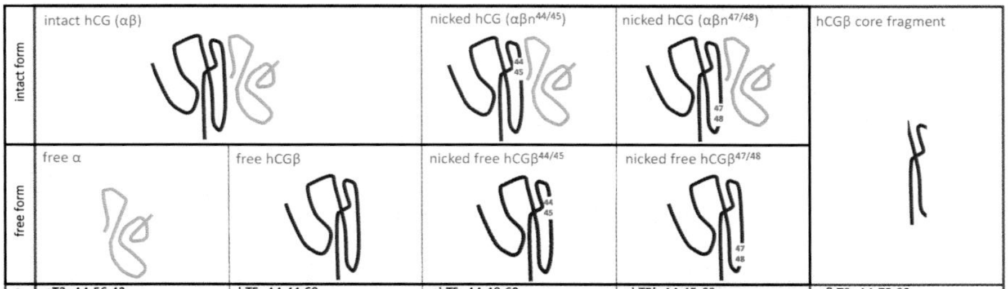

	intact hCG (αβ)		nicked hCG (αβn[44/45])	nicked hCG (αβn[47/48])	hCGβ core fragment
intact form					
free form	free α	free hCGβ	nicked free hCGβ[44/45]	nicked free hCGβ[47/48]	

a	aT2: *AA 56-42*	bT5: *AA 44-60*	nbT5: *AA 48-60*	nbT5': *AA 45-60*	cfbT9: *AA 75-92*
b	AYPTPLR	VLQGVLPQVVCNYR	VLPALPQVVCNYR	LQGVLPQVVCNYR	GVNPVVSYAVALSQCAL
c	MRM***:	SIM*:	SIM*:	SIM*:	SIM*:
d	409.3^{2+} → 584.4^{+}	1927^{+} or 964^{2+} MRM**: 964.3^{2+} → 1036.4^{+} → 891.5^{+} → 610.3^{+} MRM***: 964.2^{2+} → 1036.3^{+} → 1317.8^{+} MRM****: 642^{3+} → 518.3^{2+} → 711.4^{*+}	1529.8^{+}, 765.4^{2+} or 510.6^{3+} MRM***: 765.7^{2+} → 1036.3^{+} → 659.2^{2+} → 519.1^{2+}	1828.0^{+}, 914.5^{2+} or 610.0^{3+} MRM***: 914.7^{2+} → 1036.3^{+} → 1317.8^{+}	1909.9^{+}, 955.5^{2+} or 637.3^{3+} MRM***: 955.7^{2+} → 924.1^{+} → 740.0^{+} → 610.3^{+} cfbT5: *AA 55-60* VVNYR MRM****: 405.7^{2+} → 711.3^{+} → 612.3^{+}

FIGURE 2.5.2

Overview of the studied isovariants, both the intact forms (upper part) and free forms (middle part), their observed signature peptides and m/z values. (A) tryptic peptide code and numbers of the amino acid. The tryptic code is written as follows, the first letter indicates the origin of the peptide (α- or β-subunit), the second letter indicates the enzyme used (T for trypsin) and the first number is the position of the proteolytic peptide in the amino acid chain, (B) amino acid sequence of the signature peptides, (C) mode in which the MS is used for quantitation, (D) m/z values and transitions used for quantitation.

*From publication Ref. [37], **from publication Ref. [36], ***from publications Refs. [38,39,41–45], ****from publications Refs. [46–49].

production of multiple charged ions during electrospray ionization, which can be challenging for accurate mass determination on a low-resolution instrument. The latter was addressed by other groups using high-resolution mass spectrometers like LTQ-FT [18] and high-resolution TOF [19,20] coupled to capillary electrophoresis and interfaced with electrospray ionization.

In most of the abovementioned studies, untreated variants of hCG were determined thus focusing on the heterogeneity due to glycosylation.

The use of enzymes in the analytical workflow for hCG determination

There are two purposes for using enzymes in mass spectrometric determination of hCG: proteolysis of the protein backbone to produce peptides (analysis using the bottom-up approach) and removal of N- and O-linked glycans to study either the nonglycosylated peptide or the released glycan.

Enzymes for bottom-up approach

In the bottom-up approach for the determination of proteins in general and the protein backbone of hCG in particular, proteolytic enzymes are incorporated in the sample preparation to produce proteolytic peptides. Due to their properties, proteolytic peptides usually are easily determined by mass spectrometry [21]. In case of the hCG studies described in more detail below, both trypsin and Glu-C were used as proteolytic enzymes. While trypsin cleaves specifically on the C-terminus of the basic amino acids, arginine (Arg, R) and lysine (Lys, K) with the exception when followed by proline [22], Glu-C cleaves specifically on the C-terminus of glutamic acid (Glu, E) and aspartic acid (Asp, D) [23]. Especially the use of trypsin in the bottom-up approach is beneficial as it mainly yields doubly charged peptides with a mass between 700 and 1500, making them good candidates for mass spectrometric detection. The uses of other enzymes such as pepsin (which cleaves many different peptide bonds but with a preference for hydrophobic and aromatic residues) and Asp-N (cleaving at the N-terminal side of Asp residues) in hCG determination have only been reported once and were used for qualitative purposes [24,25].

Fig. 2.5.1 shows both the amino acid sequence of the hCG α and hCG β (both present in the intact form as heterodimer as well as in the free form as monomer) and the sites where trypsin, Glu-C, and Asp-N cut.

Enzymes for glycan removal

As can be seen from Fig. 2.5.1, hCG have several N- and O-glycosylation sites. Glycosylation causes both a positive mass deviation of the proteolytic peptide compared with its nonglycosylated form and it causes heterogeneity in m/z values for the protein and hence also for a proteolytic peptide containing the glycosylation site as the composition of the glycans varies [15,17,18,24,26−30]. To be able to make hCG more accessible to proteolysis, to produce the nonglycosylated protein or peptide, to study glycoform patterns, or to confirm the glycosylation sites, glycosidases are used to cleave off the glycans. N-glycans and O-glycans are removed using different strategies.

N-glycans in hCG are coupled to asparagine (Asn, N) at the 13th and 30th positions (β−chain in regular hCG) and the 52nd and 78th positions (α-chain regular hCG) [31] and are cleaved off by using PNGase F (or glycopeptidase F) [24−27,30,32]. The consequence of this treatment is that Asn is converted into aspartic acid (Asp, D), causing a mass increase of +0.98,402 Da when the deglycosylated peptide is measured in its singly charged form [33,34].

O-linked glycans in hCG are coupled to serine (Ser, S) at the 121st, 127th, 132nd, and 138th positions (β-chain in regular hCG, there are no O-linked glycans on the α-chain) [31] and the cleavage of O-glycans is often a multistep approach. In literature on hCG, both acid hydrolysis and neuraminidase [30,32,34] have been reported to remove sialic acids before O-glycanase [32,34] or β-(1−3,4) galactosidase and β-N-acetylglucosaminidase [30] are used to cleave off the part of the O-glycan remaining after the first treatment. This treatment is challenging as not always the bare peptides are measured [32], in other cases, partial O-glycan removal is carried out, yielding glyco peptides containing one GalNAc residues on the serine sites resulting in a mass difference of +203.09 compared with the bare peptide [30].

Isovariant determination through bottom-up approaches
Identification and differentiation of hCG isovariants

The first bottom-up mass spectrometric determination of hCG with focus on the protein backbone was carried out as early as 1995. By using trypsin, hCG was digested into its tryptic peptides. Using MALDI-TOF, 59% coverage of the α-backbone and 52% coverage of the β-backbone (both coverages based on both glycosylated and nonglycosylated peptides) of intact hCG could be observed. This was at that moment regarded to be an unambiguous legal identification of hCG [6]. Liu et al. [12,32,34] were the first to chromatographically separate proteolytic peptides (produced after both trypsin and Glu-C treatment) of hCG and in such way differentiate directly and indirectly between some of the variations in the hCG backbone. The ability to differentiate between these isovariants is based on the specificity of proteolytic peptides generated in a bottom-up approach. The differentiation was possible as tryptic cleavage of the hCG isovariants yield so-called signature peptides (or proteotypic peptides, surrogate peptides) with isovariant-specific amino acid sequences which exhibit a specific *m/z* value and MS/MS fragmentation pattern [35]. Presence of these specific peptides in a sample after tryptic cleavage indicates presence of the isovariant they originate from.

Up until now, several mass spectrometric methods for the bottom-up determination of intact hCG [6,12,14,36—40], hCG free β [32,37,39], nicked variants [34,37—39] of the β-chain at 44—45 and at 47—48 (which can occur as heterodimer as well as their free forms) and hCG β-core fragment [37—39] have been developed. Determination can be done using mass fingerprinting in the single MS mode as well as using peptide fragments in the tandem MS mode. For the single MS mode MALDI-TOF (both low and high resolution) [6,14], single quadrupole MS operated in the full scan mode and SIM mode [12,32,34,37], ion-trap MS [36], and high-resolution orbitrap MS have been used [40]. Identity confirmation using fragment spectra or mass transitions was performed on ion-trap MS [36,37,40] and triple quadrupole MS [38,39]. Fig. 2.5.2 shows an overview of the isovariants, their reported signature peptides, and *m/z* values and the most reported transitions.

Quantitation of hCG isovariants

Production of signature peptides by tryptic cleavage is reproducible and can thus be used for quantitative purposes [35]. For hCG, most focus was initially on the determination of the β-chain of hCG as only the β-chain is specific for hCG. For this purpose, βT5 emerged to be a reliable signature peptide (for nomenclature explanation, see legend to Fig. 2.5.2). Gam et al. [36] were the first to publish a method to quantify the β-chain of hCG in urine for doping analysis by means of this particular peptide using SIM (single MS). Lund et al. developed a fully validated MRM method (on a triple quadrupole MS) for the determination of intact hCG and free hCG-β in both serum and urine [38]. This method used the isotopically labeled form of βT5 for quantitation and has been evaluated for diagnostic purposes [38] and doping analyses [41,42]. Lately, efforts have been made to determine intact hCG and free hCG-β in dried blood spots (DBS) [43,50−52]. Although these DBS studies were in an exploratory phase to investigate if paper could serve as carrier for blood samples for protein determination using hCG as a model compound, they showed the power of using mass spectrometry as a tool for selective signature peptide determination.

In all the abovementioned studies, it is important to notice that βT5, although specific for the β-chain, occurs in both intact hCG and free hCG-β. In other words, the measure of βT5 is a measure of the sum of intact hCG and free hCG-β. The methods were not able to differentiate between the sources of βT5. Both Egeland et al. [45] and Butch et al. [46] addressed this challenge by developing smart monoclonal antibody (mAb)-based sample preparation involving dual extractions. How these were constructed is discussed under *Use of mAb for mass spectrometric hCG determination*. The validated dual extraction method by Butch et al. [46−49] allows differentiation between and quantitation of the free hCG-β chain, intact hCG, and βcf in urine at levels as low as 0.2 IU/L. With this method, urinary reference values for the free hCG-β chain (20 mIU/L or 0.47 pM), intact hCG (40 mIU/L or 0.94 pM), and βcf (70 mIU/L or 0.16 pM) were determined [49] as well as its use in doping analysis investigated [46,48]. For the quantitative purposes, they used isotopic labeled βT5 and βT5cf peptides. The method proposed by Egeland et al. allowed determination and differentiation of intact hCG and free hCG-β down to 10 pM (corresponding to 3.5 IU/L [53]), the two nicked forms of hCG and their corresponding free nicked forms of hCG-β down to 100 pM as well as the β-core fragment of hCG. In this case, the isotopic labeled βT5 and αT2 were used for quantitative purposes. The method was shown to perform in both urine and serum, and its potential for diagnostic purposes in testicular cancer was evaluated in a small population [45].

All the qualitative and quantitative methods for hCG were mainly based on the use of trypsin as proteolytic enzyme, and although the use of trypsin is very well established, evaluation and optimization of in-house procedures are of great importance. Not only presence of missed cleavages can happen [40] but also variabilities either caused by variation in trypsin quality or by peptide instability occur [44]. In the latter study, the positive effect of an increasing trypsin-to-protein ratio on the production of signature peptides for hCG-a and hCG-β was shown, allowing for better detection limits and shorter pretreatment times. However, it also led to signature peptide instability (especially for βT9) as increased amounts of trypsin also increased the amount of the contaminant chymotrypsin, which in its turn cleaves βT9 to smaller peptides. This did not occur for the αT2 or the βT5 peptide, making them the best candidates for quantitation using this accelerated pretreatment [44].

Use of monoclonal antibodies for mass spectrometric hCG determination

Monoclonal antibodies have been used for various purposes in the mass spectrometric determination of hCG molecules. The following section distinguishes between the use of mAbs for simple sample clean-up for quantitative determination of hCG, the use of the mass spectrometer to allow mAb specificity analysis, and the innovative combinations of mAbs to allow differentiation between signature peptides originating from an intact hCG form or a free hCGβ form.

Sample clean-up and enrichment

Inclusion of antibodies in the analytical workflow for hCG determination improves both the quantitation and differentiation. As hCG and its isovariants mainly are determined in biological matrices like serum and urine and occur in low concentrations, it is of importance to do a selective clean-up before proteolytic treatment and subsequent analysis. This is to overcome the limiting dynamic range of the mass spectrometer and to prevent sensitivity loss due to matrix effects. The antibodies are used to capture hCG molecules on the protein level after which hCG is proteolyzed using trypsin. Only the signature peptides are then determined to quantitate the parent protein. A general workflow is shown in Fig. 2.5.3.

For the studies which only investigated the presence and amount of intact hCG and free hCGβ by means of βT5, antibodies with the capability to capture several isovariants of hCG could be used. These antibodies were either coupled to Sepharose 4B

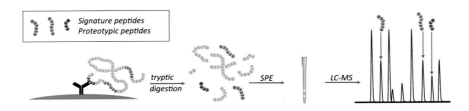

FIGURE 2.5.3

General workflow of sample clean-up using mAbs followed by tryptic digestion. mAbs are covalently coupled to a support (96-well plate, Sepharose 4B, magnetic beads) allowing extraction of hCG. Tryptic digestion can be carried out after elution of the protein or in the presence of the mAb. An SPE step is often required to desalt and enrich the sample before LC-MS determination.

beads [12,36], 96-well plates [37], or magnetic beads [38,41–43]. The digestion was carried out either after elution of the hCG molecules from the antibody [12,36] or in the presence of the antibody, omitting the elution step [37,38]. Although both approaches gave satisfactory results, Levernæs et al. [40] found that for hCG it was slightly beneficial to elute the molecule from the antibody before performing the digestion. However, this depends very much on the nature of the mAb used and the signature peptide measured. Regardless on the presence of tryptic products from the antibodies or the nature of the isovariant or other cross-reacting species captured, in all cases the specificity of the mass spectrometer was used to determine only the hCG isovariant of interest. Additionally it has been shown that with this procedure matrix effects which could disturb the determination of βT5 were not found [38].

Monoclonal antibody specificity analysis using mass spectrometry

There is an overwhelming amount of commercial and academic in-house produced mAbs available targeting hCG. Sixty-nine of these mAbs have been investigated on their specificity in several workshops on hCG and related molecules organized by "International Society of Oncology and BioMarkers (ISOBM)" [54–56]. In these workshops, a workflow mainly based on immunometric assays was used to determine the position of the epitopes. The workflow consisted of three steps: first the main specificity was determined (a, b, or c type mAb—see Fig. 2.5.4), second the epitope recognition and spatial arrangement was confirmed using sandwich assays, and third these findings were cross-referenced.

Lund et al. showed the added value of mass spectrometry in the specificity determination of the mAbs and confirmation of the epitopes they were targeting [39]. In this study, a selection of 30 mAbs which represented the most relevant epitope groups was investigated. The nomenclature of these hCG epitope groups is shown in Fig. 2.5.4.

Reference reagents for hCG were used to standardize the results: intact hCG (99/688), hCGn (99/642), hCGβ (99/650), hCGβn (99/692), hCGβcf (99/708), and hCGα (99/720) obtained from the National Institute of Biological Standards and Controls (NIBSC) [57]. The MS results were compared with results of a direct binding radioimmunoassay (DB-RIA). The DB-RIA measured the fraction of the hCG molecule bound to the mAb and was expressed as percent net binding of the maximum binding of the antigen. The mass spectrometric method used mAb-modified magnetic beads for extraction of a mixture of all reference standards, followed by mass spectrometric detection of the signature peptides of each of the isovariants. The signal intensity after extraction was normalized against their internal standard. The comparison resulted in Fig. 2.5.5. This shows the applicability of mass spectrometry to investigate the specificity of the mAbs and to confirm the position of the epitopes. An additional advantage is that due to the selectivity of the mass spectrometer, one can carry out the experiments with a mixture of hCG standards decreasing the labor intensity as it is not needed to investigate each isovariant separately for each mAb. A disadvantage for this approach is that the mass

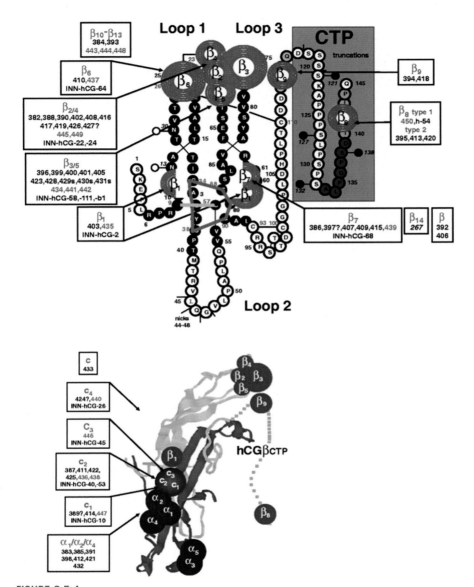

FIGURE 2.5.4

Graphic representations of hCG with a, b, and c epitope groups as well as the ISOBM code of the mAbs with affinity to the designated epitopes.

Figure reproduced from Berger, P.; Paus, E.; Hemken, P. M.; Sturgeon, C.; Stewart, W. W.; Skinner, J. P.; Harwick, L. C.; Saldana, S. C.; Ramsay, C. S.; Rupprecht, K. R.; Olsen, K. H.; Bidart, J.-M.; Stenman, U.-H.; Members of the ISOBM TD-7 Workshop on hCG and Related Molecules, Candidate epitopes for measurement of hCG and related molecules: the second ISOBM TD-7 workshop. 2013, 34 (6), 4033–4057.

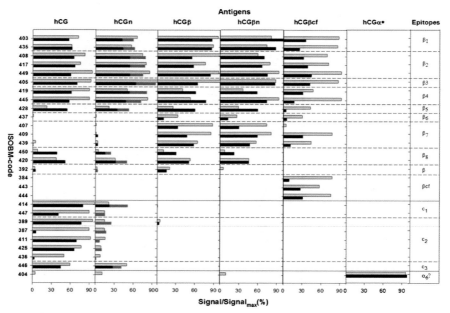

FIGURE 2.5.5

Comparative classification of ISOBM-mAbs by DB-RIA and immuno-LC-MS/MS. ISOBM-mAb code is published in the second ISOBM TD-7 workshop [56]. The results for the classification of mAbs according to their main epitope specificities by DB-RIA (gray bars) are from the workshop report [56]. The normalized MS signal intensity is the ratio of the signals for the detected hCG variants divided by that of the internal standard (black bars). LC-MS/MS signals generated by immunoextraction of the hCGn preparation showed contamination with intact hCG (red bars).

Modified and reproduced from Lund, H.; Paus, E.; Berger, P.; Stenman, U. H.; Torcellini, T.; Halvorsen, T. G.; Reubsaet, L., Epitope analysis and detection of human chorionic gonadotropin (hCG) variants by monoclonal antibodies and mass spectrometry. Tumor Biol 2014, 35 (2), 1013–1022 with permission.

spectrometer is not able to distinguish between signature peptides originating from the intact hCG and the free subunit [39].

Differentiation between signature peptides originating from intact hCG isovariants and free hCGβ isovariants using dual immunoextraction

Although mass spectrometric detection of either the signature peptide mass or their fragments is highly specific, it does not have the ability to separate between a tryptic peptide generated from the β-chain in intact hCG or from the β-chain in its free form. Including monoclonal antibodies in an innovative manner in the analytical workflow allows to separate intact hCG from the free forms. Both Butch et al.

[47] and Egeland et al. [45] constructed dual extraction workflows in which two different antibodies coupled to magnetic beads were used for sequential extraction of hCG isovariants from the same sample (see Fig. 2.5.6). The two extracts were then treated, digested, and analyzed by mass spectrometry separately resulting in two runs for each sample. Although the principle of both dual extractions was similar, the order of extraction was different (see Fig. 2.5.6).

Butch et al. [46] carried out extraction of hCGβ and hCGβcf as the first step (using mAb INN-hCG-68, ISOBM 439 (this mAb did not extract the intact hCG)) followed by extraction of the intact hCG (using INN-hCG-2, ISOBM 435 (this mAb is less specific and extracts hCGβ, hCGβcf, and the intact hCG)). Egeland et al. [45] carried out extraction of the intact hCG isovariants in the first step (using ISOBM 414 (this mAb extracts intact hCG as well as both intact hCG nicked variants)) followed by extraction of the free β-subunit isovariants (using ISOBM 419 (this mAb is also less specific and extracts free hCGβ, the free hCGβ nicked variants and the hCGβcf as well as intact forms of hCG)).

The dual extraction setup for hCG might in this sense be a model to follow for the bottom-up determination of other proteins which consist of multiple subunits.

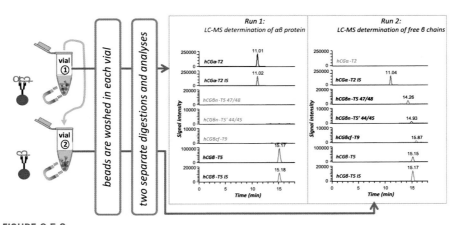

FIGURE 2.5.6

General principle of the dual extraction as described in Ref. [45] for the differentiation between signature peptides originating from the intact hCG isovariants and the free hCGβ isovariants. In the first step, the magnetic beads with mAbs against isovariants of intact hCG are incubated with serum in vial 1. After incubation, the serum aliquot is transferred to vial 2 for incubation. The magnetic beads from vial 1 and vial 2 are treated separately (wash, reduce/alkylate and digest) and analyzed on the LC-MS as run 1 (vial 1) and run 2 (vial 2).

Concluding remarks

Mass spectrometry has extensively been used with various purposes to determine hCG and related molecules. It has been proven to be a powerful tool to study variations in hCG glycoforms to map anti-hCG mAb affinities as well as to differentiate and quantify hCG isovariants. Although top-down determinations have been described, most research on the use of mass spectrometry for hCG has been performed using bottom-up approaches. Here proteolytic and deglycosylating enzymes in the analytical workflow are necessary and allows to determine intact hCG, hCGβ, hCGβ-core fragment, and hCGβ-nicked variants by means of signature peptides.

The use of reagent mAbs to clean-up and enrich seems to be inevitable when aiming at very low detection limits. They provide an additional dimension in the differentiation between the hCG isovariants and contribute in the efforts to determine all isovariants with fewer mass spectrometric analyses. Nevertheless, still at least two separate runs are needed to be able to determine all hCG variants from a sample. However, with the current proteomic labeling techniques, it should be possible to perform full isovariant profiling in one single mass spectrometric run.

References

[1] Butler SA, Burczynska BB, Iles RK. 3 — the molecular genetics of hCG. In: Cole LA, Butler SA, editors. Human chorionic gonadotropin (HGC). 2nd ed. San Diego: Elsevier; 2015. p. 19—31.

[2] Tiitinen A, Alfthan H, Valmu L, Stenman U-H. The classification, functions and clinical use of different isoforms of HCG. Hum Reprod Update 2006;12(6):769—84.

[3] Thevis M, Thomas A, Schanzer W. Detecting peptidic drugs, drug candidates and analogs in sports doping: current status and future directions. Expert Rev Proteom 2014;11(6):663—73.

[4] van den Broek I, Blokland M, Nessen MA, Sterk S. Current trends in mass spectrometry of peptides and proteins: application to veterinary and sports-doping control. Mass Spectrom Rev 2015;34(6):571—94.

[5] Fan J, Wang M, Wang CY, Cao Y. Advances in human chorionic gonadotropin detection technologies: a review. Bioanalysis 2017;9(19):1509—29.

[6] Laidler P, Cowan DA, Hider RC, Keane A, Kicman AT. Tryptic mapping of human chorionic-gonadotropin BY matrix-assisted laser-desorption ionization mass-spectrometry. Rapid Commun Mass Spectrom 1995;9(11):1021—6.

[7] Halvorsen TG, Reubsaet L. Antibody based affinity capture LC-MS/MS in quantitative determination of proteins in biological matrices. Trac Trends Anal Chem 2017;95: 132—9.

[8] Politi L, Groppi A, Polettini A. Applications of liquid chromatography — mass spectrometry in doping control. J Anal Toxicol 2005;29(1):1—14.

[9] Kicman AT, Parkin MC, Iles RK. An introduction to mass spectrometry based proteomics — detection and characterization of gonadotropins and related molecules. Mol Cell Endocrinol 2007;260:212—27.

[10] van den Broek I, Niessen WMA, van Dongen WD. Bioanalytical LC-MS/MS of protein-based biopharmaceuticals. J Chromatogr B Analyt Technol Biomed Life Sci 2013;929:161—79.

[11] Reubsaet L, Halvorsen TG. Determination of very low-abundance diagnostic proteins in serum using immuno-capture LC-MS-MS. LC GC Eur 2016;29(7):352.

[12] Liu CL, Bowers LD. Immunoaffinity trapping of urinary human chorionic gonadotropin and its high-performance liquid chromatographic-mass spectrometric confirmation. J Chromatogr B 1996;687(1):213—20.

[13] Gervais A, Hammel YA, Pelloux S, Lepage P, Baer G, Carte N, Sorokine O, Strub JM, Koerner R, Leize E, Van Dorsselaer A. Glycosylation of human recombinant gonadotrophins: characterization and batch-to-batch consistency. Glycobiology 2003;13(3): 179—89.

[14] Durgaryan A, Rundlof T, Laven M, Amini A. Identification of human chorionic gonadotropin hormone in illegally distributed products by MALDI-TOF mass spectrometry and double-injection capillary zone electrophoresis. Anal Methods 2016;8(21): 4188—96.

[15] Jacoby ES, Kicman AT, Laidler P, Iles RK. Determination of the glycoforms of human chorionic gonadotropin beta-core fragment by matrix-assisted laser desorption/ionization time-of-flight mass spectrometry. Clin Chem 2000;46(11):1796—803.

[16] Neubert H, Jacoby ES, Bansal SS, Iles RK, Cowan DA, Kicman AT. Enhanced affinity capture MALDI-TOF MS: orientation of an immunoglobulin G using recombinant protein G. Anal Chem 2002;74(15):3677—83.

[17] Toll H, Berger P, Hofmann A, Hildebrandt A, Oberacher H, Lenhof HP, Huber CG. Glycosylation patterns of human chorionic gonadotropin revealed by liquid chromatography-mass spectrometry and bioinformatics. Electrophoresis 2006;27(13): 2734—46.

[18] Thakur D, Rejtar T, Karger BL, Washburn NJ, Bosques CJ, Gunay NS, Shriver Z, Venkataraman G. Profiling the glycoforms of the intact alpha subunit of recombinant human chorionic gonadotropin by high-resolution capillary electrophoresis-mass spectrometry. Anal Chem 2009;81(21):8900—7.

[19] Camperi J, Combes A, Guibourdenche J, Guillarme D, Pichon V, Fournier T, Delaunay N. An attempt to characterize the human Chorionic Gonadotropin protein by reversed phase liquid chromatography coupled with high-resolution mass spectrometry at the intact level. J Pharm Biomed Anal 2018;161:35—44.

[20] Camperi J, De Cock B, Pichon V, Combes A, Guibourdenche J, Fournier T, Vander Heyden Y, Mangelings D, Delaunay N. First characterizations by capillary electrophoresis of human Chorionic Gonadotropin at the intact level. Talanta 2019;193:77—86.

[21] Aebersold R, Mann M. Mass spectrometry-based proteomics. Nature 2003;422:198.

[22] Olsen JV, Ong S-E, Mann M. Trypsin cleaves Exclusively C-terminal to arginine and lysine residues, vol. 3; 2004. p. 608—14.

[23] Stennicke HR, Breddam K. Chapter 561 — glutamyl endopeptidase I. In: Rawlings ND, Salvesen G, editors. Handbook of proteolytic enzymes. 3rd ed. Academic Press; 2013. p. 2534—8.

[24] Li DY, Zhang P, Li F, Chi LQ, Zhu DY, Zhang QY, Chi LL. Recognition of N-glycoforms in human chorionic gonadotropin by monoclonal antibodies and their interaction motifs. J Biol Chem 2015;290(37):22715—23.

[25] Thennati R, Singh SK, Nage N, Patel Y, Bose SK, Burade V, Ranbhor RS. Analytical characterization of recombinant hCG and comparative studies with reference product. Biologics 2018;12:23—35.

[26] Valmu L, Alfthan H, Hotakainen K, Birken S, Stenman UH. Site-specific glycan analysis of human chorionic gonadotropin beta-subunit from malignancies and pregnancy by liquid chromatography-electrospray mass spectrometry. Glycobiology 2006; 16(12):1207—18.

[27] Blanchard V, Gadkari RA, Gerwig GJ, Leeflang BR, Dighe RR, Kamerling JP. Characterization of the N-linked oligosaccharides from human chorionic gonadotropin expressed in the methylotrophic yeast Pichia pastoris. Glycoconj J 2007;24(1):33—47.

[28] Nana K, Satsuki I, Noritaka H, Akira H, Daisuke T, Teruhide Y. Mass spectrometric analysis of carbohydrate heterogeneity for the characterization of glycoprotein-based products. Trends Glycosci Glycotechnol 2008;20(112):97—116.

[29] Malatos S, Luttoo MJ, Trivedi D, Butler S, Cole L, Iles RK. Analysis of hCG beta cf glycosylation in normal and aberrant pregnancy by matrix-assisted laser desorption/ ionization time-of-flight mass spectrometry. Amino Acids 2009;37(1):124.

[30] Bai X, Li DY, Zhu J, Guan YD, Zhang QY, Chi LL. From individual proteins to proteomic samples: characterization of O-glycosylation sites in human chorionic gonadotropin and human-plasma proteins. Anal Bioanal Chem 2015;407(7):1857—69.

[31] Cole L. Human chorionic gonadotropin and associated molecules AU — Cole, Laurence A. Expert Rev Mol Diagn 2009;9(1):51—73.

[32] Liu CL, Bowers LD. Mass spectrometric characterization of the beta-subunit of human chorionic gonadotropin. J Mass Spectrom 1997;32(1):33—42.

[33] Gonzalez J, Takao T, Hori H, Besada V, Rodriguez R, Padron G, Shimonishi Y. A method for determination of N-glycosylation sites in glycoproteins by collision-induced dissociation analysis in fast atom bombardment mass spectrometry: identification of the positions of carbohydrate-linked asparagine in recombinant α-amylase by treatment with peptide-N-glycosidase F in 18O-labeled water. Anal Biochem 1992; 205(1):151—8.

[34] Liu CL, Bowers LD. Mass spectrometric characterization of nicked fragments of the beta-subunit of human chorionic gonadotropin. Clin Chem 1997;43(7):1172—81.

[35] Geng M, Ji J, Regnier FE. Signature-peptide approach to detecting proteins in complex mixtures. J Chromatogr A 2000;870(1):295—313.

[36] Gam LH, Tham SY, Latiff A. Immunoaffinity extraction and tandem mass spectrometric analysis of human chorionic gonadotropin in doping analysis. J Chromatogr B Analyt Technol Biomed Life Sci 2003;792(2):187—96.

[37] Lund H, Torsetnes SB, Paus E, Nustad K, Reubsaet L, Halvorsen TG. Exploring the complementary selectivity of immunocapture and MS detection for the differentiation between hCG isoforms in clinically relevant samples. J Proteome Res 2009;8(11): 5241—52.

[38] Lund H, Lovsletten K, Paus E, Halvorsen TG, Reubsaett L. Immuno-ms based targeted proteomics: highly specific, sensitive, and reproducible human chorionic gonadotropin determination for clinical diagnostics and doping analysis. Anal Chem 2012;84(18): 7926—32.

[39] Lund H, Paus E, Berger P, Stenman UH, Torcellini T, Halvorsen TG, Reubsaet L. Epitope analysis and detection of human chorionic gonadotropin (hCG) variants by monoclonal antibodies and mass spectrometry. Tumor Biol 2014;35(2):1013—22.

[40] Levernaes MCS, Broughton MN, Reubsaet L, Halvorsen TG. To elute or not to elute in immunocapture bottom-up LC-MS. J Chromatogr B Analyt Technol Biomed Life Sci. 2017;1055:51−60.

[41] Lund H, Snilsberg AH, Paus E, Halvorsen TG, Hemmersbach P, Reubsaet L. Sports drug testing using immuno-MS: clinical study comprising administration of human chorionic gonadotropin to males. Anal Bioanal Chem 2013;405(5):1569−76.

[42] Lund H, Snilsberg AH, Halvorsen TG, Hemmersbach P, Reubsaet L. Comparison of newly developed immuno-MS method with existing DELFIA (R) immunoassay for human chorionic gonadotropin determination in doping analysis. Bioanalysis 2013;5(5): 623−30.

[43] Rosting C, Gjelstad A, Halvorsen TG. Water-soluble dried blood spot in protein analysis: a proof-of-concept study. Anal Chem 2015;87(15):7918−24.

[44] Egeland SV, Reubsaet L, Halvorsen TG. The pros and cons of increased trypsin-to-protein ratio in targeted protein analysis. J Pharm Biomed Anal 2016;123:155−61.

[45] Egeland SV, Reubsaet L, Paus E, Halvorsen TG. Dual-immuno-MS technique for improved differentiation power in heterodimeric protein biomarker analysis: determination and differentiation of human chorionic gonadotropin variants in serum. Anal Bioanal Chem 2016;408(26):7379−91.

[46] Woldemariam GA, Butch AW. Immunoextraction-tandem mass spectrometry method for measuring intact human chorionic gonadotropin, free beta-subunit, and beta-subunit core fragment in urine. Clin Chem 2014;60(8):1089−97.

[47] Nerenz RD, Butch AW, Woldemariam GA, Yarbrough ML, Grenache DG, Gronowski AM. Estimating the hCG beta cf in urine during pregnancy. Clin Biochem 2016;49(3):282−6.

[48] Butch AW, Woldemariam GA. Urinary human chorionic gonadotropin isoform concentrations in doping control samples. Drug Test Anal 2016;8(11−12):1147−51.

[49] Butch AW, Ahrens BD, Avliyakulov NK. Urine reference intervals for human chorionic gonadotropin (hCG) isoforms by immunoextraction-tandem mass spectrometry to detect hCG use. Drug Test Anal 2018;10(6):956−60.

[50] Rosting C, Tran EV, Gjelstad A, Halvorsen TG. Determination of the low-abundant protein biomarker hCG from dried matrix spots using immunocapture and nano liquid chromatography mass spectrometry. J Chromatogr B Analyt Technol Biomed Life Sci 2018;1077:44−51.

[51] Skjærvø Ø, Solbakk EJ, Halvorsen TG, Reubsaet L. Paper-based immunocapture for targeted protein analysis. Talanta 2019;195:764−70.

[52] Browne JL, Schielen P, Belmouden I, Pennings JLA, Klipstein-Grobusch K. Dried blood spot measurement of pregnancy-associated plasma protein A (PAPP-A) and free beta-subunit of human chorionic gonadotropin (beta-hCG) from a low-resource setting. Prenat Diagn 2015;35(6):592−7.

[53] Stenman U-H, Alfthan H. Determination of human chorionic gonadotropin. Best Pract Res Clin Endocrinol Metabol 2013;27(6):783−93.

[54] Sturgeon CM, Berger P, Bidart J-M, Birken S, Burns C, Norman RJ, Stenman U-H, On behalf of the, I. W. G. o. H.. Differences in recognition of the 1st WHO international reference reagents for hCG-related isoforms by diagnostic immunoassays for human chorionic gonadotropin. Clin Chem 2009;55(8):1484−91.

[55] Berger P, Sturgeon C, Bidart JM, Paus E, Gerth R, Niang M, Bristow A, Birken S, Stenman UH. The ISOBM TD-7 workshop on hCG and related molecules. Tumor Biol 2002;23(1):1−38.

[56] Berger P, Paus E, Hemken PM, Sturgeon C, Stewart WW, Skinner JP, Harwick LC, Saldana SC, Ramsay CS, Rupprecht KR, Olsen KH, Bidart J-M, Stenman U-H, Members of the ISOBM TD-7 Workshop on hCG and Related Molecules. Candidate epitopes for measurement of hCG and related molecules: the second ISOBM TD-7 workshop. Tumor Biol 2013;34(6):4033−57.

[57] Birken S, Berger P, Bidart J-M, Weber M, Bristow A, Norman R, Sturgeon C, Stenman U-H. Preparation and characterization of new WHO reference reagents for human chorionic gonadotropin and metabolites. Clin Chem 2003;49(1):144.

hCGβcf as a quality control marker for urine mass spectrometry analysis

2.6

Ricardo J. Pais, Raminta Zmuidinaite, Ray K. Iles, Stephen A. Butler

Human chorionic gonadotropin β-core fragment (hCGβcf) is a polypeptide considered to be ubiquitously present in urine regardless of race, sex, and age [1−3]. This fragment is mainly produced by the degradation of human chorionic gonadotropin (hCG) in the kidney and excreted in the urine, representing around 80% of total hCG in urine [2]. The presence of hCGβcf in urine has been extensively used for noninvasive clinical diagnostics assays associated with pregnancy. Matrix-Assisted Laser Desorption Ionization (MALDI) Time of Flight (ToF) mass spectrometry (MS) is a rapid, affordable, and powerful diagnostic technique that is starting to find an increasing presence in clinical laboratories [4−7]. hCGβcf has been used as biomarker of pregnancy and cancer, and, in this chapter, we discuss its potential as quality control marker for urine analysis using MALDI-ToF mass spectrometry. We focus on hCGβcf spectral properties and discuss the advantages and disadvantages to its use as quality control calibrator for MS analysis of urine. Further, we will present how can hCGβcf be implemented as a quality control measure in a routine laboratory analysis and in high-throughput analysis of mass spectral data.

Detection of hCGβcf in urine

MALDI-ToF is a rapid and accurate mass spectrometry technique that uses a laser to generate and detect ions from large molecules such as proteins and peptides with little fragmentation based on their mass charge ratio (m/z) [4,8,9]. This technique is suitable to detect hCGβcf on a complex mixture of proteins, peptides, lipids and sugar-based moieties due to its unique mass [3,8,10]. Indeed, this is the case of urine, where its composition may vary according to many confounding factors such as water intake, metabolism, genetics, pathologies, and pregnancy [11,12] and containing a proteome composed of a complex mixture of proteins excreted from kidney and urinary tract [12]. Thus, the analysis of urine mass spectra is complex due to the abundance of molecules with distinct masses (Fig. 2.6.1). However, hCGβcf is quite

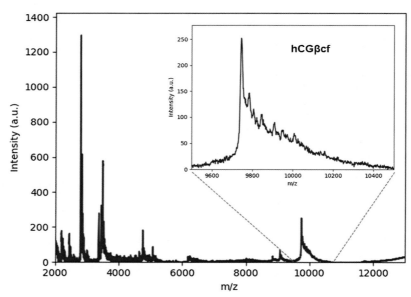

FIGURE 2.6.1 Typical urine mass spectrum generated by MALDI-ToF and hCGβcf identification.

The inset figure denotes the spectral region of hCGβcf detection.

easy to distinguish in urine using MALDI-ToF due to its characteristic mass (9.7 kDa) and its glycosylated forms which have been well described before [2,3]. In MALDI-ToF mass spectrometry of urine, these hCGβcf characteristics render asymmetrically distributed peaks in the mass region between 9500m/z and 10,400 m/z (see inset in Fig. 2.6.1). Typically, hCGβcf mass spectrum shows a sharp maximum peak around 9750 m/z, followed by several others with reduced intensity. The peak with the maximum intensity corresponds to the nonglycosylated form of hCGβcf (~9750 m/z), whereas the subsequent peaks with higher masses correspond to the respective glycosylated forms [3]. In general, the characteristic peaks associated with hCGβcf is further characterized by its broad and skewed right distribution, observed from 9750 m/z to 10,400 m/z. Together, these spectral characteristics assign to hCGβcf a classical spectral signature in urine, which can be seen as its unique "fingerprint."

Problems in hCGβcf detection

The characteristic spectral features of hCGβcf may not be always observed due to extrinsic and/or intrinsic problems associated to the urine sample being analyzed using MALDI-ToF mass spectrometry [8]. In some cases, this is the result of poor-quality spectra that can arise from bad instrument calibration, which in turn is pointed as the main extrinsic source. This can either result in very noisy spectra or spectra with poor signal-to-noise ratios (SNRs) which depend on MALDI-ToF instrument parameters such as laser power, pulse extraction, and number of cumulated laser shots [8,13,14]. Sample dilution is another potential source of problems in detecting hCGβcf, which can simply be because the abundance of biological material is not enough to obtain an adequate signal for correct identification. Other intrinsic problems may also result in missing hCGβcf detection, where sample preparation and storage may cause proteins to precipitate, aggregate, denature or polypeptide side chains can be removed by chemical reactions that result in mass shifts. Thus, accessing the mass spectra quality is a critical step before conducting any analysis on urine samples.

hCGβcf as a reference signature

As previously described, the detection of hCGβcf in MALDI-ToF-based urine analysis is advantageous because it can be easily identified in high-quality spectra and represents a good choice as a marker for quality control when compared against other possible biological markers present in urine. The obvious advantage lies on the fact that it is the most frequently observed protein fragment signal in many urine mass spectra (Fig. 2.6.2). hCGβcf signal is not the strongest in the spectrum but still can be placed on the top 10 strongest signals in urine. This makes hCGβcf more suitable to be used as a representative reference for the urine spectrum containing proteins excreted from kidney. In addition, it can be easily quantified by other techniques, such as immunoassay, to check the signal (peak) actually arises from molecular hCGβcf.

Importantly, the characteristic spectral signature of hCGβcf has a much higher degree of conservation in comparison with other protein signals (see region I to III in Fig. 2.6.3). From the hCGβcf spectral signature, it is visible that its maximum peak at ~9750 m/z does not change, making this a huge advantage for its identification on the mass spectrum. In addition, the asymmetric nature of hCGβcf spectral signature is more specific than most protein signals observed in urine mass spectra, which is advantageous for preventing false detection of hCGβcf (Fig. 2.6.2). Moreover, hCGβcf signal location is distant from other protein signals in the spectrum (>100 m/z) which facilitates the correct detection by the absence of interfering signals from neighboring peaks. This is not the case of many other protein signals between the range of 2000 m/z and 7000 m/z (Fig. 2.6.2). In these regions, multiple proteins have signals that overlap due to proximity in terms of their molecular mass. Some signals do show a substantial degree of isolation and reasonable signal intensity, placing them as possible candidates to indicate a good-quality urine mass spectrum (Fig. 2.6.2). However, the variability associated with the intensity on these mass regions, together with the lack of consistency in the observed signature, favors the choice of hCGβcf as reference peak.

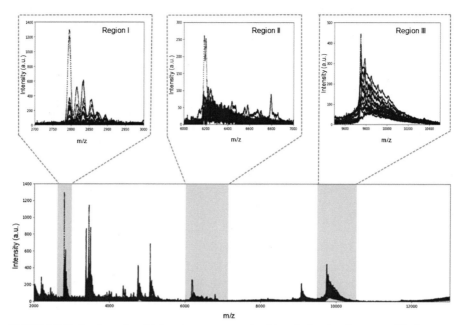

FIGURE 2.6.2 Overlap of multiple urine mass spectra (down) showing three amplified regions (up).

Regions in gray denote possible biomarkers for quality control. Overlap was produced with 30 urine samples from pregnant women from the UK. Depicted regions I, II, and III show the three best candidate protein signals that could represent urine spectra. Region III denotes the hCGβcf characteristic signature.

While the spectral signature of hCGβcf has these significant advantages for quality control, it also has some limitations. The main limitation lies in its inherent variability in terms of its signal intensity due to variability in the concentration in urine. For example, if we compare good quality and concentrated pregnancy urine MS, one order of magnitude in variation is expected (see inset of hCGβcf in Fig. 2.6.2). Variation could actually increase up to two orders of magnitude if we compare pregnant women with nonpregnant women and men. Another limitation is the potential for hCGβcf to display chemical changes such as glycosylation due to diseases independent of the sample collection [3,8]. This would actually cause a shift in the peak location and possible changes in the asymmetric signature peak leading to misleading interpretation in terms of sample quality. Thus, utilizing hCGβcf detection for quality control in mass spectral analysis should be considered in a qualitative manner and possible deviations should be taken into account due to pathological interference which affect concentration and structure.

Relation of hCGβcf to spectral quality

In mass spectrometry, the quality of spectra is frequently accessed through measuring the instrument resolution by calculating the SNR [13,15]. Additionally, the detection power is also measured by simply calculating the total ion current (sum of all ion count). However, for the analysis of urine by mass spectrometry, these two measures are not enough since they do not cover the biological quality of the spectra. One reason lies on the fact that MALDI-ToF technology is very sensitive and well-resolved spectra may be achieved only due to proteins from the urinary tract. These proteins are not necessarily metabolically relevant and would simply mislead the biological interpretation of urine mass spectra. For this purpose, hCGβcf is an ideal candidate as a quality control marker to detect if proteins excreted from kidney are present in the urine proteome since they are ubiquitously excreted from kidney regardless of age, sex, health, and ethnicity [2,10,16]. In this section, we illustrate the informative capacity of hCGβcf for quality using four analyzed cases, where all mass spectra were accepted by high SNR and total ion current (Fig. 2.6.3).

Ideally, a fresh, early morning, concentrated urine sample will have a well-resolved spectrum detecting a perfect hCGβcf signature (see example in Fig. 2.6.3A). This would give the indication that other proteins, if present, with concentrations above hCGβcf will also have good resolution, and thus we have a representative sample of metabolic relevance in urine. In addition, the detection of a hCGβcf spectral signature can also provide an additional qualitative indication of instrument resolution since it is characterized by several well-defined peaks (Fig. 2.6.3A). The typical hCGβcf signature is gradually lost with dilution even when the mass spectra are at an acceptable SNR (Fig. 2.6.3). In these cases, the loss of hCGβcf signature follows a reduction of the SNR of hCGβcf peak and does not correlate with the SNR of the mass spectra using the highest signal. This property is particularly important for rejecting mass spectra that are too dilute in proteins metabolized in the kidney avoiding misleading conclusions, especially in clinical diagnostic applications. Another interesting property of hCGβcf dilution is the mass shift of its peak to higher mass value (Fig. 2.6.3). This further places the location of hCGβcf peak as a good indicator of the sample quality in terms of protein concentration excreted by the kidney.

Sample storage conditions and sample aging can also cause misleading interpretations of urine mass spectra. For example, several cycles of freezing and thawing of urine samples can result in substantial changes in the spectra due to chemical reactions during the process of freezing and thawing. In this case, the SNR of hCGβcf is frequently high, but the typical hCGβcf spectral signature is lost showing a shift of its maximum isotopic peak to higher mass (Fig. 2.6.2C). This can be interpreted as a molecular change in the hCGβcf polypeptide side chain by the addition of molecules that resulted from chemical reactions with other components present in the urine. Precipitation and decomposition are also two possibilities that may occur in the case of very old samples. In this case, it is possible to observe a substantial reduction

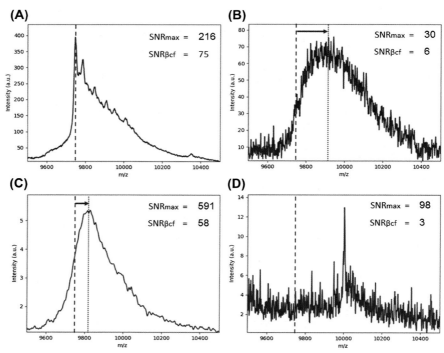

FIGURE 2.6.3 **Mass spectral comparison in the hCGβcf mass region of well-resolved spectra in different conditions.**

(A) Fresh and highly concentrated urine sample. (B) Fresh and very diluted urine samples. (C) Highly concentrated urine sample with 7-weeks-old sample under seven freeze and thaw cycles (D) Highly concentrated urine sample with 7-weeks-old sample stored at 4° and exposed to air. All urine samples were from pregnant women, and spectra were generated with Shimadzu MALDI-ToF instrument. SNR was calculated for the highest peak in the spectrum (SNR_{max}) and the highest peak in the mass range for hCGβcf detection ($SNR_{hCGβcf}$).

or even complete loss of the hCGβcf signature (Fig. 2.6.2D). Taken all together, the changes in the hCGβcf mass spectral signature, in particular the presence and the location of peak, gives important information regarding the biological quality of the urine spectra as well as indicating good spectral resolution.

Implementation of hCGβcf in quality control: a new concept

Several research studies are now starting to use the detection of hCGβcf as a quality control marker to select urine mass spectra that are biologically interpretable, discarding the ones which may cause misleading conclusion. This current practice started with research studies on hCGβcf detection and alterations in mass spectral profiles of urine from pregnant women, which have been correlated with fetal aneuploidies and other abnormalities [3,16]. The hCGβcf spectral signature can be easily checked in urine mass spectra by simply visualizing the spectra between 9500 m/z and 10,500 m/z and checking for the presence of the characteristic peak at ~ 9750 m/z. For this visual inspection, freely available software such as mMass provides a user-friendly interface that can easily zoom the spectra into the range of hCGβcf [17]. At the same time, it is possible to check for the SNR, which can also be estimated visually on the spectra, as described above.

For more systematic analysis, the identification of the hCGβcf signature can be easily programed toward the development of fully automated bioinformatic pipelines. In python, the code is straightforward as it is shown in following example:

```
=====================================================================
# mzpks is a list with m/z values of all peaks detected in MS
# Ipks is a list with I values of all peaks detected in MS
# LNoise is a list with local noise values in MS
BCpk = "not detected"
for k, mz in enumerate(mzpks):
        if mz > 9700 and mz < 9800:
                SNRbc  =  float ( Ipks [ k ] ) / LNoise [ k ]
                if SNRbc >= 5:
                        BCpk = "peak detected in range"
    print BCpk
=====================================================================
```

Programing an automated search for hCGβcf signature on mass spectral data can be much more advanced and detailed, embedded in nested loops to tackle multiple mass spectra. A recent computational and fully automated workflow has successfully applied hCGβcf detection for quality control decisions on large datasets, rendering a precise identification of hCGβcf absent of human bias and error [18]. Importantly, this computational approach demonstrated advantages in comparison with strictly manual approaches, namely in terms of data processing time (up to 100-fold faster), saving human resources and increasing of accuracy in quality control decisions [18]. This computational approach made it possible to use MALDI-ToF spectrometry as an ultrahigh-throughput technique [19]. Moreover, filtering data by searching for hCGβcf also contributed to a better identification of mass spectral patterns of fetal aneuploidies on urine from pregnant women [18].

Perspectives

As highlighted in this chapter, hCGβcf is an ideal marker for detecting good-quality urine mass spectra and improving the discriminatory power of the tests developed based on MALDI-ToF technology when analyzing urine. This has already been used in clinical proteomics applications since the quality of the data is fundamental for extracting accurate diagnostic information. Because MALDI-ToF technology is a noninvasive, rapid, accurate, and economical laboratory technique, this could result in a positive impact on healthcare systems [6,7]. Currently, MALDI-ToF mass spectrometry is only used in microbiology for detecting distinct types of bacteria [4,9,20]. In principle, having hCGβcf detection as a standard control reference would facilitate the future development of other types of diagnostic tests, particularly of urine, generalizing this type of diagnostic method in clinics. These would be particularly important for the diagnostics of pathologies in obstetrics and reproductive medicine, where hCGβcf is more concentrated and gives rise to better spectral signatures. The fact that is now possible to check for hCGβcf in an automated way that opens the possibility of tackling ultrahigh-throughput data from MALDI-ToF instruments [19]. This further facilitates the possibility of screening huge populations with rapid and affordable tests based on the analysis of urine data from high-throughput MALDI-ToF instruments. It now remains for the development of fully automated diagnostic software tools, coupled with MALDI-ToF analytical instruments, to bring MS diagnostics to clinics and advancing mass population screening.

References

[1] Iles RK, Lee CL, Howes I, Davies S, Edwards R, Chard T. Immunoreactive β-core-like material in normal postmenopausal urine: human chorionic gonadotrophin or LH origin? Evidence for the existence of LH core. J Endocrinol 1992;133:459−66.

[2] Lee CL, Iles RK, Shepherd JH, Hudson CN, Chard T. The purification and development of a radioimmunoassay for beta-core fragment of human chorionic gonadotrophin in urine: application as a marker of gynaecological cancer in premenopausal and postmenopausal women. J Endocrinol 1991;130:481−9. Available: http://www.ncbi.nlm.nih.gov/pubmed/1719119.

[3] Iles RK, Cole LA, Butler SA. Direct analysis of hCGβcf glycosylation in normal and aberrant pregnancy by matrix-assisted laser desorption/ionization time-of-flight mass spectrometry. Int J Mol Sci 2014;15:10067−82. https://doi.org/10.3390/ijms150610067.

[4] Angeletti S. Matrix assisted laser desorption time of flight mass spectrometry (MALDI-TOF MS) in clinical microbiology. J Microbiol Methods 2017;138:20−9. https://doi.org/10.1016/j.mimet.2016.09.003.

[5] Nomura F. Proteome-based bacterial identification using matrix-assisted laser desorption ionization-time of flight mass spectrometry (MALDI-TOF MS): a revolutionary shift in clinical diagnostic microbiology. Biochim Biophys Acta 2015;1854:528−37. https://doi.org/10.1016/j.bbapap.2014.10.022.

[6] Gaillot O, Blondiaux N, Loïez C, Wallet F, Lemaître N, Herwegh S, et al. Cost-effectiveness of switch to matrix-assisted laser desorption ionization-time of flight

mass spectrometry for routine bacterial identification. J Clin Microbiol 2011;49:4412. https://doi.org/10.1128/JCM.05429-11.

[7] Tan KE, Ellis BC, Lee R, Stamper PD, Zhang SX, Carroll KC. Prospective evaluation of a matrix-assisted laser desorption ionization-time of flight mass spectrometry system in a hospital clinical microbiology laboratory for identification of bacteria and yeasts: a bench-by-bench study for assessing the impact on time to identification and cost-effectiveness. J Clin Microbiol 2012;50:3301−8. https://doi.org/10.1128/JCM.01405-12.

[8] Duncan MW, Nedelkov D, Walsh R, Hattan SJ. Applications of MALDI mass spectrometry in clinical chemistry. Clin Chem 2015;62:1−10. https://doi.org/10.1373/clinchem.2015.239491.

[9] De Carolis E, Vella A, Vaccaro L, Torelli R, Spanu T, Fiori B, et al. Application of MALDI-TOF mass spectrometry in clinical diagnostic microbiology. J Infect Dev Ctries 2014;8:1081−8. https://doi.org/10.3855/jidc.3623.

[10] Trivedi DK, Iles RK. Do not just do it, do it right: urinary metabolomics−establishing clinically relevant baselines. Biomed Chromatogr 2014;28:1491−501. Wiley Online Library.

[11] Bouatra S, Aziat F, Mandal R, Guo AC, Wilson MR, Knox C, et al. The human urine metabolome. PLoS One 2013;8:e73076. https://doi.org/10.1371/journal.pone.0073076. Public Library of Science.

[12] González-Buitrago JM, Ferreira L, Lorenzo I. Urinary proteomics. Clin Chim Acta 2007;375:49−56. https://doi.org/10.1016/j.cca.2006.07.027.

[13] Monchamp P, Andrade-Cetto L, Zhang JY, Henson R. Signal processing methods for mass spectrometry. Systems Bioinformatics 2007:101−24.

[14] Diao L, Clarke CH, Coombes KR, Hamilton SR, Roth J, Mao L, et al. Reproducibility of seLDI spectra across time and laboratories. Cancer Inform 2011;10:45−64. https://doi.org/10.4137/CIN.S6438.

[15] Galleani L, Cohen L, Nelson D. Local signal to noise ratio, vol. 6313; 2006. https://doi.org/10.1117/12.684026. 63130Q−9.

[16] Iles RK, Shahpari ME, Cuckle H, Butler SA. Direct and rapid mass spectral fingerprinting of maternal urine for the detection of Down syndrome pregnancy. Clin Proteomics 2015;12:9. https://doi.org/10.1186/s12014-015-9082-9.

[17] Strohalm M, Hassman M, Kosata B, Kodíček M. mMass data miner: an open source alternative for mass spectrometric data analysis. Rapid Commun Mass Spectrom 2008;22:905−8. https://doi.org/10.1002/rcm.3444.

[18] Pais RJ, Zmuidinaite R, Butler SA, Iles RK. An automated workflow for MALDI-ToF mass spectra pattern identification on large data sets: an application to detect aneuploidies from pregnancy urine. Informatics Med Unlocked 2019;16:100194. https://doi.org/10.1016/J.IMU.2019.100194. Elsevier.

[19] Haslam C, Hellicar J, Dunn A, Fuetterer A, Hardy N, Marshall P, et al. The evolution of MALDI-TOF mass spectrometry toward ultra-high-throughput screening: 1536-well format and beyond. J Biomol Screen 2016;21:176−86. https://doi.org/10.1177/1087057115608605.

[20] Lo CI, Fall B, Sambe-Ba B, Diawara S, Gueye MW, Mediannikov O, et al. MALDI-tof mass spectrometry: a powerful tool for clinical microbiology at Hôpital principal de Dakar, Senegal (West Africa). PLoS One 2015;10:e0145889. https://doi.org/10.1371/journal.pone.0145889. Mischak H, editor.

Pregnancy and fertility

How hCG was used as tool to study LH action

3.1

Ilpo Huhtaniemi

My research career started about 50 years ago at the University of Helsinki with the Ph.D. project on steroid metabolism in the human fetus (e.g., Ref. [1]). After completing the thesis, I moved for postdoctoral training to the University of California San Francisco where my supervisor, Dr. Robert B. Jaffe, gave me the task to study the regulation of testosterone production in human fetal testis. This is when I first came across hCG as a tool to study gonadotropin action. It was natural to use hCG because the purest gonadotropin preparations at that time, in the mid-1970s, were the R. Canfield CR preparations provided by the NIH. hCG was also the apparent fetal gonadotropin, with orders of magnitude higher than pituitary LH in fetal circulation.

I used hCG first to detect LH receptors in fetal testis. The hormone preparation was [^{125}I]-radioiodinated. The proportion of label bound to bioactive hCG molecules was assessed by incubation in excess of LH receptors in rat testis homogenate. It was typically 30%−50%, which was quite good taken that the biological activity of the starting material was 10,000 IU/mg, i.e., about two-thirds of 100% pure hormone. It was possible to quantitate LH/hCG receptors in very small samples of tissue (≈ 1 mg). Another part of the study was to incubate testis slices in the presence of hCG and to demonstrate that it stimulated testosterone production. The experiments worked, and we were able to show that human fetal testis tissue expresses high-affinity receptors for hCG and that hCG stimulates testosterone production [2]. In light of today's knowledge, this study sounds trivial, but it was novel information in those days.

After San Francisco, I moved to the Mecca of gonadotropin receptor research, the laboratory of Dr. Kevin J. Catt, at the NIH (Bethesda, MD). Similar techniques were used there to study the physiology of rat gonadotropin receptor regulation. Downregulation of LH receptor had just been discovered, and my task was to study how rat fetal Leydig cells respond to strong gonadotropin stimulation, using again hCG. Surprisingly, we found that downregulation does not work in fetal testis [3]; the molecular mechanism of this finding still remains unclear. Industrial quantities of various endocrine tissues were homogenized and incubated with radiolabeled hCG for receptor measurements. The work was technically quite robust and we used to call it "grinding and binding." Nevertheless, lots of useful information was produced, and hCG was the key reagent in all experiments. All of this was done in the premolecular time, before we knew anything about the structure of LH receptor or had access to pure recombinant hCG.

100 Years of Human Chorionic Gonadotropin. **https://doi.org/10.1016/B978-0-12-820050-6.00013-8**

References

[1] Huhtaniemi I, Ikonen M, Vihko R. Presence of testosterone and other neutral steroids in human fetal testes. Biochem Biophys Res Commun 1970;38:715−20.

[2] Huhtaniemi IT, Korenbrot CC, Jaffe RB. hCG binding and stimulation of testosterone biosynthesis in the human fetal testis. J Clin Endocrinol Metab 1977;44:963−7.

[3] Huhtaniemi IT, Katikineni M, Catt KJ. Regulation of luteinizing-hormone-receptors and steroidogenesis in the neonatal rat testis. Endocrinology 1981;109:588−95.

The role of hCG in endometrial receptivity and embryo implantation

3.2

Jemma Evans

Introduction

The role of hCG and specific hCG isoforms in human endometrial receptivity and embryo implantation is difficult to define. A large number of in vitro and in vivo studies conducted in primates and humans strongly suggest a role for hCG in endometrial receptivity. However, the findings of these studies have not translated to clinical studies where the efficacy of intrauterine hCG delivery has not supported benefit on pregnancy outcome, this may be partially due to suboptimal study design. The scene is further complicated when the source of hCG is taken into account. Studies have variously used urinary hCG preparations, which are known to be contaminated with growth factors, or recombinant hCG, which is representative of one form of hCG only. The characterization of a hyperglycosylated form of hCG which accounts for up to 40% of hCG released by hatched blastocysts has never been directly investigated for its role in endometrial receptivity and embryo implantation. What then is the true impact of hCG in the endometrium with respect to receptivity? This chapter will summarize current knowledge and highlight avenues for future study in this area.

The composition of hCG is all important

There are five isoforms of hCG [2]; these isoforms have differing activities as indicated by the different tissues which predominantly produce each form. HCG is a dimer consisting of an α- and a β-subunit. The α-subunit is identical to that of other gonadotropin hormones (e.g., LH and FSH), with the β-subunit providing specificity. "Hormonal" or "regular" hCG is produced by the syncytiotrophoblast cells of the placenta during pregnancy. This form acts to maintain progesterone production by the corpus luteum which supports maintenance of the pregnancy until placental progesterone production is sufficient at around 8—12 weeks of pregnancy. Sulfated hCG, is produced by the gonadotrope cells within the pituitary. This form of hCG is also proposed to mediate endocrine functions; however, little is truly known about its function. Hyperglycosylated hCG (hCG-H), a form of the glycoprotein with excessive branching and complexity of the hCG oligosaccharide side chains, is produced by the invasive extravillous cytotrophoblasts in the placenta during the first trimester of pregnancy and by the malignant cells of hCG producing cancers. Its release by the preimplantation embryo has also been characterized recently [3]. This hyperglycosylated form of hCG is thought to act in an autocrine manner similar to a cytokine. The free β-subunit and hyperglycosylated β-subunit have also been described, but seem mainly to characterize malignancy and may be less important in endometrial receptivity. With reference to embryo-maternal communication during embryo implantation, hCG gene expression has been detected from the eight-cell stage of embryo development before embryo hatching [4]. However, hCG-β is predominantly released by unhatched embryos [3]. The release of hCG isoforms by human embryos has been quantified, revealing that around 50% of hCG produced by hatched blastocysts is regular hCG, 40% is HCG-H, and 10% is hCG-β [3]. This confirmed the findings of an earlier study which demonstrated that acidic forms of hCG were released by early embryos; glycosylation changes the pI resulting in a relatively acidic molecule [5]. Given that the hatched blastocyst enters into a dialogue with the maternal endometrium to achieve implantation, these three forms are prime candidates for influencing endometrial function. Indeed, altered levels of hCG and hCG-H have been associated with early pregnancy loss [6−8]. The composition of hCG used for in vitro, in vivo, and clinical studies [9] is therefore critical in assessing the relevance of the resulting data to endometrial receptivity and embryo implantation.

A recent study by Butler and Cole [9] demonstrated the large variation in composition of commercially available hCG preparations commonly used in a variety of studies. Recombinant hCG (Serono Ovidrel) contained 100% "regular" hCG with normal glycosylation. This has been used extensively in studies of endometrial function and embryo implantation; however, as suggested above, this does not represent the unique hCG milieu at the time of implantation. Indeed, none of the hCG preparations examined, accurately represent the hCG composition released by the human preimplantation embryo, with proportions of hCG-H falling significantly short of the ~40% identified in embryo culture media. The situation is further complicated when considering the urinary hCG preparations conventionally used in such studies. Growth factors including EGF and TGFβ have been found in hCG preparations [10−12] and may partially account for the activation of the TGFβ receptor attributed to hCG-H [10]. No currently commercially available preparations of hCG are representative of the milieu produced by the hatched preimplantation blastocyst (described above). The current body of data examining its role in endometrial receptivity and embryo implantation may not, therefore, be directly physiologically relevant.

Endometrial receptivity

The endometrium becomes ready or "receptive" for implantation by an embryo for around 4 days each menstrual cycle between cycle days 20—24 (of an ideal 28-day cycle [13], Fig. 3.2.1). The ovarian steroid hormones play key roles in preparing the endometrium for embryo implantation. After ovulation of an oocyte from the dominant ovarian follicle, around day 14 of the menstrual cycle, the resultant corpus luteum produces progesterone which promotes secretory transformation of the

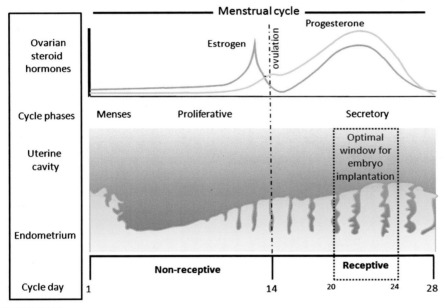

FIGURE 3.2.1

After menses (designed as day 1 of the menstrual cycle), the endometrium undergoes repair and, under the influence of increasing levels of estrogen, regeneration during the proliferative phase of the menstrual cycle. The estrogen surge from the dominant ovarian follicle triggers LH production from the anterior pituitary leading to ovulation of the oocyte around day 14 of the cycle. The empty follicle forms the corpus luteum which predominantly produces progesterone. Progesterone induces a secretory transformation within the endometrium, preparing the endometrium for implantation of the embryo during a conception cycle. The time at which the endometrium is optimally receptive to an embryo falls between days 20—24 of the 28-day menstrual cycle, termed the window of implantation. For a short time, either side of this window, the endometrium can allow implantation but pregnancy outcomes are less optimal [1]. The endometrial cells become terminally differentiated by the action of progesterone and, in the absence of conception, must be shed at menses to allow appropriate development of the tissue in subsequent cycles.

endometrium during the second half of the cycle. The endometrial epithelial cells become highly secretory and produce a large number of soluble proteins, glycoproteins, and lipids along with extracellular vesicles containing cargo [13,14]. All are

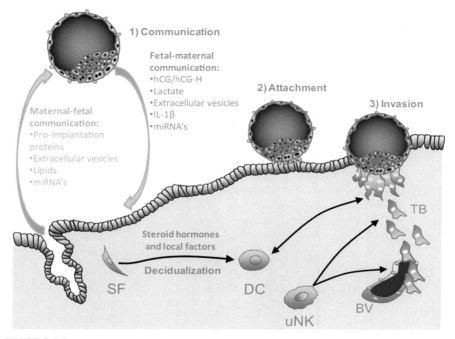

FIGURE 3.2.2

(1) During the peri-implantation phase, the maternal endometrium releases factors which enter into a communication with the embryo to facilitate implantation. Similarly the hatched embryo releases factors which communicate with the endometrium to further enhance implantation likelihood. At this time the stromal fibroblasts (SF) undergo progesterone-mediated terminal differentiation known as decidualization, resulting in production of decidualized cells (DC). (2) After two-way preimplantation communication, the trophectoderm cells of the embryo adhere to the maternal endometrial luminal epithelium to establish implantation. (3) The trophectoderm cells of the embryo then differentiate into trophoblast (TB) cells and invade further into the maternal endometrium to establish full implantation. The trophoblast cells continue to release factors which influence function of the endometrial cells, with specific endometrial cells types, including the DC's and uterine natural killer cells (uNK) similarly communicating with the trophoblast cells and also influencing blood vessel (BV) function to establish appropriate hemochorial placentation.

Adapted from Salamonsen LA, Nie G, Hannan NJ, Dimitriadis E. Society for Reproductive Biology Founders' Lecture 2009. Preparing fertile soil: the importance of endometrial receptivity. Reprod Fertil Dev. 2009;21(7): 923–934.

released into the uterine cavity where they can enter into a dialogue with the embryo to facilitate embryo implantation, establishing maternal-fetal communication (Fig. 3.2.2). Combined estrogen and progesterone, in addition to local factors within the endometrium, promote the terminal differentiation of the endometrial stromal fibroblasts into epithelial-like cells in a process known as decidualization, a critical maternal adaptation for human pregnancy. Specific immune cells resident within the endometrium, including uterine natural killer cells and T-regulatory cells, are also critical in endometrial receptivity and the embryo implantation process. It is now known that signals produced by the hatched embryo and released in close proximity to the endometrium can further promote endometrial receptivity and facilitate the implantation process, establishing fetal-maternal communication (Fig. 3.2.2). The impact of hCG on endometrial receptivity has been extensively investigated and is one of the most well-characterized embryonic factors in terms of fetal-maternal communication. However, as summarized below, there is still considerable scope for understanding the full impact of blastocyst-derived hCG with the data of some studies cast into doubt by their use of urinary-derived hCG potentially contaminated with a large number of other factors.

Does hCG facilitate endometrial receptivity?
In vivo studies

The most relevant studies in this area have used humans and the baboon as a model of endometrial receptivity. Seminal studies performed by Licht and colleagues used an intrauterine microdialysis device in a loop, to infuse 500 IU urinary hCG (Predalon, Organon) into the uterine cavity during the secretory phase of the menstrual cycle (LH+5−12) for 5 hours followed by collection of uterine effluent [15]. They demonstrated differential effects of hCG on IGFBP-1, depending on the specific time within the cycle that hCG perfusion was performed. During the estimated time of the implantation window, hCG had no effect on uterine IGFBP-1 concentrations. However, later in the cycle, close to the time of menstruation, hCG inhibited IGFBP-1. This is likely reflective of the physiology of the tissue at this time of the cycle; IGFBP-1 is a marker of the decidual transformation of endometrial stromal cells which only manifests in the nonpregnant endometrium toward the end of the menstrual cycle. It was proposed that this may be a mechanism whereby the hCG-secreting embryo may extend the opening of the window of endometrial receptivity and thus facilitate embryo implantation. Following the same experimental protocol, the investigators also demonstrated that hCG (1) increased vascular endothelial growth factor (VEGF) production; (2) increased leukemia inhibitory factor (LIF) production; (3) inhibited macrophage colony stimulating factor (M-CSF); and (4) promoted tissue remodeling by inducing MMP-9 with no effect observed on TIMP-1 [16]. Caution must be used in extrapolation of these results to human embryo implantation. Although this work was performed in vivo in humans, the hCG used (Predalon) is considered to be a relatively crude preparation in which the relative proportions of the relevant hCG forms and the potential contaminating factors are unknown.

The baboon provides a valuable model to examine endometrial changes in a nonhuman primate that exhibits menstruation. Examining changes in such models is critical as features of endometrial remodeling for receptivity and pregnancy are unique to menstruating species. These changes include spontaneous stromal cell decidualization (terminal hormone-mediated differentiation of the endometrial stromal cells) and unique changes in cell populations to enable the highly invasive hemochorial placentation exhibited by these species. Treatment of baboons with recombinant hCG into the uterus via oviductal cannulation mediated a large number of changes important for receptivity. Morphological changes including formation of epithelial plaques, were observed in the hCG-treated animals, in addition to expression of factors important in endometrial receptivity including glycodelin, leukemia inhibitory factor (LIF), interleukin-6 (IL-6), and the IL-6 signal transducer (gp130 receptor) [17,18]. Importantly, these changes required a synergistic interaction with hormone-mediated actions as such changes were not observed in ovariectomized animals [17]. In contrast with the human above, studies in the baboon suggested that hCG could promote decidualization [17]. However, different phases of the menstrual cycle were examined and the baboons were treated with hCG for 4 days rather than 5 hours as in the human studies suggesting that in the long term hCG may indeed facilitate decidualization. These data may be more relevant to the human in vivo situation than the studies performed in humans, as recombinant rather than urinary hCG was used. However, a remaining question is the influence of hCG biosimilar to that released by the human embryo; this is known to contain ~40% hCG-H, while the recombinant hCG used in the baboon studies contained <0.1% hCG-H [9]. We will not truly know the influence of hCG in endometrial receptivity and embryo implantation until the impact of combined hCG/hCG-H with a composition biosimilar to that released by the human embryo is determined.

In vitro studies

A number of in vitro studies using endometrial epithelial cells isolated from human or baboon endometrium, endometrial epithelial cell lines, endometrial stromal cells, endometrial uterine natural killer cells, and endometrial explants support a role for hCG in promoting endometrial receptivity. Recombinant and urinary hCG treatment of primary human endometrial epithelial cells and endometrial epithelial cell lines promotes endometrial receptivity-associated factors including VEGF, LIF, IL-11, GM-CSF, FGF-2, COX-2, and prokineticin 1 [19—23]. Indeed, hCG-mediated LIF production was dependent on prior induction of prokineticin 1, indicating a signaling cascade required for hCG-mediated endometrial receptivity [20]. In baboon endometrial epithelial cells, recombinant hCG was demonstrated to activate Gq-coupled receptor signaling leading to ERK 1/2 phosphorylation, rather than the classic Gαs coupling resulting in cAMP release as observed in the ovary [24,25]. It was proposed that activation of an alternate signal transduction pathway in endometrial cells may prevent receptor desensitization at the maternal-fetal interface [26]. However, both in vivo and in vitro studies confirm that long-term treatment of the endometrium/endometrial epithelial cells with hCG downregulates the LHCG receptor [27−29]. Treatment of endometrial explants (tissue segments ~1 mm in diameter) with urinary hCG similarly mediated expression of receptivity factors including HOXA10, VEGF, glycodelin, and decay accelerating factor [30,31]. These explant studies are interesting as both endometrial epithelial and stromal cells are present and the investigators determined that the tissue fragments were viable throughout the term of the experiment. hCG also impacts the function of endometrial stromal cells. As indicated above, endometrial stromal cells undergo hormone-mediated decidualization in each menstrual cycle; hCG both promotes and inhibits decidualization and the discrepancies between studies may be due to the different sources of hCG utilized. Urinary hCG appears to promote decidualization of endometrial stromal cells [32] while recombinant hCG inhibits decidualization [33−36]. Indeed, the impact of both urinary hCG and recombinant hCG on endometrial stromal cells has been directly compared [35]. In this study, recombinant hCG protected decidualized endometrial cells against oxidative damage, while in the same experimental paradigm urinary hCG induced cell death factors [35]. These data suggest that while hCG can modulate the maternal environment, its true impact in endometrial receptivity cannot be determined from the in vitro studies as neither recombinant nor urinary hCG is biosimilar with that released from the human preimplantation embryo. However, urinary hCG does contain between 2.2% and 12% hCG-H and may be considered marginally more physiologically representative of the preimplantation blastocyst hCG milieu.

Within the peri-implantation environment, local immune cells, particularly uterine natural killer cells, are important as they release factors which facilitate both trophoblast invasion [37,38] and remodeling of the uterine spiral arteries which is critical for appropriate placental development [39]. Treatment of uterine natural killer cells isolated from human first trimester decidua tissues (endometrium of pregnancy) with urinary hCG stimulated their proliferation [40], suggesting that the embryo can enhance the maternal environment for its own implantation. Interestingly, deglycosylation of hCG, abrogated this proliferation, again indicating that specific hCG glycoforms are important for this effect. This proliferation was proven to be mediated via the mannose receptor rather than the LHCG receptor, suggesting, along with the impact of deglycosylation, that hCG-H may be responsible for uterine natural killer cell proliferation. More recent studies have examined the global impact of hCG on endometrial epithelial cells, demonstrating that hCG superimposed on an estrogen and progesterone primed environment, differentially regulates both cellular expression and secretion of proteins [41]. Recombinant hCG-mediated upregulation of 67 and downregulation of 126 cellular proteins compared with estrogen/progesterone treatment alone, regulating cellular functions including metabolism, basement membrane and cell connectivity, and proliferation/differentiation.

Furthermore hCG's influence on secreted proteins was to upregulate 35 and down-regulate eight proteins that mediate cellular functions including cell adhesion, regulation of development, cytoskeletal/ECM remodeling, and immune response [41]. This important study provides a more global view of how hCG may modulate endometrial receptivity, implicating critical cellular functions during receptivity and implantation, such as cell adhesion and remodeling, as regulated by this embryonic factor. However, as recombinant hCG is not fully representative of the natural embryonic environment, this study should be followed up with use of a biosimilar formulation of hCG.

Clinical studies

The above studies generally examined short-term treatment of endometrial cells with hCG before determination of its downstream targets. Indeed, this is logical when we consider that the endometrium would be exposed to hCG for only a short period around the time of peri-implantation, when the blastocyst has hatched in close proximity to the endometrial epithelium. Since the hatched blastocyst completes implantation within 24—48 hours in a natural conception cycle, the endometrium would be exposed to hCG for a maximum of 2 days before implantation was initiated. This situation is complicated in IVF cycles when embryo transfer is in the same cycle as oocyte retrieval. In IVF cycles, systemically administered hCG is commonly used for final oocyte maturation, resulting in exposure of the body, and the endometrium, to hCG around 5—7 days prior to embryo transfer into the uterine cavity (Fig. 3.2.3). However, when frozen embryos are transferred during natural cycle, the body is not exposed to precocious hCG. A number of clinical studies have used the in vitro and in vivo data described above, as a rationale for exposing the endometrium to hCG via intrauterine infusion prior to embryo transfer, in an attempt to improve endometrial receptivity, and thereby implantation/pregnancy rates, with mixed results.

A recent Cochrane review of 12 randomized controlled trials [42] found insufficient evidence to support the use of such intrauterine hCG to support embryo implantation. Indeed, 75% of the studies were at a high risk of bias with unclear descriptions of study methods and lack of blinding. These conclusions were further supported by a meta-analysis of eight randomized controlled trials [43] in which no beneficial effect of intrauterine hCG could be demonstrated for live birth rates or spontaneous abortion rates. Indeed, two studies investigating intrauterine hCG administration between 5 and 17 days prior to embryo transfer or intrauterine insemination were discontinued early due to a detrimental effect on implantation and pregnancy rates [44,45]. Further investigations examined the impact of administering intrauterine hCG immediately prior (4—10 minutes) to embryo transfer [46—50]. All used urinary hCG in doses between 100 and 1000 IU, and only two of the five studies [47,48] found a beneficial effect of intrauterine hCG on implantation and pregnancy rate at a dose of 500IU. The remaining three studies either found no effect [46] or a negative effect [49,50] on implantation and pregnancy rates. Many of these

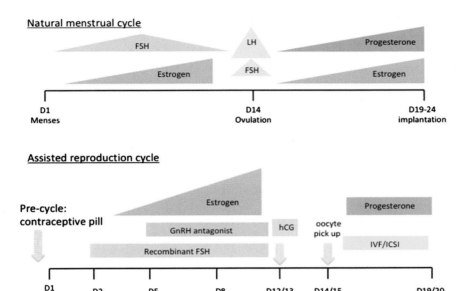

FIGURE 3.2.3

In a natural menstrual cycle, the body is exposed to gradually increasing concentrations of follicle-stimulating hormone (FSH) during the proliferative phase of the cycle followed by declining levels as increasing estrogen released by the dominant ovarian follicle repress GnRH-mediated FSH production by the anterior pituitary. The large increase in estrogen by the rapidly growing dominant ovarian follicle mediates positive feedback on hypothalamic GnRH resulting in a surge of luteinizing hormone (LH) and FSH which results in ovulation. Increasing levels of both estrogen and progesterone production by the corpus luteum during the secretory phase of the cycle act in a negative feedback loop to inhibit GnRH-mediated gonadotropin release. During the window of optimal receptivity (days 19–24), the endometrium may be exposed to hCG for a short period of time in a conception cycle. In an assisted reproduction cycle, the GnRH-mediated control of reproduction is downregulated to allow control of ovarian follicle development by administration of exogenous hormones, the aim being to develop multiple ovarian follicle for ovulation rather than a single follicle as in most natural cycles. The natural hormonal control is often overridden by use of the combined oral contraceptive pill (combination of estrogen/progesterone) followed by administration of set doses of FSH, to stimulate ovarian follicle development, rather than the gradually increasing levels observed in natural cycles. Development of multiple follicles can lead to supraphysiological levels of estrogen. Ovulation, as induced by these high levels of estrogen, is suppressed by use of a GnRH antagonist (or an agonist, not illustrated here). Final oocyte maturation/ovulation is then triggered by injection of a bolus of hCG resulting in precocious exposure to hCG outside the normal implantation window. Oocyte pick up is performed around 36 hours later followed by exogenous administration of progesterone to support the secretory phase of the cycle. In a fresh cycle, the embryo is placed into the uterine cavity around 7 days after hCG induced ovulation.

peri-transfer hCG studies were prospective clinical trials and contained relatively small patient numbers. However, Volovsky et al. [49] performed a retrospective analysis of 9720 embryo transfers with intrauterine hCG infusion used in 458 subjects based on clinical advice, patient wishes, and the proposed benefits of intrauterine hCG infusion at the time of treatment (2011−15). In this large population study, peri-transfer intrauterine hCG had no beneficial effect on pregnancy rates in frozen embryo transfers or women with recurrent implantation failure (RIF) but exerted a negative effect on pregnancy rates in women without RIF and in fresh embryo transfer cycles. This observation of a negative effect in women undergoing fresh embryo transfer cycles is in line with previous in vitro and baboon in vivo studies which suggest that prolonged exposure to hCG downregulates the LHCG receptor thus abrogating/reducing hCG-mediated cellular signaling [18,27,28]. Women undergoing fresh embryo transfer are exposed to hCG for final oocyte maturation around 5 days before embryo transfer, therefore further exogenous hCG exposure may additionally compromise the response to blastocyst hCG. Additional investigations have examined the impact of intrauterine hCG infusion 2−3 days prior to embryo transfer/endometrial biopsy, again with mixed results. Infusion of hCG into the uterine cavity of fertile oocyte donors 2 days before endometrial biopsy appeared to benefit some measures of endometrial receptivity (stromal cell differentiation, progesterone receptor, and complement C3 expression), but no benefit on overall receptivity, as assessed by the endometrial receptivity gene array (ERA), was observed [51]. This study was in fertile women, rather than the infertile population usually examined in ART studies: these women may be relatively "protected" against the detrimental impact of exogenous hormonal stimulation. Indeed, we previously demonstrated that the endometrial histology of oocyte donors is less disturbed than that of infertile women following hormonal stimulation for ART cycles [52].

Overall, it appears that there is little benefit in performing intrauterine hCG administration during IVF cycles and in some cases, during IVF cycles with fresh embryo transfers, and in women without RIF, exogenous hCG administration exerts a negative effect on pregnancy outcomes. However, despite these mixed results, hCG may be beneficial in some groups of women. As demonstrated by Tesarik et al. [53], oocyte recipients with low endogenous gonadotropin levels appeared to benefit from midcycle hCG, resulting in improved pregnancy rates. Therefore, the subjects to whom hCG is administered must be carefully chosen if this intervention is to be used.

Conclusions and future directions

That hCG plays an important role in fetal-maternal communication is clear from in vivo human and nonhuman primate investigations and in vitro studies utilizing human endometrial cells. As one of the early embryonic products, hCG maximizes endometrial receptivity and therefore, a "good" embryo producing appropriate amounts of hCG can likely facilitate its own implantation. Acute stimulation of the endometrium with hCG, mimicking the timing of blastocyst implantation (over 24−48 hours) may be beneficial to pregnancy success. However, clinical studies, supported by nonhuman primate and in vitro data, appear to reinforce the idea that chronic or precocious exposure to hCG, as experienced in an IVF cycle when a bolus of hCG is used for final oocyte maturation, may be detrimental for endometrial responses to the subsequent acute hCG released by the blastocyst at implantation. It is clear that intrauterine hCG should not be used as an adjunct in IVF cycles except in specifically selected populations, e.g., oocyte recipients with low endogenous gonadotropins. A major issue in all work to date examining hCG in endometrial receptivity, centers on the composition or source of hCG used for such studies. In vivo, in vitro, and clinical studies have used either urinary hCG from a variety of sources which contain not only a number of hCG forms but also growth factor contaminants, or recombinant hCG which represents a "pure" source but only one form of hCG. Understanding of hCG forms representative of those released by the hatched blastocyst at peri-implantation is urgently needed if we are to understand the true impact of hCG in endometrial receptivity and embryo implantation. Thus studies using a hCG preparation comprising 50% "regular" hCG, 40% hCG-H, and 10% hCG-β would provide more physiological evidence of its role.

References

[1] Wilcox AJ, Baird DD, Weinberg CR. Time of implantation of the conceptus and loss of pregnancy. N Engl J Med 1999;340(23):1796−9.
[2] Cole LA. hCG, five independent molecules. Clin Chim Acta 2012;413(1−2):48−65.
[3] Butler SA, Luttoo J, Freire MO, Abban TK, Borrelli PT, Iles RK. Human chorionic gonadotropin (hCG) in the secretome of cultured embryos: hyperglycosylated hCG and hCG-free beta subunit are potential markers for infertility management and treatment. Reprod Sci 2013;20(9):1038−45.
[4] Woodward BJ, Lenton EA, Turner K. Human chorionic gonadotrophin: embryonic secretion is a time-dependent phenomenon. Hum Reprod 1993;8(9):1463−8.
[5] Lopata A, Oliva K, Stanton PG, Robertson DM. Analysis of chorionic gonadotrophin secreted by cultured human blastocysts. Mol Hum Reprod 1997;3(6):517−21.
[6] Kovalevskaya G, Birken S, Kakuma T, Ozaki N, Sauer M, Lindheim S, et al. Differential expression of human chorionic gonadotropin (hCG) glycosylation isoforms in failing and continuing pregnancies: preliminary characterization of the hyperglycosylated hCG epitope. J Endocrinol 2002;172(3):497−506.
[7] O'Connor JF, Ellish N, Kakuma T, Schlatterer J, Kovalevskaya G. Differential urinary gonadotrophin profiles in early pregnancy and early pregnancy loss. Prenat Diagn 1998; 18(12):1232−40.
[8] Puget C, Joueidi Y, Bauville E, Laviolle B, Bendavid C, Lavoue V, et al. Serial hCG and progesterone levels to predict early pregnancy outcomes in pregnancies of uncertain viability: a prospective study. Eur J Obstet Gynecol Reprod Biol 2018;220:100−5.
[9] Butler SA, Cole LA. Evidence for, and associated risks with, the human chorionic gonadotropin supplemented diet. J Diet Suppl 2016;13(6):694−9.

[10] Koistinen H, Hautala L, Koli K, Stenman UH. Absence of TGF-beta receptor activation by highly purified hCG preparations. Mol Endocrinol 2015;29(12):1787—91.

[11] Malatos S, Neubert H, Kicman AT, Iles RK. Identification of placental transforming growth factor-beta and bikunin metabolites as contaminants of pharmaceutical human chorionic gonadotrophin preparations by proteomic techniques. Mol Cell Proteom 2005;4(7):984—92.

[12] Yarram SJ, Jenkins J, Cole LA, Brown NL, Sandy JR, Mansell JP. Epidermal growth factor contamination and concentrations of intact human chorionic gonadotropin in commercial preparations. Fertil Steril 2004;82(1):232—3.

[13] Salamonsen LA, Nie G, Hannan NJ, Dimitriadis E. Society for Reproductive Biology Founders' Lecture 2009. Preparing fertile soil: the importance of endometrial receptivity. Reprod Fertil Dev 2009;21(7):923—34.

[14] Nguyen HP, Simpson RJ, Salamonsen LA, Greening DW. Extracellular vesicles in the intrauterine environment: challenges and potential functions. Biol Reprod 2016;95(5):109.

[15] Licht P, Russu V, Lehmeyer S, Moll J, Siebzehnrubl E, Wildt L. Intrauterine microdialysis reveals cycle-dependent regulation of endometrial insulin-like growth factor binding protein-1 secretion by human chorionic gonadotropin. Fertil Steril 2002;78(2):252—8.

[16] Licht P, Fluhr H, Neuwinger J, Wallwiener D, Wildt L. Is human chorionic gonadotropin directly involved in the regulation of human implantation? Mol Cell Endocrinol 2007;269(1—2):85—92.

[17] Fazleabas AT, Donnelly KM, Srinivasan S, Fortman JD, Miller JB. Modulation of the baboon (*Papio anubis*) uterine endometrium by chorionic gonadotrophin during the period of uterine receptivity. Proc Natl Acad Sci USA 1999;96(5):2543—8.

[18] Sherwin JR, Sharkey AM, Cameo P, Mavrogianis PM, Catalano RD, Edassery S, et al. Identification of novel genes regulated by chorionic gonadotropin in baboon endometrium during the window of implantation. Endocrinology 2007;148(2):618—26.

[19] Bourdiec A, Shao R, Rao CV, Akoum A. Human chorionic gonadotropin triggers angiogenesis via the modulation of endometrial stromal cell responsiveness to interleukin 1: a new possible mechanism underlying embryo implantation. Biol Reprod 2012;87(3):66.

[20] Evans J, Catalano RD, Brown P, Sherwin R, Critchley HO, Fazleabas AT, et al. Prokineticin 1 mediates fetal-maternal dialogue regulating endometrial leukemia inhibitory factor. FASEB J 2009;23(7):2165—75.

[21] Paiva P, Hannan NJ, Hincks C, Meehan KL, Pruysers E, Dimitriadis E, et al. Human chorionic gonadotrophin regulates FGF2 and other cytokines produced by human endometrial epithelial cells, providing a mechanism for enhancing endometrial receptivity. Hum Reprod 2011;26(5):1153—62.

[22] Perrier d'Hauterive S, Charlet-Renard C, Berndt S, Dubois M, Munaut C, Goffin F, et al. Human chorionic gonadotropin and growth factors at the embryonic-endometrial interface control leukemia inhibitory factor (LIF) and interleukin 6 (IL-6) secretion by human endometrial epithelium. Hum Reprod 2004;19(11):2633—43.

[23] Zhou XL, Lei ZM, Rao CV. Treatment of human endometrial gland epithelial cells with chorionic gonadotropin/luteinizing hormone increases the expression of the cyclooxygenase-2 gene. J Clin Endocrinol Metab 1999;84(9):3364—77.

[24] Banerjee P, Sapru K, Strakova Z, Fazleabas AT. Chorionic gonadotropin regulates prostaglandin E synthase via a phosphatidylinositol 3-kinase-extracellular regulatory kinase pathway in a human endometrial epithelial cell line: implications for endometrial responses for embryo implantation. Endocrinology 2009;150(9):4326—37.

[25] Srisuparp S, Strakova Z, Brudney A, Mukherjee S, Reierstad S, Hunzicker-Dunn M, et al. Signal transduction pathways activated by chorionic gonadotropin in the primate endometrial epithelial cells. Biol Reprod 2003;68(2):457—64.

[26] Filicori M, Fazleabas AT, Huhtaniemi I, Licht P, Rao CV, Tesarik J, et al. Novel concepts of human chorionic gonadotropin: reproductive system interactions and potential in the management of infertility. Fertil Steril 2005;84(2):275—84.

[27] Cameo P, Szmidt M, Strakova Z, Mavrogianis P, Sharpe-Timms KL, Fazleabas AT. Decidualization regulates the expression of the endometrial chorionic gonadotropin receptor in the primate. Biol Reprod 2006;75(5):681—9.

[28] Evans J, Salamonsen LA. Too much of a good thing? Experimental evidence suggests prolonged exposure to hCG is detrimental to endometrial receptivity. Hum Reprod 2013;28(6):1610—9.

[29] Sherwin JR, Hastings JM, Jackson KS, Mavrogianis PA, Sharkey AM, Fazleabas AT. The endometrial response to chorionic gonadotropin is blunted in a baboon model of endometriosis. Endocrinology 2010;151(10):4982—93.

[30] Fogle RH, Li A, Paulson RJ. Modulation of HOXA10 and other markers of endometrial receptivity by age and human chorionic gonadotropin in an endometrial explant model. Fertil Steril 2010;93(4):1255—9.

[31] Palomino WA, Argandona F, Azua R, Kohen P, Devoto L. Complement C3 and decay-accelerating factor expression levels are modulated by human chorionic gonadotropin in endometrial compartments during the implantation window. Reprod Sci 2013; 20(9):1103—10.

[32] Han SW, Lei ZM, Rao CV. Treatment of human endometrial stromal cells with chorionic gonadotropin promotes their morphological and functional differentiation into decidua. Mol Cell Endocrinol 1999;147(1—2):7—16.

[33] Fluhr H, Carli S, Deperschmidt M, Wallwiener D, Zygmunt M, Licht P. Differential effects of human chorionic gonadotropin and decidualization on insulin-like growth factors-I and -II in human endometrial stromal cells. Fertil Steril 2008;90(4 Suppl. l): 1384—9.

[34] Fluhr H, Krenzer S, Deperschmidt M, Zwirner M, Wallwiener D, Licht P. Human chorionic gonadotropin inhibits insulin-like growth factor-binding protein-1 and prolactin in decidualized human endometrial stromal cells. Fertil Steril 2006;86(1):236—8.

[35] Kajihara T, Tochigi H, Uchino S, Itakura A, Brosens JJ, Ishihara O. Differential effects of urinary and recombinant chorionic gonadotropin on oxidative stress responses in decidualizing human endometrial stromal cells. Placenta 2011;32(8):592—7.

[36] Salker M, Teklenburg G, Molokhia M, Lavery S, Trew G, Aojanepong T, et al. Natural selection of human embryos: impaired decidualization of endometrium disables embryo-maternal interactions and causes recurrent pregnancy loss. PLoS One 2010; 5(4):e10287.

[37] Hanna J, Goldman-Wohl D, Hamani Y, Avraham I, Greenfield C, Natanson-Yaron S, et al. Decidual NK cells regulate key developmental processes at the human fetal-maternal interface. Nat Med 2006;12(9):1065—74.

[38] Lash GE, Otun HA, Innes BA, Percival K, Searle RF, Robson SC, et al. Regulation of extravillous trophoblast invasion by uterine natural killer cells is dependent on gestational age. Hum Reprod 2010;25(5):1137—45.

[39] Robson A, Harris LK, Innes BA, Lash GE, Aljunaidy MM, Aplin JD, et al. Uterine natural killer cells initiate spiral artery remodeling in human pregnancy. FASEB J 2012; 26(12):4876—85.

[40] Kane N, Kelly R, Saunders PT, Critchley HO. Proliferation of uterine natural killer cells is induced by human chorionic gonadotropin and mediated via the mannose receptor. Endocrinology 2009;150(6):2882−8.

[41] Greening DW, Nguyen HP, Evans J, Simpson RJ, Salamonsen LA. Modulating the endometrial epithelial proteome and secretome in preparation for pregnancy: the role of ovarian steroid and pregnancy hormones. J Proteomics 2016;144:99−112.

[42] Craciunas L, Tsampras N, Coomarasamy A, Raine-Fenning N. Intrauterine administration of human chorionic gonadotropin (hCG) for subfertile women undergoing assisted reproduction. Cochrane Database Syst Rev 2016;5:CD011537.

[43] Osman A, Pundir J, Elsherbini M, Dave S, El-Toukhy T, Khalaf Y. The effect of intrauterine HCG injection on IVF outcome: a systematic review and meta-analysis. Reprod Biomed Online 2016;33(3):350−9.

[44] Fatemi HM, Kyrou D, Bourgain C, Van den Abbeel E, Griesinger G, Devroey P. Cryopreserved-thawed human embryo transfer: spontaneous natural cycle is superior to human chorionic gonadotropin-induced natural cycle. Fertil Steril 2010;94(6): 2054−8.

[45] Prapas N, Tavaniotou A, Panagiotidis Y, Prapa S, Kasapi E, Goudakou M, et al. Low-dose human chorionic gonadotropin during the proliferative phase may adversely affect endometrial receptivity in oocyte recipients. Gynecol Endocrinol 2009;25(1):53−9.

[46] Hong KH, Forman EJ, Werner MD, Upham KM, Gumeny CL, Winslow AD, et al. Endometrial infusion of human chorionic gonadotropin at the time of blastocyst embryo transfer does not impact clinical outcomes: a randomized, double-blind, placebo-controlled trial. Fertil Steril 2014;102(6):1591−1595 e2.

[47] Mansour R, Tawab N, Kamal O, El-Faissal Y, Serour A, Aboulghar M, et al. Intrauterine injection of human chorionic gonadotropin before embryo transfer significantly improves the implantation and pregnancy rates in in vitro fertilization/intracytoplasmic sperm injection: a prospective randomized study. Fertil Steril 2011;96(6):1370−1374 e1.

[48] Santibanez A, Garcia J, Pashkova O, Colin O, Castellanos G, Sanchez AP, et al. Effect of intrauterine injection of human chorionic gonadotropin before embryo transfer on clinical pregnancy rates from in vitro fertilisation cycles: a prospective study. Reprod Biol Endocrinol 2014;12:9.

[49] Volovsky M, Healey M, MacLachlan V, Vollenhoven BJ. Should intrauterine human chorionic gonadotropin infusions ever be used prior to embryo transfer? J Assist Reprod Genet 2018;35(2):273−8.

[50] Wirleitner B, Schuff M, Vanderzwalmen P, Stecher A, Okhowat J, Hradecky L, et al. Intrauterine administration of human chorionic gonadotropin does not improve pregnancy and life birth rates independently of blastocyst quality: a randomised prospective study. Reprod Biol Endocrinol 2015;13:70.

[51] Strug MR, Su R, Young JE, Dodds WG, Shavell VI, Diaz-Gimeno P, et al. Intrauterine human chorionic gonadotropin infusion in oocyte donors promotes endometrial synchrony and induction of early decidual markers for stromal survival: a randomized clinical trial. Hum Reprod 2016;31(7):1552−61.

[52] Evans J, Hannan NJ, Hincks C, Rombauts LJ, Salamonsen LA. Defective soil for a fertile seed? Altered endometrial development is detrimental to pregnancy success. PLoS One 2012;7(12):e53098.

[53] Tesarik J, Hazout A, Mendoza C. Luteinizing hormone affects uterine receptivity independently of ovarian function. Reprod Biomed Online 2003;7(1):59−64.

Qualitative analysis of hCG variants and glycoforms in urine, using matrix-assisted laser desorption ionization time-of-flight mass spectrometry: a potential companion diagnostic tool to immunoassays in pregnancy and cancer

3.3

Raminta Zmuidinaite, Jameel Luttoo, Ray K. Iles, Fady I. Sharara, Thommas Kwenko Abban, Laurence A. Cole, Stephen A. Butler

Introduction

Human chorionic gonadotropin (hCG) is a very heterogeneous molecule which has been employed as a diagnostic marker in pregnancy for almost a century and to a lesser extent as a biomarker in cancer where it has found particular use in the diagnosis and monitoring of gestational trophoblastic disease (GTD) and testicular cancer. Generally, hCG is an α/β heterodimeric glycoprotein hormone with eight glycosylation sites containing four N-linked oligosaccharides and four O-linked oligosaccharides. The mass of hCG is often reported as around 36 kDa, in reality the mass range of the intact holo-hormone ranges between 34 and 40 kDa. As such, the term hCG is a collective term encompassing a range of heterogeneous molecules with both subtle and more extensive peptide and oligosaccharide variation. Variants of hCG recognized by the IFCC include hCG (the hormone sometimes referred to as intact hCG), hCGβ (the free hCGβ subunit of hCG), hCGα (the free α subunit of hCG, which is common to all glycoprotein hormones), hCGn (nicked hCG, any hCG which is cleaved in loop 2—the Keutman loop—of hCG), and hCGβcf (the urinary breakdown product of hCG, the hCG β-core fragment or β core; also known as UGP or UGF—urinary gonadotropic peptide and fragment, respectively. Other variants which are not formally recognized (because no international standard has ever been produced) include hCGh or hCGH (a hyperglycosylated form of hCG defined by the ability of one antibody, B152, to recognize a portion of the β-subunit hyperglycosylated at the carboxyl end of the molecule), hCGs, sulfated hCG or pituitary hCG (a form of hCG produced by the pituitary most noticeably after menopause). hCGf or familial hCG (a short form of hCG produced in low concentration by men and women in some families), hCGt, truncated hCG (a smaller variant of hCG identified in patients suffering from hyperemesis gravidarum), hCGq or quiescent hCG (a low level hCG produced in patients following treatment of, or prior to, treatment for GTDs or choriocarcinoma and more recently the term extravillous cytotrophoblast hCG has also been coined for the hCG produced at the leading edge of implantation and invasion in cancer (see Chapter 3.6). Finally and certainly the most common term, is β-hCG, which is a misleading term often used to mean a hCG assay which may or may not be used to describe any of the above variants. This confusion stems from the very first specific hCG assays that were used to distinguish hCG from LH. Where the first assays cross-reacted with LH (because of common epitopes in both α and β subunits) the new "β hCG" assays were specific, the name is now synonymous with hCG assays. The term total hCG is sometimes used to describe the detection of *any* form of hCG which contains a hCGβ subunit and includes assays which recognize one or two epitopes common to *all* variants of hCG, effectively an "all hCG" assay [1].

Despite significant efforts by both the IFCC and ISOBM working groups to standardize hCG measurement, there is still some debate as to the most appropriate hCG assay to use in some situations. The IFCC working group assigned nomenclature and quantified the standards using molar concentration [2], but IU/L and mIU/mL persist in the literature. To date the structure of hCG (intact hCG) has been characterized by HPLC-mass spectrometry and by crystallographic analysis. Using trypsin digestion, peptide mass mapping of hCG and its subunits has also been carried out using matrix-assisted laser desorption/ionization time-of-flight mass spectrometry (MALDI-ToF MS) [3—6].

Carbohydrate heterogeneity within hCG has been reported previously with variable mono-, bi-, and triantennary carbohydrate structures being found in normal and abnormal pregnancies [7]. In earlier studies, we described the purification of hCGβcf from pregnancy urine which was reduced by dithiothreitol (DTT) reduction and analyzed by MALDI-ToF MS. It was concluded that the mass spectrum of DTT-reduced hCGβcf, while not precisely defining hCGβcf glycosylation, would appear to result in distinctive fingerprint [8]. Recently, we demonstrated that variability in hCGβcf could be seen using a direct MALDI-ToF MS approach [9] and is also very useful as an internal calibrant (Chapter 2.6). It should be stated that it is now possible to detect picomolar concentrations using this method, and the identification of hCG variants produced by embryos in culture have been described this way [10]. Additionally, by analyzing certain m/z regions including those adjacent to hCG on MALDI spectra it is possible to accurately diagnose Down syndrome from the urine of pregnant women [11] and predict embryos with best chance of implantation from noninvasive analysis of the culture fluid [11a].

There are practical limitations in MALDI-ToF MS as a quantitative technique; however, the ability to quantify has been demonstrated in several studies [12−14]. Nevertheless, it comes with limitations, where the raw mass spectra produced cannot be used directly to produce comparative data for diagnostic tests. However, hCG is an abundant molecule in the urine of patients who are pregnant or have cancer and are comparative within sample analysis by MALDI, this presents an opportunity to identify both qualitative and quantitative changes in hCG, which may be indicative of clinical disorders (see Chapter 2.2).

It is therefore possible to demonstrate the applicability of MALDI-ToF MS as a companion diagnostic tool to identify qualitative changes in hCG molecule and its variants, being equally sensitive to all hCG forms and without tedious sample pretreatment.

hCG and hCGβ standards and samples

The hCG and hCGβ standards and samples are indicated in Table 3.3.1. Briefly, hCG from Sigma (C0684 and C6322) and Abcam (ab51782) were purchased for this study. hCG C0684 was produced from pregnancy urine with a potency of 14 000 IU/mg; hCG C6322 was recombinant hCG expressed from mouse cell line

Table 3.3.1 Indicating the name of the hCG and hCGβ standards used including supplier and source.

Name	Molecule	Supplier	Source
C0684	hCG	Sigma Aldrich	Pregnancy urine
C6322	hCG	Sigma Aldrich	Recombinant hCG expressed from mouse cell line
ab51782	hCG	Abcam	Postmenopausal women sterile urine
CR127	hCG	Prof. Laurence Cole	Purified from propriety crude extracts of pooled normal pregnancy urine
C0419	hCGβ	Sigma Aldrich	Pregnancy urine
ab61032	hCGβ	Abcam	Pregnancy urine
325−11	hCGβ	Lee BioSolution	Pregnancy urine

(lyophilized, 10,000 IU/mg vial); and hCG ab51782 was produced from a sterile preparation of urine of postmenopausal women with a biological activity of 5000 IU/mg. Additionally, CR127 is a standard preparation of hCG purified from propriety crude extracts of pooled normal pregnancy urine and was a gift from Professor Laurence A. Cole. Standards of hCGβ from Sigma Aldrich (C0419), Abcam (ab61032), and Lee BioSolution (325-11) were also purchased for this study, and these were all produced from pregnancy urine. Lyophilized samples were reconstituted using HPLC grade water at a concentration of 0.1 μg/μL, and a summary of the standards can be seen in Table 3.3.1. Unprocessed urine samples (n = 109) were derived from the normal pregnancy from women attending a fertility clinic, gestational age 6 to 10 weeks, provided by Dr Sharara.

MALDI-ToF mass spectrometry

Reconstituted standards and thawed urine samples were subjected to MALDI-ToF mass spectrometry. Using the precoat method and sinapinic acid as MALDI matrix (20 mg/mL in acetonitrile/0.1% trifluoroacetic acid, 2:1 (v/v)), 0.5 μL of each standard or sample was applied directly onto the MALDI target plate, and allowed to air dry. Sinapinic acid was the matrix of choice due to the intense spectra it produces for ions in the protein mass range (i.e., above 10 kDa). Mass spectrometric analysis was carried out on a MALDI-ToF mass spectrometer (Shimadzu, Axima CFR plus), using a pulsed nitrogen laser (λmax = 337 nm) which was used to desorb ions from each sample in regular pulses. The ions were accelerated by a 20-kV electrical field up a 1.2 m linear tube and detected by a microchannel plate detector at a sampling rate of 500 MHz. Spectra were generated by summing 300 laser shots in positive ion linear mode. A laser power of 90 arbitrary units (a.u.) was used and the peaks were processed by smoothing at 500 channels. A threshold of 25% centroid was used to determine the peak mass in each spectrum. During standardization, the laser firing and data acquisition was automated (using the raster and auto experiment software tools) in order to keep consistency and in keeping with a standardized approach not influenced by user bias. A six-point mass calibration was performed externally (nearest well for each sample) using single and doubly charged ions of the following standards: horse heart cytochrome C ([M+H]+ = 12 361 Da and [M+2H] 2+ = 6181 Da); trypsinogen ([M+H]+ = 23 981 Da and [M+2H]2+ = 11 991 Da; and aldolase ([M+H]+ = 39 211 Da and [M+2H]2+ = 19 606 Da). Each was at a concentration of 10 pmol/μL, all purchased from Sigma Aldrich.

In silico data processing

The spectra generated from the analysis of the urine obtained from early pregnancy was subjected to additional in silico processing using mMass software [15] and comparative summary analysis performed in R [16].

Qualitative hCG analysis by direct MALDI-ToF mass spectrometry

The mass spectra of hCGβ from Abcam, BioSolution, and Sigma gave rise to similar profiles with mean m/z of centroid peaks at 23,715, 23,527, and 23,433, respectively, following analysis of 33 replicates for each (Table 3.3.2). Further analysis of difference indicated that while there was no significant difference between hCGβ from Abcam and BioSolution (P-value = .101), there was indeed a difference between hCGβ Sigma and hCGβ BioSolution (P-value $<$.0001). No other isoform of hCG was seen in these samples except the respective masses of 46,780, 46,843, and 46,906 Da which were likely to be the dimers of corresponding hCGββ as published previously [17]. Typical spectra of recombinant hCGβ have also been published previously [10].

Unlike hCGβ, the mass spectra of intact hCG clearly indicated differences between the inferred masses of the samples. The mean m/z for centroid peaks of hCG from Abcam, Sigma C0684, Sigma C0890, and CR127 were 36,279, 37,145, 37,164, and 36,685, respectively (Table 3.3.2).

The differences between the masses from the four sources indicate clear separation of the mass data of hCG Abcam from either Sigma C0684 or Sigma C0809 (P value $<$ .0001 each in two sample t test) and from CR127 (P- value $<$ 0.0001) when compared with 2-sample t test. Similarly, CR127 showed significant mass separation

Table 3.3.2 The masses and descriptive statistical data of intact hCG and hCGβ analyzed from different standard preparations which are commercially available. Also shown are data for hCG and hCGβ, as well as hCGβcf from pregnancy urine analyzed as neat unprocessed urine by MALDI.

Preparation and molecule	Number of samples	Mean (m/z) +1	SD	CV (%)
hCGβ				
Sigma	33	23,433	203	0.8
Lee Biosolution	33	23,527	254	1.0
Abcam	33	23,715	176	0.7
Neat Pregnancy Urine	109	23,764	467	2
Intact hCG				
CR127	50	36,685	237	0.6
Abcam	50	36,279	132	0.3
Sigma (C0684)	50	37,145	129	0.3
Sigma (C6322)	50	37,164	146	0.2
Neat Pregnancy Urine	109	36,520	822	2.2
hCGβcf				
Neat Pregnancy Urine	109	9751	20	0.2

from both Sigma samples (p- value of <0.0001). In contrast, there was no difference between the two Sigma products hCG C0684 and hCG C6322 (*P*-value = .186) despite one being sourced from urine and the other a recombinant protein; they were both significantly larger than CR127. It has been shown that the levels of pituitary hCG appears to be higher in postmenopausal than in premenopausal women and are clearly present in preparations of human urinary menopausal gonadotropins [18−20]. The pituitary hCG molecular form has an altered carbohydrate structure, which often results in a faster disappearance from the bloodstream [21]. This postmenopausal sample had a significantly lower mass due to variable sugar moieties of hCG produced by the pituitary. No other peaks relating to hCG were observed in these spectra. Typical spectra of recombinant hCG, recombinant hCGβ, and hCGh are easily resolvable and have been published previously [10] (Chapter on MALDI from hCG second edition).

Unprocessed urine samples

109 urine samples from normal gestations gave rise to visibly different spectra indicating both hCG and hCGβ peaks. Mass spectral profiles of 12 unprocessed urine samples were selected for illustrative purposes to show the possible variations in hCG masses and in some cases molecular variants in common hCG mass spectra (Fig. 3.3.1). All spectra were aligned on a common m/z axis to illustrate molecular mass shifts commonly seen in urine samples from pregnant women. Molecules hCG and hCGβ are shown together with peak "shoulders" that tail off toward higher masses and represent the extent of variability in glycosylation moieties present on the peptides. It is tempting to refer to these shoulders as separate molecules and consider that the species to the right of hCGβ or hCG may be due to hyperglycosylated variants of hCGβ (hCGβh) or hCG (hCGh) such as those which have been suggested as occurring in pregnancy and cancer. In the case of hCGh (or a large form hCG as identified here), it has been possible to achieve baseline separation between hCG and what appears to be hCGh. While these peaks are still broad and clearly contain mass variation due to their own heterogeneity in glycosylation, the baseline separation between the two species suggests independent molecules. In the case of hCGβ, the larger secondary "shoulder" forms may only be part of the gross heterogeneity in glycosylation rather than an entirely separate molecular species, although this cannot be completely discounted.

This mass variability can be seen across all urine samples analyzed (n = 109) and the masses of hCG variants in particular is very broad even when a secondary hCG species, which is probably what we refer to as hCGh, is regarded as a variant in its own right (Fig. 3.3.2).

The urinary hCG breakdown product, hCGβcf, is always present (Chapter 2.6) and was clearly identified in all 109 urine samples here, and the percentage variation in the masses observed indicates that there is very little mass change in hCGβcf across all pregnancies with only 117 Da difference between the smallest and largest

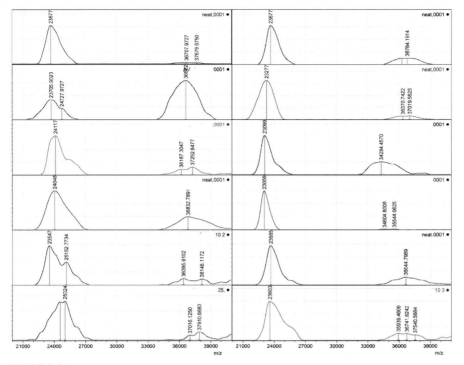

FIGURE 3.3.1

Mass spectral profiles of 12 selected urine samples, aligned based on m/z, showing hCGβ and hCG peaks, their mass shifts and variability in the profile of different hCG species.

form of the molecule (Fig. 3.3.2A). This perfectly illustrates the potential clinical utility of hCGβcf as a calibrant (as described in Chapter 2.6) when analyzing hCG directly from unprocessed urine on MALDI-ToF MS.

The mean mass size for each of the molecules was 9751 m/z for hCGβcf, 23,764 m/z for hCGβ, and 36,520 m/z for hCG, and the mass distribution for each molecular species can be seen in Fig. 3.3.2. In contrast to hCGβcf, hCG has a range of 34,480−40,561 m/z and hCGβ has a range of 22,956−26,215 m/z, the extremes of this range can be seen in Fig. 3.3.3. Finally, hCGh, identified here as an entirely different species as a baseline separated peak from hCG, ranges from a mass of 40,210−41,080 m/z (mean = 40,588 m/z). These values have been compared with the standard samples in Table 3.3.2, where urinary hCGβ, is similar in mass to the standard preparations, but urinary hCG while similar to CR127 and Abcam preparations is lower in mass than either of the Sigma preparations.

In addition to these common mass species, it is also possible to occasionally see single mass outliers with extreme masses. These outliers, which are as yet unexplained, are probably due to extreme variation in glycovariation which are otherwise

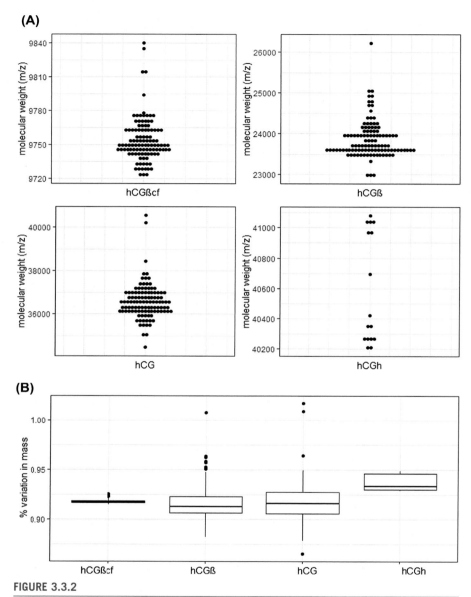

FIGURE 3.3.2

(A) Dot plots of hCGβcf, hCGβ, hCG, and hCGh, where molecular weight variation for each sample in a data set is observed across 109 samples for the gestational weeks of pregnancy studied here (gestational weeks 6–10). (B) The comparison of variability of the spread of these masses. Each sample is normalized to the sum of all masses of each molecule, rendering data comparable. In the case of hCGβcf, hCGβ, and hCG, molecular species were observed in all urine samples. In the case of hCGh, it was only observed in 16 of the 109 samples studied.

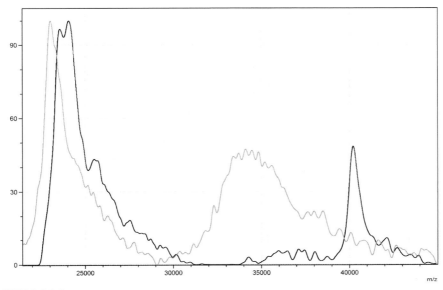

FIGURE 3.3.3

The sample with the largest hCGβ and hCG forms (black) compared with that of the smallest forms of hCGβ and hCG (gray) seen in the cohort tested.

rarely observed. In general, the variation in the smaller molecules is less than those of the larger molecules which may be more than just a feature of percentage variation. While there are only the remnants of two sugar residues from complex biantennary sugar units on hCGβcf, hCG, and to a greater extent hCGh, both have eight complex branched oligosaccharide moieties, thus enabling higher variation in molecular mass and the overall mass range for these two molecules.

It is tempting to hypothesize that a urine sample containing large forms of hCG or hCGh during pregnancy will also include large forms of hCGβ or hCGβcf, indeed this is suggested by Fig. 3.3.3 and has been postulated before, in particular the relationship between hCG and hCGβcf [9]. However, this is not exactly what was observed across the urine samples studied here. In fact, there was a degree of correlation between the masses of hCG and hCGβ ($R = 0.79$) but no correlation at all between the masses of hCG and hCGβcf ($R = 0.58$) or the masses of hCGβ and hCGβcf ($R = 0.42$) as seen in Fig. 3.3.4. There were insufficient data points for hCGh (n = 16) to make any correlations with confidence.

It has also been suggested that certain, larger, molecular forms of hCG exist earlier in pregnancy, but we found no evidence of this in this study, and while there is a significant variation in masses of hCG between individuals there is no general trend from small to large forms or large to small forms in any of the hCG species throughout gestation in any of the samples studied here (Fig. 3.3.5). Greater variability seen in hCGh may be due to the smaller sample set (n = 16) and while the

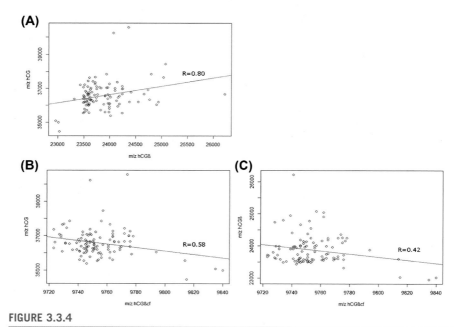

FIGURE 3.3.4

Pearson correlation plots of the three hCG molecular species in relation to one another. Each panel shows relationship between (A) hCG with hCGβ, (B) hCG with hCGβcf, and (C) hCGβ with hCGβcf. The R squared values for each plot of 0.80, 0.58, and 0.42 are indicated, respectively.

molecular mass does appear to be highly variable within each gestational week, the variability from week to week is not likely to be significant and further studies are required to examine this trend.

Summary

MALDI-TOF MS has great potential in standardizing a qualitative approach to documenting hCG molecular variation which has been challenging using immunoassays. MALDI can easily assign each hCG species to a specific mass range which would allow a qualitative reference to each standard sample preparation and thus guide selection for international standards for different applications. Furthermore, the simplicity of the MALDI technique, which now involves a rapid benchtop analyzer, makes it easy to analyze urine, directly, without the need for any pre-preparation, and quickly obtain qualitative information about hCG.

One drawback of analyzing hCG by MALDI-TOF MS is the presence of broad peaks, covering a mass range, rather than a single sharp mass peak; this is caused by the extensive glycovariation and consequent microheterogeneity in the molecule. While this problem can be overcome by performing enzymatic digests of the hCG

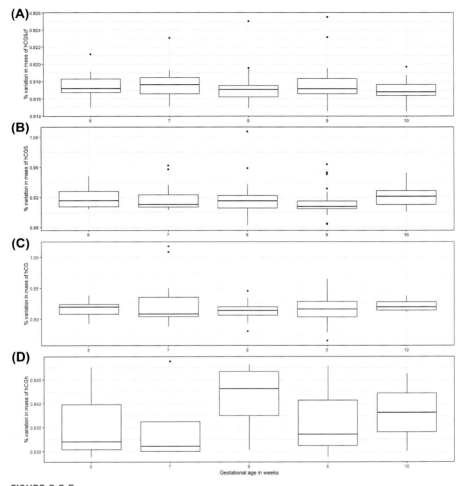

FIGURE 3.3.5

Variation in the molecular mass shown in m/z ratio across the gestational ages studied in this cohort of 109 urine samples. Molecular species shown include hCGβcf, hCGβ, hCG, and hCGh for panels A, B, C, and D, respectively. No trend in increasing or decreasing molecular mass relative to gestational age is observed in any of the molecular species studied.

prior to mass spectrometry, it would be more attractive, and more practical, to analyze hCG in urine without preprocessing. Therefore, direct analysis of urine by MALDI, in combination with quantitative data, which is now also possible by MALDI (see Chapter 2.2) as well as traditional immunoassays, could lead to a better-informed diagnosis and management of pregnancy and also in cancers where hCG is produced.

References

[1] Gronowski AM, Grenache DG. Characterization of the hCG variants recognized by different hCG immunoassays: an important step toward standardization of hCG measurements. Clin Chem 2009.

[2] Bristow A, et al. Establishment, value assignment, and characterization of new WHO reference reagents for six molecular forms of human chorionic gonadotropin. Clin Chem 2005;51(1):177−82.

[3] Birken S, et al. The heterogeneity of human chorionic gonadotropin (hCG). II. Characteristics and origins of nicks in hCG reference standards. Endocrinology 1991; 129(3):1551−8. Oxford University Press.

[4] Kardana A, et al. The heterogeneity of human chorionic gonadotropin (hCG). I. Characterization of peptide heterogeneity in 13 individual preparations of hCG. Endocrinology 1991;129(3):1541−50. Oxford University Press.

[5] Laidler P, et al. Tryptic mapping of human chorionic gonadotropin by matrix-assisted laser desorption/ionization mass spectrometry. Rapid Commun Mass Spectrom 1995; 9(11):1021−6. Wiley Online Library.

[6] Valmu L, et al. Site-specific glycan analysis of human chorionic gonadotropin β-subunit from malignancies and pregnancy by liquid chromatography—electrospray mass spectrometry. Glycobiology 2006;16(12):1207−18. Oxford University Press.

[7] Elliott MM, et al. Carbohydrate and peptide structure of the α- and β-subunits of human chorionic gonadotropin from normal and aberrant pregnancy and choriocarcinoma. Endocrine 1997;7(1):15−32. https://doi.org/10.1007/BF02778058. Humana Press.

[8] Jacoby ES, et al. Determination of the glycoforms of human chorionic gonadotropin β-core fragment by matrix-assisted laser desorption/ionization time-of-flight mass spectrometry. Clin Chem 2000;46(11):1796−803.

[9] Iles RK, Cole LA, Butler SA. Direct analysis of hCGβcf glycosylation in normal and aberrant pregnancy by matrix-assisted laser desorption/ionization time-of-flight mass spectrometry. Int J Mol Sci 2014;15(6):10067−82. https://doi.org/10.3390/ijms150610067. Multidisciplinary Digital Publishing Institute (MDPI).

[10] Butler SA, et al. Human chorionic gonadotropin (hCG) in the secretome of cultured embryos. Reprod Sci 2013;20(9):1038−45. https://doi.org/10.1177/1933719112472739. SAGE PublicationsSage CA: Los Angeles, CA.

[11] Iles RK, et al. Direct and rapid mass spectral fingerprinting of maternal urine for the detection of Down syndrome pregnancy. Clin Proteomics 2015;12(1):9. https://doi.org/10.1186/s12014-015-9082-9.

[11a] Iles RK, et al. Secretome profile selection of optimal IVF embryos by matrix-assisted laser desorption ionization time-of-flight mass spectrometry. J Assist Reprod Genet 2019 Jun;36(6):1153−60. https://doi.org/10.1007/s10815-019-01444-7. Epub 2019 May 15.

[12] Bucknall M, Fung KYC, Duncan MW. Practical quantitative biomedical applications of MALDI-TOF mass spectrometry. J Am Soc Mass Spectrom 2002;13(9):1015−27. https://doi.org/10.1016/S1044-0305(02)00426-9.

[13] Timm W, et al. Peak intensity prediction in MALDI-TOF mass spectrometry: a machine learning study to support quantitative proteomics. BMC Bioinformatics 2008; 9(1):443. https://doi.org/10.1186/1471-2105-9-443.

[14] Lange C, et al. 'Quantitative matrix-assisted laser desorption ionization−time of flight mass spectrometry for rapid resistance detection. J Clin Microbiol 2014;52(12): 4155−62.

[15] Strohalm M, et al. mMass data miner: an open source alternative for mass spectrometric data analysis. Rapid Commun Mass Spectrom 2008;22(6):905−8. https://doi.org/10.1002/rcm.3444.

[16] Team RC. A language and environment for statistical computing. Vienna, Austria2014': R Foundation for Statistical Computing; 2014. https://www.R-project.org.

[17] Butler SA, et al. The beta-subunit of human chorionic gonadotrophin exists as a homodimer. J Mol Endocrinol 1999;22:185−92.

[18] Armstrong EG, et al. Use of a highly sensitive and specific immunoradiometric assay for detection of human chorionic gonadotropin in urine of normal, nonpregnaiit, and pregnant individuals*. J Clin Endocrinol Metab 1984;59(5):867−74. https://doi.org/10.1210/jcem-59-5-867. Oxford University Press.

[19] Akar AH, et al. Human chorionic gonadotrophin-like and β-core-like materials in postmenopausal urine. J Endocrinol 1990;125(3):477−84. https://doi.org/10.1677/joe.0.1250477.

[20] Rodgers M, et al. Human chorionic gonadotrophin contributes to the bioactivity of Pergonal. Clin Endocrinol 1992;37(6):558−64. https://doi.org/10.1111/j.1365-2265.1992.tb01488.x. John Wiley & Sons, Ltd (10.1111).

[21] Braunstein GD. False-positive serum human chorionic gonadotropin results: causes, characteristics, and recognition. Am J Obstet Gynecol 2002;187(1):217−24. https://doi.org/10.1067/MOB.2002.124284. Mosby.

Phenotypic characterization of transgenic mouse models overproducing hCG

3.4

Susana B. Rulli, Matti Poutanen, Ilpo T. Huhtaniemi

Introduction

It is presently known that the human chorionic gonadotropin (hCG) is a hormone produced by a variety of human organs, existing in various forms and exerting vital biological functions, whereas it is not produced in most other mammalian species including the rodents. hCG is structurally and functionally related to luteinizing hormone (LH) of the pituitary gland, and the two hormones share a high degree of sequence homology, both being heterodimeric glycoproteins composed of a common α-subunit and a hormone-specific β-subunit. Both LH and hCG interact with the same LH/hCG receptor (LHCGR) and are essential for sexual development and reproduction. hCG acts as a potent LH agonist by inducing gonadal steroidogenesis and ovulation. However, also many other biological functions are attributed to hCG, and the physiologic roles of these two hormones are characterized by differences in expression pattern, biopotency, and regulation [1,2].

In addition to gonads, low level of LHCGR expression has been detected in numerous nongonadal tissues, such as in the brain, adipose tissue, endometrium, endothelial cells, as well as in tumor tissues. In certain organs, such as the liver, kidney, lung, and intestine, LHCGRs disappear at birth, suggesting a role in the growth and differentiation in the fetus [3–5]. However, the physiological relevance of these extragonadal LHCGRs is not completely clarified [6]. Their functional significance is undermined by findings that both mice and humans with LHCGR knockout or inactivating mutation, respectively, can maintain normal pregnancy following transplantation of wild-type (WT) ovarian tissue [7] or ovum donation [8].

There are many physiological and pathological conditions where the LH/hCG levels and/or actions are elevated. One such situation is the first trimester of pregnancy in women when hCG is produced by placental trophoblasts in very high

100 Years of Human Chorionic Gonadotropin. https://doi.org/10.1016/B978-0-12-820050-6.00016-3

amounts, being essential for the maintenance of progesterone production by corpus luteum gravidarum, for preparing the uterus for implantation and for placental development [9]. hCG also stimulates fetal testicular testosterone production, which is needed for masculinization of the male fetus [10]. Another physiological condition is the secretion of small amounts of hCG by the human pituitary gland, which increases during menopause [11]. The exposure to elevated gonadotropins after menopause or following infertility treatments is proposed to be a risk factor for ovarian tumors [12–14]. In contrast, reduced risk for ovarian cancer is associated with multiple pregnancies, breast-feeding, oral contraceptive use, and estrogen replacement therapy, all of which lead to lower levels and reduced exposure to gonadotropins. Ectopic expression of hCGβ/hCG has been demonstrated in different cancers, such as lung, colon, bladder, pancreas, breast, gonads, prostate, and stomach, usually associated with neoplastic diseases in advanced stages [15,16]. Finally, activating mutations of LHCGR represents a situation of chronic elevation of gonadotropin action, hallmarked by the dramatic early-onset male-limited precocious puberty [17,18]. It remains unclear whether such conditions have other effects than providing inappropriate gonadal stimulation.

Our understanding of the gonadotropic hormone biology has been greatly enhanced by the generation of genetically modified mouse models. These techniques provide *in vivo* models to study the role of a hormone throughout life from very early developmental stages. Gain-of-function approaches involve the overexpression of gonadotropins that may mimic the effects of hypersecretion syndromes and activating mutations in humans [17,19–21]. We, therefore, developed transgenic (TG) mice producing persistently high levels of bioactive hCG. In this way, we aimed to amplify certain actions and regulatory mechanisms that otherwise would remain unnoticed. Indeed, multiple reproductive alterations and tumorigenesis were observed in these mice. The purpose of this chapter is to summarize the main findings of these studies.

Generation of transgenic mice producing hCG

To generate TG mice with persistent production of hCG, we used the human ubiquitin C promoter that displays ubiquitous, low level, expression from midpregnancy onwards [22]. Two different TG mouse lines were generated using the same promoter: mice expressing the hCGβ subunit [23] and mice expressing the common α-subunit [24]. The TG mouse lines were generated by the conventional pronuclear microinjection technique and were maintained by breeding the TG males with WT FVB/n females [23]. Crossbreeding the mice expressing the hCGβ-subunit (hCGβ+ mice) with those expressing the common α-subunit (hCGα+ mice) was necessary to obtain double TG (hCGαβ+ mice), which expresses both subunits in a chronic and ubiquitous fashion [24] (Fig. 3.4.1).

The hCGβ+ mice produce biologically active heterodimers due to association of the TG hCGβ-subunit with the endogenous common α-subunit produced in excess by the mouse pituitary. The dimerization process is expected to occur mainly in gonadotropes and thyrotropes [25], but possibly also in some extrapituitary tissues, such as the ovary, where the α-subunit gene has been shown to be expressed [26]. Transgene expression results in a 40-fold increase in circulating hCG/LH bioactivity in hCGβ+ females and a three- to fourfold elevation of hCG/LH bioactivity in hCGβ+ males. This difference between males and females appear to be the

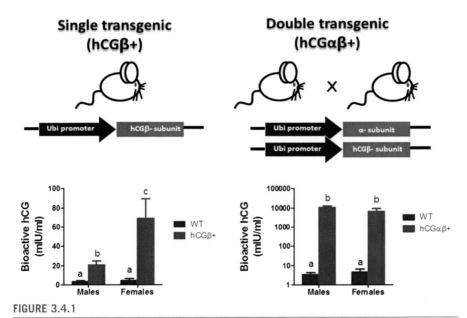

FIGURE 3.4.1

Representative figure showing the transgenic mouse models with overexpression of hCG subunits: hCGβ+ mice express the hCGβ-subunit under the Ubiquitin C promoter; the hCGαβ+ mice express both the common α- and the hCGβ-subunit under the same promoter. Bars (±SEM) represent the circulating levels of bioactive hCG in males and females (determined by testicular interstitial cell *in vitro* bioassay; [23]). Bars with different superscript letters are significantly different ($P < .05$, ANOVA).

Data adapted from Rulli SB, Kuorelahti AI, Karaer O, Pelliniemi L, Poutanen M, Huhtaniemi IT Reproductive disturbances, pituitary lactotrope adenomas, and mammary gland tumors in transgenic female mice producing high levels of human chorionic gonadotropin. Endocrinology 143: 4084–4095, 2002; Rulli SB, Ahtiainen P, Makela S, Toppari J, Poutanen M, Huhtaniemi IT Elevated steroidogenesis, defective reproductive organs and infertility in transgenic male mice overexpressing human chorionic gonadotropin. Endocrinology 144: 4980–4990, 2003.

result of the sex steroid-feedback regulation of the α-subunit in the pituitary gland [23,24].

In the double TG hCG$\alpha\beta$+ mice, hCG rises in both sexes to pharmacological levels 100-fold higher than detected in the hCGβ+ mice [24,27−29]. TG mice expressing the common α-subunit were indistinguishable from their WT littermates, confirming that free α-subunit is devoid of detectable bioactivity.

Phenotype of transgenic hCGβ+ mice
Females

The hCGβ+ females exhibit precocious puberty, constant diestrus-type pattern in their estrous cycle from 45 days onwards, and infertility in adulthood. As a consequence of the increased hCG synthesis, the steroid profile of hCGβ+ females is altered. A transient increase in estradiol level is detected at peripuberty, but it declines to normal in adulthood. From 2 months of age onwards, serum progesterone and testosterone levels are increased, with progesterone being the primary steroid hormone produced [23]. The ovarian morphology of young adult hCGβ+ mice shows the presence of occasional hemorrhagic cysts and luteinized unruptured follicles. Furthermore, enlarged ovaries with massive luteinization resembling luteomas are developed after 6 months of age [23].

The hCGβ+ females are also hyperprolactinemic, reaching up to 600-fold increased serum prolactin concentration by the age of 10−12 months. The luteotropic action of prolactin in rodents is well known, and it is responsible for progesterone production and corpus luteum maintenance in murine pregnancy [30]. The excessive luteinization observed in TG females due to the elevated levels of hCG and prolactin cause a constant progesterone overproduction. High hCG/LH levels are also related to increased androgens concentration, and this may be a cause for follicular cyst development [31].

The hCGβ+ females show hyperplastic pituitary lactotrope cells. The hyperplasia is evidenced from the age of 2 months onward, and it progresses gradually into pituitary adenomas. By the age of 12 months, large prolactinomas with suprasellar expansion, distorted architecture, and dilated blood-filled spaces are observed with 100% penetrance [23]. The neoplastic foci show breakdown of the reticulin fiber network, being a diagnostic sign of adenoma, and immunostaining for prolactin confirmed the lactotrope origin for the adenomas. Interestingly, ovariectomy prevented the development of prolactinomas, indicating that ovarian factors are responsible for this pathological response.

Estrogens are well-established stimulators of pituitary adenomas [32,33]. Since in hCGβ+ females, pituitary adenomas develop in the presence of normal estrogen but constantly elevated progesterone levels, the role of progesterone, and its possible cooperative action with estrogens in promoting prolactinomas was studied in these mice [34]. We showed that long-term treatment with tamoxifen and mifepristone (estrogen and progesterone antagonists, respectively) effectively inhibited the tumor growth and hyperprolactinemia. A combined postgonadectomy estradiol/progesterone treatment was more effective than estrogen alone in inducing tumor growth. The studies demonstrated that the growth of these estrogen-dependent pituitary adenomas is amplified by progesterone [34]. It appears that in the presence of normal estradiol levels, the Cyclin D1 (Ccdn1)/Cyclin-dependent kinase 4 (CDK4)/retinoblastoma protein (pRB)/E2F1 pathway can be directly enhanced by progesterone, with concomitant activation of several oncogenes, including *Hmga2* and *E2f1*, and downregulation/inactivation of *retinoblastoma protein (RB)* [34].

A reduced TGFβ-1 activity in prolactinomas has been proposed to be involved in tumor development, since TGFβ-1 is an inhibitor of lactotrope function. The expression of different components of the pituitary TGFβ-1 system was compared in males and females in this model [35]. Reduced pituitary TGFβ-1 levels and expression of TGFβ-1 target genes, TGFβ-1 receptors, *Ltbp1*, Smad4, and Smad7 were found in hCGβ+ females. No differences were found between the pituitaries of TG and WT males.

In addition to prolactinomas, the mammary gland of hCGβ+ female mice exhibit lobuloalveolar growth, resembling the prelactating state [23]. This is followed by the appearance of mammary gland adenocarcinomas by the age of 12 months. These tumors are metastatic to several organs and have similar histopathology as those observed in TG mice with the activation of the Wnt/β-catenin signaling pathway, showing accumulation of β-catenin accompanied by abnormal expression of the *Wnt* genes [36]. Thus, TG hCG production along with increased estrogen, progesterone, and prolactin levels results in proliferation and dedifferentiation of the mammary gland epithelium in the hCGβ+ mice. Ovariectomy abolishes this tumorigenic phenotype, indicating the dependence of tumorigenesis on ovarian endocrine activity.

Hyperprolactinemia appears to be essential for the phenotypic defects in the hCGβ+ females, since most of them are reversed by treatment with dopamine agonists, with proven efficacy to treat hyperprolactinemia [37]. In line with this, a long-term bromocriptine treatment of adult hCGβ+ females, from 2 to 6 months of age, effectively reduced the obesity, pituitary growth, and disturbances in the hormone profile. Additionally, a 1-week administration of cabergoline to young hCGβ+ females (5-week-old) also effectively normalized their phenotype and recovered their fertility [37]. The development of ovarian cysts and the presence of massive luteinization of hCGβ+ females are also prevented by cabergoline. This is accompanied by normalized progesterone and testosterone synthesis, and normalized gene expression of *Lhcgr* and *Akr1c18* (the enzyme 20α-hydroxysteroid dehydrogenase responsible for converting progesterone into biologically inactive 20α-dihydroprogesterone).

The cabergoline treatment abolishes the main proliferative stimulus responsible for the pituitary growth and prolactinoma development. Thus, once the prolactin secretion is properly controlled by cabergoline, the massive luteinization of the ovary and the progesterone overproduction is prevented. In this regard, lactotrope proliferation may be suppressed both by a direct action on the pituitary by increasing the dopaminergic tone and by an indirect effect by reducing the progesterone-induced tumorigenic signaling pathways. The short-term treatment with cabergoline leads to persistent elimination of hyperprolactinemia and prolactinoma (even at old mice) but only when administered to young females [37]. This shows that chronically elevated hCG levels are able to induce persistent alterations of the pituitary—gonadal axis that are not reversed once the dysfunctional phenotype is established at adulthood.

Crossbreeding of the hCGβ+ mice with prolactin receptor—deficient mice ($Prlr^{-/-}$) confirmed the importance of prolactin in promoting the phenotypic alterations of hCGβ+ females [38]. In these double mutant females, the lack of $Prlr$ in the presence of high bioactive hCG levels prevented the massive luteinization of the ovaries and the mammary tumor development during adulthood. These studies emphasize the permissive role of prolactin as a regulator of hCG/LH action on the ovary and on its secondary extragonadal effects [38].

The endocrine alterations induced by chronic hCG production lead to significant metabolic dysfunctions in females. Adult hCGβ+ females are obese, mainly with abdominal fat accumulation [23]. The obese phenotype is associated with hyperinsulinemia, glucose intolerance, and impaired glucose-stimulated insulin secretion that precedes or accompanies the development of insulin resistance [39]. The failure of β-cell function in this model is evident, since despite hyperinsulinemia, basal glucose ranges within the normal values, but not after an i.p. glucose load. Besides, hypertriglyceridemia and high triglyceride/HDL-C index were found in adult female mice [39]. Interestingly, cabergoline treatment applied on 5-week-old hCGβ+ mice effectively prevents the metabolic alterations. These data indicate a key role of the hyperprolactinemia-induced gonadal dysfunction in the metabolic disturbances of hCGβ+ females [39].

In summary, extragonadal phenotypes are observed in females: obesity [23], glucose intolerance and insulin resistance [39], pituitary macroprolactinoma [23,34,35], mammary gland adenocarcinoma [23,36,38], and elevated bone density [40]. However, all the extragonadal phenotypes of the hCGβ+ females are abolished by gonadectomy despite maintaining a persistent and high secretion of hCG, indicating that ovarian stimulation and abnormal gonadal hormone production, rather than direct extragonadal hCG effects was responsible for the extragonadal phenotypes observed in the hCGβ+ females.

Males

Phenotypic characterization of the hCGβ+ males revealed no obvious alterations; these were fertile with full spermatogenesis and normal sperm quality despite reduced testis size and serum FSH [24].

Phenotype of double transgenic hCGαβ+ mice
Females

The double TG females overexpressing both Cα- and hCGβ-subunits (hCGαβ+) also show precocious puberty, infertility, and enhanced steroidogenesis [41]. The regulation of the hypothalamic-pituitary unit is also affected in TG hCGαβ+ females [29]. These females show a transient surge of estradiol at peripuberty. In addition, testosterone levels are elevated at least from postnatal day 14 onward. In immature hCGαβ+ females, the early FSH surge is suppressed, together with reduced expression of *Fshb*, *Lhb*, and *Gnrhr* genes at the pituitary level; these effects are reversed by ovariectomy. This suggests that the negative feedback regulation of the gonadotropin axis occurs prematurely in these females [29]. Transgenic females also exhibit elevated hypothalamic aromatization in the preoptic area (POA), which is the sexually differentiated area that controls the LH surge in adulthood. When the antiandrogen flutamide was administered to hCGαβ+ females from postnatal day 6 until puberty, CYP19A1 expression was normalized. These results suggest that early postnatal exposure of females to androgen action induces permanent alterations on the sex-specific organization of the brain and determines the masculinization/defeminization of the aromatase expression in the POA in females at the onset of puberty [29].

Young adult hCGαβ+ females develop ovarian germ cell tumors that are phenocopies of human teratomas [28]. These tumors are characterized by the presence of a wide variety of tissue types including ectodermal, mesodermal, and endodermal derivatives, like keratinizing squamous epithelium, hair follicles, sebaceous glands, neural tissue, cartilage, digestive or respiratory epithelia. These tumors are one of the most frequent types of ovarian tumors in women, representing around 20% of all ovarian neoplasm. They are benign, however, displaying malignant transformation with an incidence of approximately 1.4%–2% [42,43]. The molecular pathogenesis of this neoplasm in humans has not been fully clarified. Consequently, our transgenic hCGαβ+ mouse model provides a novel resource to reveal the molecular mechanisms involved in the formation of ovarian germ-cell-derived tumors and to allow a better understanding of their treatment and prevention.

Males

As with hCGβ+ males, precocious puberty is not detected in the double transgenic hCGαβ+ males. The serum testosterone is elevated and testicular steroidogenesis is enhanced, despite downregulation of the LHCGR. The timing of the balanopreputial separation and onset of spermatogenesis are indistinguishable from WT males [27]. It may therefore be that the postnatal sexual maturation is already maximal in males with physiological gonadotropin stimulation and cannot be accelerated by elevated LH/hCG stimulation.

The hypothalamic—pituitary function of prepubertal hCGαβ+ males is affected, as manifested by the high hypothalamic GnRH concentration and accelerated GnRH pulse frequency, which induces downregulation of the GnRH receptor and reduction of FSH synthesis and secretion at the pituitary level [41]. A profound and persistent malfunction of the neuroendocrine feedback control of the gonadotropin axis is evident, with persistently low FSH levels throughout life. These are reestablished by blockade of the androgen action perinatally [41]. These findings suggest that androgen excess during a critical window between gestational day 18 and postnatal day 14 is able to disrupt the developmental programming of the male hypothalamic-pituitary-gonadal axis. A direct testosterone-dependent regulation of hypothalamic CYP19A1 expression is apparent, indicating that locally produced estrogens might play a key role in the hypothalamic-pituitary phenotype of hCGαβ+ males [41].

Young hCGαβ+ males first show full spermatogenesis and normal sperm quality, but progressive tubular degeneration occurs as the animals grow older. This event correlates with the appearance of epididymal structural abnormalities and altered sperm structure with bent tails. Testis size is smaller with enlarged seminal vesicles and prostate, dilated vasa deferentia and bladder, as well as kidney defects at adulthood [24]. Foci of degenerative seminiferous tubules are characteristic of the hCGαβ+ phenotype, but absent in hCGβ+ mice. Infertility of young hCGαβ+ males appears to be mechanical and/or behavioral in origin. hCGαβ+ males also display aggressive behavior toward females and present with impaired mating ability, as evidenced by the lack of vaginal plugs during breeding. This suggests that the problem is at the level of copulatory or ejaculatory function, and not in sperm production.

Interestingly, immature hCGαβ+ males develop Leydig cell adenomas. These reach their maximum size at 10 days postpartum but disappear by puberty, when normal regression of fetal Leydig cells occurs. Studying the expression of fetal and adult Leydig cell markers suggested that the Leydig cell adenomas originated from the fetal population, providing evidence that the adult-type Leydig cells may be resistant to development of gonadotropin-induced adenomas [27].

Concluding remarks

TG technologies have proven fundamental to provide novel information on the role of gonadotropins in reproductive pathophysiology. As part of such studies, our work with TG mice presenting with hCG hypersecretion has provided insight into a great number of anomalies at different levels of the endocrine regulatory axis. These studies have helped to identify regulatory mechanisms affected by disruptive gonadotropin stimuli, such as hypersecretion, also unraveling new therapeutic strategies to interfere with certain endocrine pathologies. Our studies have indicated that chronic hypersecretion of hCG promotes manifold endocrine anomalies that are accompanied by gonadal and extragonadal tumors. Those in gonads are considered as primary effects, whereas those found in the female pituitary and mammary glands are due to secondary effects of the altered gonadal function. On the basis of the evidence gathered it seems that the female reproductive system is more vulnerable to gonadotropin dysregulation than the one in males.

Acknowledgments

We thank all our collaborators from the University of Turku (Turku, Finland) and the Institute of Biology and Experimental Medicine (IBYME-CONICET, Buenos Aires, Argentina) that were involved in the project all along these years.

References

[1] Choi J, Smitz J. Luteinizing hormone and human chorionic gonadotropin: distinguishing unique physiologic roles. Gynecol Endocrinol 2014;30:174–81.

[2] Casarini L, Santi D, Brigante G, Simoni M. Two hormones for one receptor: evolution, biochemistry, actions, and pathophysiology of LH and hCG. Endocr Rev 2018;39: 549–92.

[3] Abdallah MA, Lei ZM, Li X, Greenwold N, Nakajima ST, Jauniaux E, Rao CV. Human fetal nongonadal tissues contain human chorionic gonadotropin/luteinizing hormone receptors. J Clin Endocrinol Metab 2004;89:952–6.

[4] Cole LA. Biological functions of hCG and hCG-related molecules. Reprod Biol Endocrinol 2010;8:102.

[5] Rao CV, Lei ZM. The past, present and future of nongonadal hCG/LH actions in reproductive biology and medicine. Mol Cell Endocrinol 2007;269:2–8.

[6] Pakarainen T, Ahtiainen P, Zhang FP, Rulli S, Poutanen M, Huhtaniemi I. Extragonadal LH/hCG action–not yet time to rewrite textbooks. Mol Cell Endocrinol 2007;269:9–16.

[7] Pakarainen T, Zhang FP, Poutanen M, Huhtaniemi I. Fertility in luteinizing hormone receptor-knockout mice after wild-type ovary transplantation demonstrates redundancy of extragonadal luteinizing hormone action. J Clin Investig 2005;115:1862–8.

[8] Mitri F, Bentov Y, Behan LA, Esfandiari N, Casper RF. A novel compound heterozygous mutation of the luteinizing hormone receptor -implications for fertility. J Assist Reprod Genet 2014;31:787–94.

[9] Jameson JL. Hollenberg AN Regulation of chorionic gonadotropin gene expression. Endocr Rev 1993;14:203–21.

[10] Huhtaniemi I. Fetal testis—a very special endocrine organ. Eur J Endocrinol 1994;130: 25–31.

[11] Cole LA, Sasaki Y, Muller CY. Normal production of human chorionic gonadotropin in menopause. N Engl J Med 2007;356:1184–6.

[12] Riman T, Nilsson S. Persson IR Review of epidemiological evidence for reproductive and hormonal factors in relation to the risk of epithelial ovarian malignancies. Acta Obstet Gynecol Scand 2004;83:783–95.

[13] Filicori M, Fazleabas AT, Huhtaniemi I, Licht P, Rao CV, Tesarik J, Zygmunt M. Novel concepts of human chorionic gonadotropin: reproductive system interactions and potential in the management of infertility. Fertil Steril 2005;84:275–84.

[14] Konishi I. Gonadotropins and ovarian carcinogenesis: a new era of basic research and its clinical implications. Int J Gynecol Cancer 2006;16:16–22.

[15] Iles RK, Delves PJ, Butler SA. Does hCG or hCGβ play a role in cancer cell biology? Mol Cell Endocrinol 2010;329:62–70.

[16] Cole LA, Butler S. Hyperglycosylated hCG, hCGβ and Hyperglycosylated hCGβ: interchangeable cancer promoters. Mol Cell Endocrinol 2012;349:232–8.

[17] Themmen APN, Huhtaniemi IT. Mutations of gonadotropins and gonadotropin receptors: elucidating the physiology and pathophysiology of pituitary-gonadal function. Endocr Rev 2000;21:551–83.

[18] Huhtaniemi IT, Themmen AP. Mutations in human gonadotropin and gonadotropin-receptor genes. Endocrine 2005;26:207–17.

[19] Burns KH, Matzuk MM. Minireview: genetic models for the study of gonadotropin actions. Endocrinology 2002;143:2823–35.

[20] Rulli SB, Huhtaniemi I. What have gonadotrophin overexpressing transgenic mice taught us about gonadal function? Reproduction 2005;130:283—91.

[21] Huhtaniemi I, Ahtiainen P, Pakarainen T, Rulli SB, Zhang FP. Poutanen M Genetically modified mouse models in studies of luteinising hormone action. Mol Cell Endocrinol 2006;252:126—35.

[22] Schorpp M, Jager R, Schellander K, Schenkel J, Wagner EF, Weiher H, Angel P. The human ubiquitin C promoter directs high ubiquitous expression of transgenes in mice. Nucleic Acids Res 1996;24:1787—8.

[23] Rulli SB, Kuorelahti AI, Karaer 0, Pelliniemi L, Poutanen M. Huhtaniemi IT Reproductive disturbances, pituitary lactotrope adenomas, and mammary gland tumors in transgenic female mice producing high levels of human chorionic gonadotropin. Endocrinology 2002;143:4084—95.

[24] Rulli SB, Ahtiainen P, Makela S, Toppari J, Poutanen M. Huhtaniemi IT Elevated steroidogenesis, defective reproductive organs and infertility in transgenic male mice overexpressing human chorionic gonadotropin. Endocrinology 2003;144:4980—90.

[25] Kendall SK, Gordon DF, Birkmeier TS, Petrey D, Sarapura VD, O'Shea KS, Wood WM, Lloyd RV, Ridgway EC, Camper SA. Enhancer-mediated high level expression of mouse pituitary glycoprotein hormone alpha-subunit transgene in thyrotropes, gonadotropes, and developing pituitary gland. Mol Endocrinol 1994;8:1420—33.

[26] Markkula M, Kananen K, Klemi P, Huhtaniemi I. Pituitary and ovarian expression of the endogenous follicle-stimulating hormone (FSH) subunit genes and an FSH beta-subunit promoter-driven herpes simplex virus thymidine kinase gene in transgenic mice; specific partial ablation of FSH-producing cells by antiherpes treatment. J Endocrinol 1996;150:265—73.

[27] Ahtiainen P, Rulli S, Pelliniemi LJ, Toppari J, Poutanen M, Huhtaniemi I. Fetal but not adult Leydig cells are susceptible to adenoma formation in response to persistently high hCG level; a study on hCG overexpressing transgenic mice. Oncogene 2005;24:7301—9.

[28] Huhtaniemi I, Rulli S, Ahtiainen P, Poutanen M. Multiple sites of tumorigenesis in transgenic mice overproducing hCG. Mol Cell Endocrinol 2005;234:117—26.

[29] Gonzalez B, Ratner LD, Scerbo MJ, Di Giorgio NP, Poutanen M, Huhtaniemi IT, Calandra RS, Lux-Lantos VA, Cambiasso MJ, Rulli SB. Elevated hypothalamic aromatization at the onset of precocious puberty in transgenic female mice hypersecreting human chorionic gonadotropin: effect of androgens. Mol Cell Endocrinol 2014;390:102—11.

[30] Ben-Jonathan N, LaPensee CR, LaPensee EW. What can we learn from rodents about prolactin in humans? Endocr Rev 2008;29:1—41.

[31] Beloosesky R, Gold R, Almog B, Sasson R, Dantes A, Land-Bracha A, et al. Induction of polycystic ovary by testosterone in immature female rats: modulation of apoptosis and attenuation of glucose/insulin ratio. Int J Mol Med 2004;14:207—15.

[32] Colao A, Di Sarno A, Cappabianca P, Di Somma C, Pivonello R, Lombardi G. Withdrawal of long-term cabergoline therapy for tumoral and nontumoral hyperprolactinemia. N Engl J Med 2003;349:2023—33.

[33] Gillam MP, Molitch ME, Lombardi G, Colao A. Advances in the treatment of prolactinomas. Endocr Rev 2006;27:485—534.

[34] Ahtiainen P, Sharp V, Rulli SB, Rivero-Muller A, Mamaeva V, Roytta, et al. Enhanced LH action in transgenic female mice expressing hCGbeta subunit induces pituitary prolactinomas; the role of high progesterone levels. Endocr Relat Cancer 2010;17:611—21.

[35] Faraoni E, Camilletti MA, Abeledo A, Ratner LD, De Pino F, Huhtaniemi IT, Rulli SB, Díaz-Torga G. Sex differences in the development of prolactinoma in mice overexpressing hCGβ: role of pituitary TGFβ1. J Endocrinol 2017;232:535−46.

[36] Kuorelahti A, Rulli S, Huhtaniemi I, Poutanen M. hCG upregulates wnt5b and wnt7b in the mammary gland and hCG{beta} transgenic female mice present with mammary gland tumors exhibiting characteristics of the Wnt/{beta}-catenin pathway activation. Endocrinology 2007;148:3694−703.

[37] Ratner LD, Gonzalez B, Ahtiainen P, Di Giorgio NP, Poutanen M, Calandra RS, Huhtaniemi IT, Rulli SB. Short-term pharmacological suppression of the hyperprolactinemia of infertile hCG overproducing female mice persistently restores their fertility. Endocrinology 2012;153:5980−92.

[38] Bachelot A, Carré N, Mialon O, Matelot M, Servel N, Monget P, et al. The permissive role of prolactin as a regulator 1 of luteinizing hormone action in the female mouse ovary and extragonadal tumorigenesis. Am J Physiol Endocrinol Metab 2013;305: E845−52.

[39] Ratner LD, Stevens G, Bonaventura MM, Lux-Lantos VA, Poutanen M, Calandra RS, Huhtaniemi IT, Rulli SB. Hyperprolactinemia induced by hCG leads to metabolic disturbances in female mice. J Endocrinol 2016;230:157−69.

[40] Yarram SJ, Perry MJ, Christopher TJ, Westby K, Brown N, Lamminen T, Rulli SB, Zhang F-P, Huhtaniemi I, Sandy JR. Mansell JP Luteinizing hormone receptor knockout (LURKO) mice and transgenic human chorionic gonadotrophin overexpressing mice have bone phenotypes. Endocrinology 2003;144:3555−64.

[41] Gonzalez B, Ratner LD, Di Giorgio NP, Poutanen M, Huhtaniemi IT, Calandra RS, Lux Lantos VA, Rulli SB. Endogenously elevated androgens alter the developmental programming of the hypothalamic-pituitary axis in male mice. Mol Cell Endocrinol 2011;332:78−87.

[42] Comerci Jr JT, Licciardi F, Bergh PA, Gregori C. Breen JL Mature cystic teratoma: a clinicopathologic evaluation of 517 cases and review of the literature. Obstet Gynecol 1994;84:22−8.

[43] Ulbright TM. Gonadal teratomas: a review and speculation. Adv Anat Pathol 2004;11: 10−23.

Role of human chorionic gonadotropin in reproductive medicine

3.5

Mazen R. Fouany, Fady I. Sharara

Introduction

Human chorionic gonadotropin (hCG) is a member of the glycoprotein hormone family also comprising the pituitary-derived follicle stimulating hormone (FSH), luteinizing hormone (LH), and thyroid-stimulating hormone (TSH). Each hormone consists of a noncovalently bound α- and β-subunits where within a species the α-subunit is identical and hormone specificity is determined by the unique β-subunit [2].

hCG has been associated with the initiation and maintenance of pregnancy and has an essential role in reproductive medicine. Both hCG and LH interact with the same receptor which is the LH/hCG receptor, and hCG and LH have both been used to stimulate events that are caused by the interaction of either hormone with the LH/hCG receptor [1]. An example of this is the use of hCG to trigger final follicle and oocyte maturation and ovulation in place of LH at the end of ovulation induction regimens.

Physiology

In assisted reproductive technologies, human chorionic gonadotropin has traditionally replaced luteinizing hormone as the molecule responsible for the crucial step in ovum meiosis and maturation, as well as in maturation of its supporting cells. Despite the advances in reproductive medicine, the actual event of ovulation is far from simple and involves multiple cascades and processes, most of which are still poorly understood.

Following the LH surge and the progesterone rise, the follicle stimulating hormone surge results in an increased response of the LH receptors to LH. Both LH and hCG bind to the same receptor; however, this does not necessarily imply an

100 Years of Human Chorionic Gonadotropin. **https://doi.org/10.1016/B978-0-12-820050-6.00017-5**

identical receptor response due to the structural differences in the β-subunit and their clearance rates from the circulation (Klement, 2017). In assisted reproduction, injected hCG has a much slower plasma metabolic clearance than LH, which consists of a rapid phase in the first 5—9 hours following its administration and a slower phase in the 1—1.3 days after administration. After 36 hours, the calculated half-life of hCG is 2.32 days, as compared with LH, for which estimates have ranged from 1 hour to 3—5 hours [3]. Even in terms of receptor exposure, one cannot conclude the same behavior, since the natural midcycle surge is characterized by three phases lasting a total of 48 hours while the induced surge follows a different pattern [4].

hCG and LH are dimeric hormones that belong to the glycoprotein hormone family. The LH/hCG receptor is a large cell-surface glycoprotein with the characteristic structure that makes it a member of the superfamily of G protein—coupled receptors. This receptor has a dynamic expression pattern throughout the menstrual cycle. It reaches maximum expression and effect in the midluteal phase and decreases with corpus luteum regression. In contrast, medicated cycles are characterized by peak biological activity at midcycle and lowest activity during the luteal phase. This is another potential explanation for the differences in LH-/hCG-mediated cascades [5].

Therapeutic use of human chorionic gonadotropin
Ovulation induction

hCG has been used in ovulation induction as well as in in vitro fertilization. In ovulation alone, induction using clomiphene, letrozole, or gonadotropins, hCG is usually given to induce ovulation as oocyte release is necessary for natural conception to occur. However, in assisted reproduction, where follicular development is usually achieved by daily administration of FSH or HMG injections, hCG induces oocyte maturation in IVF cycles. Since recombinant LH is not available in high enough doses to induce oocyte maturation, hCG has traditionally been used as a surrogate for LH [6]. Since LH/hCG receptors have been detected in the human cervix, preovulatory LH concentrations or administered hCG may also directly influence endocervical epithelial cells to affect mucus secretion, and hence, sperm transport [7].

Whether hCG should be used routinely in clomiphene ovulation induction has not been fully addressed. A recent study in subfertile couples undergoing controlled ovarian hyperstimulation and intrauterine insemination (IUI) concluded that recombinant hCG (r-hCG) administration was associated with an increased clinical pregnancy rate compared with spontaneous LH surge. When r-hCG was administered concomitantly with a serum LH surge, this benefit was amplified [8]. The effect appears to be of particular importance in recombinant FSH-medicated cycles rather than clomiphene or letrozole. IUI can be done successfully at either 24 or 36 hours after hCG in clomiphene citrate—stimulated cycles [9]. This allows more flexibility and convenience for both physicians and patients, especially during weekends. Despite this, the fact that most IVF centers in the United States and across the world have been using hCG trigger in patient undergoing controlled ovulation induction using clomiphene, letrozole, and gonadotropins, we found no trials evaluating the use of ovulation triggers in anovulatory women treated with ovulation-inducing agents and its effect on clinical pregnancy rate [19].

Oocyte maturation

A hCG dose of 5000 or 10,000 IU, administered intramuscularly or subcutaneously, has been used for oocyte maturation prior to IVF after an initial study found a significantly worse outcome with lower doses [10]. The route of administration does not seem to affect clinical outcome, and oocyte retrieval is scheduled for approximately 36 hours following hCG administration [2]. The optimal size of the developing follicle with respect to retrieving an oocyte appears to be between 18 and 20 mm [11]. LH receptor expression by the preovulatory follicle is important in natural cycles to respond to the LH surge as well as in stimulated cycles where hCG is effective in promoting oocyte maturation and ovulation [2].

The failure to retrieve oocytes form preovulatory follicles is called empty follicle syndrome and is the result of error in injecting the hCG, variation in the urinary purified form or rapid clearance of hCG. The incidence has been reported to be up to 0.5% [12].

r-hCG is now readily available and appears to be as effective as urinary-derived hCG with fewer local injection site reactions and higher endogenous serum progesterone concentrations as a result. However, there was a trend toward a higher incidence of ovarian hyperstimulation syndrome (OHSS) with the more potent rhCG. Several studies have compared the equivalence of human recombinant LH and human recombinant hCG in terms of potency, kinetics, and response. There are significant intracellular differences mainly in activating certain cascade pathways with more hCG dominance compared with the recombinant LH [13]. Therapeutically, r-hCG appears at least as effective as urinary hCG for inducing ovulation and oocyte maturation prior to IVF [20]. HCG has also been used both for in vivo priming of immature follicles and as a component of the culture system for oocyte maturation. Initial in vitro maturation success rates were poor but the introduction of in vivo hCG priming (administered 36 hours prior to retrieval) accelerated the maturation process and resulted in satisfactory pregnancy rates. Culturing oocytes in vitro was equally successful in the presence of either r-hCG or recombinant LH which supports that both hormones are effective in promoting oocyte maturation. This process has many potential benefits in reproductive medicine including future fertility preservation, eliminating OHSS, and reducing the financial costs by avoiding expensive gonadotropin preparations [7].

Additional pathophysiological roles of hCG include the following:

- Inducing angiogenesis in embryo implantation: The role of hCG in coordinating embryo implantation has been demonstrated by its extragonadal responses in multiple model systems. HCG results in the production and expression of certain proteins, which have been postulated to play a role in endometrial receptivity and embryo implantation. This will result in regulating the maternal immune response and preventing the rejection of the fetus by the mother [14].
- Trophoblastic invasion in its earlier stages: The interaction of hCG with native hCG results in facilitating the invasive activities of the trophoblastic villi. The extravillous cytotrophoblast cells are the main invasive cells of the placenta, forming fingerlike projections or villi, as a result of rapid cellular proliferation. The trophoblastic villi produce hCG, which multiplies the proliferative response exponentially, invading the villi through the decidua and driving the embryo deep into the myometrium, thus anchoring it [14]. Taken together, all of the above support the thesis that HCG demonstrates important paracrine effects on decidualization, implantation, vascularization, and tissue remodeling.

Daily administration of 200 IU of hCG in addition to recombinant FSH in patients with prior failed attempts have been shown to increase the pregnancy rate [15]. HCG addition to recombinant FSH, even in women of advanced reproductive age with higher basal FSH levels, which are often considered to have poorer ovarian reserve, may be associated with better-quality embryos and higher pregnancy rates [16]. Also, administration of hCG and progesterone during the luteal phase is associated with higher rates of live birth or ongoing pregnancy than placebo [17].

Role of hCG in ovarian hyperstimulation syndrome

OHSS is a serious iatrogenic complication of controlled ovarian hyperstimulation, exacerbated and perpetuated by the presence of circulating levels of hCG. The condition is characterized by ascites, ovarian enlargement, and increased capillary permeability. The pathophysiology of OHSS is based on the role of vascular endothelial growth factor (VEGF) as a mediator of these changes. Due to its prolonged clearance, the use of hCG in the final follicular maturation results in triggering OHSS [18]. This is explained by the ability of hCG in upregulating VEGF expression in luteinized granulosa cells. Since VEGF is already elevated during the gonadotropin stimulation phase, preceding hCG injection, it is further stimulated by hCG administration. VEGF is considered the major driving force in the hyperpermeability characterizing OHSS and is therefore a key player in its pathophysiology. Also endogenous hCG synthesis after a successful IVF and embryo transfer and specially in multiple pregnancy is associated with higher incidence of OHSS [18].

In the current ART era, the use of hCG triggering is challenged due to the risk of OHSS, and multiple clinics have reported routine, successful use of GnRH agonist triggering, and reserving the use hCG for special circumstances or for in vivo fertility cycles. GnRH agonist triggering has been proven to avoid OHSS, although it is still inferior in terms of pregnancy rate and live births when a fresh embryo transfer is performed [1]. A possible explanation of the superiority of hCG is the expression of LH/hCG receptor in the reproductive tract along with the prolonged half-life of hCG as compared with LH. Another explanation is the role of hCG on endometrial cells could explain the role of hCG in promoting pregnancy.

Conclusion

Ovulation triggering techniques have evolved throughout the era of assisted reproduction. Until the last decade, hCG was a major component of ART cycles. In order to avoid OHSS, the use of GnRH agonists has replaced hCG when OHSS is predicted. However, hCG still has an important role in ovulation induction and maturation of follicles. GnRH agonist triggering in combination with hCG provides an option to achieve better results in special circumstances and/or populations. While GnRH agonist is a better option for egg maturation, hCG is superior for luteal phase support.

References

[1] Klement AH, Shulman A. hCG triggering in ART: an evolutionary concept. Int J Mol Sci 2017;18(5):1075.

[2] Keay SD, Vatish M, Karteris E, Hillhouse EW, Randeva HS. The role of hCG in reproductive medicine. BJOG 2004;111:1218−28.

[3] Richards JS. Ovulation: new factors that prepare the oocyte for fertilization. Mol Cell Endocrinol 2005;234:75−9. https://doi.org/10.1016/j.mce.2005.01.004.

[4] Castillo JC, Humaidan P, Bernabeu R. Pharmaceutical options for triggering of final oocyte maturation in art. BioMed Res Intern 2014;2014:580171. https://doi.org/10.1155/2014/580171.

[5] Schwarz S, Krude H. The human chorionic gonadotropin (hCG) receptor: a new class within the family of GTP protein coupled receptors. Epitope mapping of receptor-bound agonistic and antagonistic forms of hCG. Wien Klin Wochenschr 1992;104(15):492.

[6] Ludwig M, Doody KJ, Doody KM. Use of recombinant human chorionic gonadotrophin in ovulation induction. Fertil Steril 2003;79:1051−9.

[7] Lin YH, Hwang JL, Huang LW, et al. Combination of FSH priming and hCG priming for in-vitro maturation of human oocytes. Hum Reprod 2003;18:1632−6.

[8] Taerk E, Hughes E, Greenberg C, Neal M, Amin S, Faghih M, Karnis M. Controlled ovarian hyperstimulation with intrauterine insemination is more successful after r-hCG administration than spontaneous LH surge. J Reprod Infert 2017;18(3):316−22.

[9] Yumusak OH, Kahyaoglu S, Pekcan MK, Isci E, Ozyer S, Cicek MN, Tasci Y, Erkaya S. Which is the best intrauterine insemination timing choice following exogenous hCG administration during ovulation induction by using clomiphene citrate treatment? A retrospective study. SpringerPlus 2016;5:1307.

[10] Abdalla HI, Ah-Moye M, Brinsden P, Howe DL, Okonofua F, Craft I. The effect of the dose of human chorionic gonadotropin and the type of gonadotropin stimulation on oocyte recovery rates in an in vitro fertilization program. Fertil Steril 1987;48:958−63.

[11] Scott RT, Hofmann GE, Muasher SJ, Acosta AA, Kreiner DK, Rosenwaks Z. Correlation of follicular diameter with oocyte recovery and maturity at the time of transvaginal follicular aspiration. J In Vitro Fertil Embryo Transf 1989;6:73−5.

[12] Quintans CJ, Donaldson MJ, Blanco LA, Pasqualini RS. Empty follicle syndrome due to human errors; its occurrence in an in-vitro fertilization programme. Hum Reprod 1998;13:2703−5.

[13] Casarini L, Lispi M, Longobardi S, Milosa F, La Marca A, Tagliasacchi D, Pignatti E, Simoni M. LH and hCG action on the same receptor results in quantitatively and qualitatively different intracellular signalling. PLoS One 2012;7:e46682. https://doi.org/10.1371/journal.pone.0046682.

[14] Banerjee P, Fazleabas A. Extragonadal actions of chorionic gonadotropin. Rev Endocr Metab Disord December 2011;12(4):323−32.

[15] Drakakis P, Loutradis D, Beloukas A, Sypsa V, Anastasiadou V, Kalofolias G, Arabatzi H, Kiapekou E, Stefanidis K, Paraskevis D, Makrigiannakis A, Hatzakis A, Antsaklis A. Early hCG addition to rFSH for ovarian stimulation in IVF provides better results and the cDNA copies of the hCG receptor may be an indicator of successful stimulation. Reprod Bio Endocrinol 2009;7:110.

[16] Partsinevelos GA, Antonakopoulos N, Kallianidis K, Drakakis P, Anagnostou E, Bletsa R, Loutradis D. Addition of low-dose hCG to rFSH during ovarian stimulation for IVF/ICSI: is it beneficial? Clin Exp Obstet Gynecol 2016;43(6):818−25.

[17] Van Der Linden M, Buckingham K, Farquhar C, Kremer JA, Metwally M. Luteal phase support for assisted reproduction cycles. Cochrane Database Syst Rev July, 2015;(7): CD009154.

[18] Wang TH, Horng SG, Chang CL, Wu HM, Tsai YJ, Wang HS, Soong YK. Human chorionic gonadotropin-induced ovarian hyperstimulation syndrome is associated with up-regulation of vascular endothelial growth factor. J Clin Endocrinol Metab 2002;87:3300−8. https://doi.org/10.1210/jcem.87.7.8651.

[19] Scott RT, Bailey SA, Kost ER, Neal GS, Hofmann GE, Illions EH. Comparison of leuprolide acetate and human chorionic gonadotropin for the induction of ovulation in clomiphene citrate-stimulated cycles. Fertil Steril 1994;61:872−9. https://doi.org/10.1016/S0015-0282(16)56699-0.

[20] The European. Induction of final oocyte maturation and early luteinization in women undergoing ovulation induction for assisted reproduction treatment-recombinant hCG versus urinary hCG. Hum Reprod 2000;15. 1446−145.

Pregnancy hCG

3.6

Laurence A. Cole

Introduction

I call this chapter human chorionic gonadotropin (hCG) 2019 because it is an update of hCG biology, or a very up-to-date review of hCG. A lot has changed in hCG biology. This is all reviewed here.

Multiple forms of hCG

There are three independent forms of hCG present in pregnancy, the nonpregnant healthy individual, cancer and as produced by the pituitary gland, the autocrine hyperglycosylated hCG, and the autocrine extravillous cytotrophoblast hCG [1,2]. Structurally, each is distinct (Fig. 3.6.1), each having a unique carbohydrate side chain structure, and each either binds the luteinizing hormone (LH)/hCG hormone receptor (the hormone hCG) or the ancestral transforming growth factor-β (TGFβ) receptor (hyperglycosylated hCG and extravillous cytotrophoblast hCG) [3–5].

As illustrated in Fig. 3.6.1, each has a common amino acid structure, and a differing carbohydrate structure [1,2]. Fig. 3.6.1 shows Butler structures of hCG, using Wu, Lapthorn, and Lustbader X-ray crystallography models [6–8] and a thermodynamic computer model of the remaining sequences. The hormone hCG has Type 1 O-linked structures on the β-subunit C-terminal peptide, and a unique C-terminal peptide that bisects the β39-58 loop, blocking it from nicking [9]. Hyperglycosylated hCG and extravillous cytotrophoblast hCG both have Type 2 O-linked oligosaccharides, and extravillous cytotrophoblast hCG has triantennary N-linked oligosaccharides (Fig. 3.6.1).

The hormone hCG is produced by syncytiotrophoblast cells in pregnancy. Hyperglycosylated hCG is made by root cytotrophoblast cells, and extravillous cytotrophoblast hCG is made by the differentiated extravillous cytotrophoblast cells in pregnancy and by cancer cells [1,2].

Considering carbohydrate structure [10], the hormone hCG is 84.5% of the hCG molecules produced in pregnancy, hyperglycosylated hCG is 1.9%, and extravillous cytotrophoblast hCG is 13.7% (six samples examined). The hormone hCG is 77% of

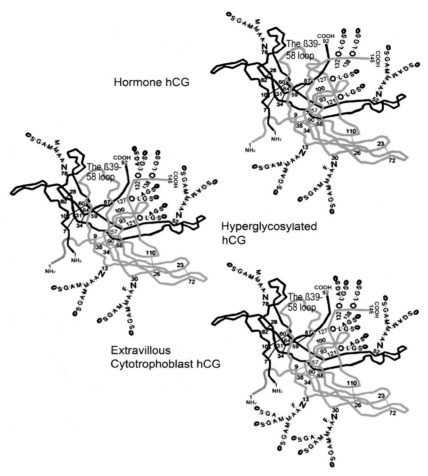

FIGURE 3.6.1

Butler structures of hCG, using Wu, Lapthorn, and Lustbader X-ray crystallography models [5—7] and a thermodynamic computer model of the remaining sequences.

the hCG molecules produced in hydatidiform mole, hyperglycosylated hCG is 0%, and extravillous cytotrophoblast hCG is 23% (three samples examined) [10]. The hormone hCG is just 25.8% of the hCG produced in choriocarcinoma, hyperglycosylated hCG is 21.9%, and extravillous cytotrophoblast hCG is 52.9% (five samples examined) [10].

The placenta differentiates with blastocyst implantation, multiple cytotrophoblast cells fuse together to make multiple nucleus syncytiotrophoblast cells [11,12] (Fig. 3.6.2), cytotrophoblast cells differentiate to make villous

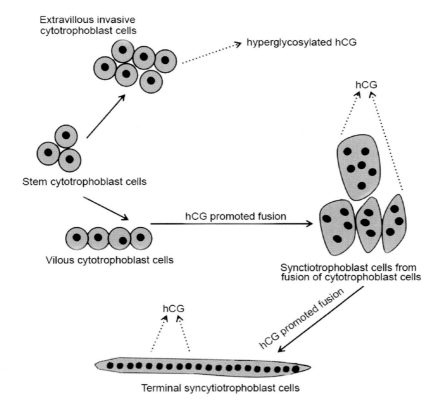

Extravillous invasive
cytotrophoblast cells

hyperglycosylated hCG

hCG

Stem cytotrophoblast cells

hCG promoted fusion

Vilous cytotrophoblast cells

Synctiotrophoblast cells from
fusion of cytotrophoblast cells

hCG

hCG promoted fusion

Terminal syncytiotrophoblast cells

FIGURE 3.6.2

Cytotrophoblast differentiation and formation of villous cytotrophoblast, extravillous
cytotrophoblast, and syncytiotrophoblast cells.

cytotrophoblast and extravillous cytotrophoblast cell [13,14] (Fig. 3.6.2). These
cells then make the hormone hCG, hyperglycosylated hCG, and extravillous cytotrophoblast hCG.

hCG processing

The hormone hCG is not rapidly nicked or cleaved at β47-48 because of the
C-terminal peptide blockage of loop β39-58 [9]. So the intact hormone hCG binds
the LH/hCG hormone receptor. The receptor has poor affinity for nicked hormones
[15]. Hyperglycosylated hCG and extravillous cytotrophoblast hCG are both immediately nicked by leukocyte elastase upon secretion. They rapidly dissociate
releasing the β-subunit which binds the autocrine TGFβ receptor (Fig. 3.6.3).

Upon entering the blood, the nonnicked hormone hCG looses its C-terminal peptide, by the action of leukocyte elastase. The hormone missing the C-terminal

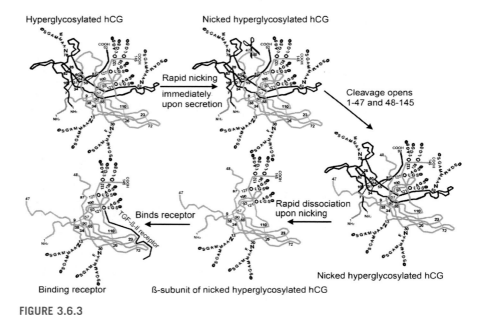

Hyperglycosylated hCG   Nicked hyperglycosylated hCG

Rapid nicking immediately upon secretion

Cleavage opens 1-47 and 48-145

Binds receptor

Rapid dissociation upon nicking

Binding receptor   ß-subunit of nicked hyperglycosylated hCG

Nicked hyperglycosylated hCG

FIGURE 3.6.3

The nicking of hyperglycosylated hCG and extravillous cytotrophoblast hCG, dissociation and release of the β-subunit which binds the TGFβ receptor.

peptide, rapidly dissociate to form the β-subunit missing the C-terminal peptide, the end product of serum and urine digestion. Nicked hyperglycosylated hCG and nicked extravillous cytotrophoblast hCG both are subject to loosing their C-terminal peptide as a result of leukocyte elastase digestion. They are then cleaved in the kidney to form β-core fragment, β6-40/β55-92 the end product of serum and urine digestion [16,17]. N-linked oligosaccharides are cleaved, loosing galactose and sialic acid (Table 3.6.1).

hCG functions

The hormone hCG has multiple functions in pregnancy. The most important as indicated by its critical role in human evolution [18,19] is clearly hemochorial placentation or generation of the fetal feeding apparatus. hCG promotes the formation of hemochorial placentation or adaption of this form of fetal feeding verses epithelio-chorial placentation [18,19]. The hormone hCG firstly forms the single cell skin of syncytiotrophoblast cells that surround the villous core [20](Fig. 3.6.4). This is the barrier that separates the maternal and fetal circulation. It secondly extends the spiral arteries so that they reach the hemochorial placentation apparatus (Fig. 3.6.4) [21]. Thirdly, it develops the internal circulation within the villous core that extends the villous core to the fetus (Fig. 3.6.4) [22].

Table 3.6.1 Urine B204 assay (cancer cutoff 3.0 pmol/mL) and supersensitive B204 assay (cancer cutoff 0.1 pmol/mL) detect β-core fragment, free β-subunit, hyperglycosylated hCG free β-subunit and nicked free β-subunit.

| | Urine B204 assay | | | Urine B204 assay | | |
| | Ultrasensitive assay, Cutoff > 0.1 pmol/mL | | | Regular assay, Cutoff >3 pmol/mL | | |
Source	#Cases	#Detected	Sensitivity	#Cases	#Positive	Sensitivity
A. Trophoblastic malignancies						
Choriocarcinoma				63	63	100%
Ovarian germ cell cancer				11	11	100%
Testicular germ cell cancer				17	17	100%
Total				**91**	**91**	**100%**
B. Nontrophoblastic malignancy						
Bladder cancer				140	62	44%
Breast cancer	130	130	100%	456	156	34%
Cervical cancer				410	197	48%
Colorectal cancer				80	29	36%
Endometrial cancer				233	103	44%
Gastric cancer				205	90	44%
Hepatic cancer				46	21	44%
Lung cancer	115	115	100%	154	38	25%
Intestinal cancer				17	8	47%
Lymphoma				41	13	32%
Ovarian cancer	56	56	100%	207	145	70%
Pancreatic cancer	40	40	100%	29	16	55%
Prostate cancer				12	9	75%
Renal cancer				66	32	48%
Uterine cancer				63	26	41%
Vulvar cancer				8	4	50%
Total	**341**	**341**	**100%**	**2167**	**949**	**44%**
C. Healthy						
NED, postcancer chemotherapy				33	2	6%
NED, postcancer surgery				21	1	5%

Continued

Table 3.6.1 Urine B204 assay (cancer cutoff 3.0 pmol/mL) and supersensitive B204 assay (cancer cutoff 0.1 pmol/mL) detect β-core fragment, free β-subunit, hyperglycosylated hCG free β-subunit and nicked free β-subunit.—*cont'd*

Source	Urine B204 assay Ultrasensitive assay, Cutoff > 0.1 pmol/mL			Urine B204 assay Regular assay, Cutoff >3 pmol/mL		
	#Cases	#Detected	Sensitivity	#Cases	#Positive	Sensitivity
Healthy female, no cancer history				72	2	3%
Healthy male, no cancer history				28	1	4%
Total				**154**	**6**	**4%**
D. Benign Disease						
Benign gynecological lesion, tumor				28	0	0%
Follicular ovarian cyst, benign				71	1	0%
Benign ovarian cyst, nonfunctional				26	0	0%
Cervical carcinoma in situ				12	0	0%
Cervical dyskaryosis				66	2	0%
Condyloma				30	0	0%
Endometriosis				16	1	0%
Myoma				27	3	0%
Total				**276**	**7**	**0%**

The hormone hCG also takes over from menstrual cycle LH in promoting progesterone production by the corpus luteum [23]. It drives progesterone production from 4 to 7 weeks of gestation, when progesterone production is taken over by syncytiotrophoblast cell.

Suppression of maternal macrophage and immune response to foreign placenta and fetal tissue is a major function of hCG [24]. The hormone hCG also stops the myometrium muscle from having contractions during pregnancy [25].

Finally, the hormone hCG also attunes growth and invasion of trophoblast tissue led by hyperglycosylated hCG and extravillous cytotrophoblast hCG [26].

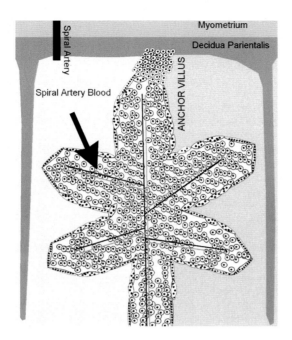

FIGURE 3.6.4

Human hemochorial placentation, a single chamber is shown.

Hyperglycosylated hCG has clear function in pregnancy. Development of the villous core of cytotrophoblast cells in hemochorial placentation apparatus [27]. The start of invasion in blastocyst implantation [28] and the growth of the placenta throughout pregnancy [29] are all promoted by hyperglycosylated hCG.

Extravillous cytotrophoblast hCG controls invasion in blastocyst implantation [28] and controls deep implantation of the hemochorial placentation apparatus [29].

Ovulation

Published research indicates that hyperglycosylated hCG or extravillous cytotrophoblast is produced in low concentrations during the menstrual cycle peaking at day 14 [30]. It was thought that maybe hCG has a role in ovulation. Maybe hyperglycosylated hCG or extravillous cytotrophoblast hCG drive the proteolytic enzyme release of the oocyte at the end of ovulation. This needs to be confirmed.

References

[1] Cole LA. The carbohydrate structure of the hormone hCG, the autocrine hyperglycosylated hCG, and the extravillous cytotrophoblast hyperglycosylated hCG. J Glycobiol 2018;7:100136.

[2] Cole LA. The 4 separate forms of hCG. Am J Obstet Gynecol 2019 (in press).

[3] Butler SA, Ikram MS, Mathieu S, Iles RK. The increase in bladder carcinoma cell population induced by the free beta subunit of hCG is a result of an anti-apoptosis effect and not cell proliferation. Br J Canc 2000;82:1553—6.

[4] Berndt S, Blacher S, Munuat C, Detilleux J, Evain-Brion D, Noel A, Fournier T, Foidart JM. Hyperglycosylated human chorionic gonadotropin stimulates angiogenesis through TGF-ß receptor activation. FASEB J 2013;12:213686.

[5] Ahmud F, Ghosh S, Sinha S, Joshi SD, Mehta VS, Sen E. TGF-ß-induced hCG-ß regulates redox homeostasis in glioma cells. Mol Cell Biochem 2015;399:105—12.

[6] Wu H, Lusbader JW, Yee L, Canfield RE, Hendrickson WA. Structure of human chorionic gonadotropin at 2.6Å resolution from MAD analysis of the selenmethionyl protein. Structure 1994;2:545—58.

[7] Lapthorn AJ, Harris DC, Littlejohn A, Lustbader JW, Canfield RE, Machin KJ, Morgan FJ, Isaacs NW. Crystal structure of human chorionic gonadotropin. Nature 1994;369:455—62.

[8] Lustbader JW, Yarmush DL, Birken S, Puett D, Canfield R. The application of chemical studies of human chorionic gonadotropin to visualize is three-dimensional structure. Endocr Rev 2013;14:291—310.

[9] Cole LA. The minute structural difference between the hormone hCG and the autocrine hyperglycosylated hCG. J Glycobiol 2017;6:1000127.

[10] Elliott MM, Kardana A, Lustbader JW, Cole LA. Carbohydrate and Peptide structure of the α- and ß-subunits of human chorionic gonadotropin from normal and aberrant pregnancy and choriocarcinoma. Endocr J 1997;7:15—32.

[11] Kolahi KS, Valent AM, Thornburg K. Cytotrophoblast, not syncytiotrophoblast, dominates glycolysis and oxidative phosphorylation in human term placenta. Sci Rep 2017; 7:42941. https://doi.org/10.1038/srep42941.

[12] Gaster M, Huppertz B. Fusion of cytotrophoblast with syncytiotrophoblast in human placenta: factors involved with synctialization. J Reproduktionsmed Endocrinol 2008; 5:76—82.

[13] Tarrade A, Kuen RL, Malassiné A, Tricottet V, Blain P, Vidaud M, Evain-Brion D. Characterization of human villous and extravillous trophoblasts isolated from first trimester placenta. Lab Investig 2001;81:1199—211.

[14] Handwerger S. New insights into the regulation of human cytotrophoblast cell differentiation. Mol Cell Endocrinol 2010;323:94—104.

[15] Cole LA. Biological function of hCG and hCG-related molecules. Reprod Biol Endocrinol 2010;8:102—16.

[16] Norman RJ, Buchholz MM, Somogyi AA, Amato F. hCGβ core fragment is a metabolite of hCG: evidence from infusion of recombinant hCG. J Endocrinol 2000;164:299—305.

[17] Birken S, Armstrong EG, Kolks MAG, Cole LA, Agosto GM, Krichevsky A, Canfield RE. The structure of the human chorionic gonadotropin ß-subunit core fragment from pregnancy urine. Endocrinology 1988;123:572—83.

[18] Cole LA, Khanlian SA, Kohorn EI. Evolution of the human brain, chorionic gonadotropin and hemochorial implantation of the placenta: origins of pregnancy failures, preeclampsia and choriocarcinoma. J Reprod Med 2008;53:449—557.

[19] Cole LA. The evolution of the primate, hominid and human brain. Primatology 2015;4: 100124.

[20] Shi QJ, Lei ZM, Rao CV, Lin J. Novel role of human chorionic gonadotropin in differentiation of human cytotrophoblasts. Endocrinology 1993;132:387—95.

[21] Burton GJ, Jauniaux E, Watson A. Maternal arterial connections to the placental inter-villous space during the first trimester of human pregnancy: the Boyd collection revisited. Am J Obstet Gynecol 1999;181:718–24.

[22] Rao CV, Li X, Toth P, Lei ZM. Expression of epidermal growth factor, transforming growth factor-alpha and their common receptor genes in human umbilical cords. J Clin Endocrinol Metab 1995;80:1012–20.

[23] Järvelä IY, Ruokonen A, Tekay A. Effect of rising hCG levels on the human corpus luteum during early pregnancy. Human Reprod 2008;23:2775–81.

[24] Akoum A, Metz CN, Morin M. Marked increase in macrophage migration inhibitory factor synthesis and secretion in human endometrial cells in response to human chorionic gonadotropin hormone. J Clin Endocrinol Metab 2005;90:2904–10.

[25] Eta E, Ambrus G, Rao V. Direct regulation of human myometrial contractions by human chorionic gonadotropin. J Clin Endocrinol Metab 1994;79:1582–6.

[26] Cole LA. hCG attenuates hyperglycosylated hCG-driven growth and invasion. J Molec Oncol Res 2018;2:13–20.

[27] Cole LA. hCG and hyperglycosylated hCG, promoters of villous placenta and hemochorial placentation. In: Nicholson R, editor. Placenta: functions, development and disease. Nova Publishers; 2013. p. 155–66. Nova Publishers.

[28] Sasaki Y, Ladner DG. Cole LA Hyperglycosylated hCG the source of pregnancy failures. Fertil Steril 2008;89. 1871-1786.

[29] Cole LA. The autocrines hyperglycosylated hCG and extravillous cytotrophoblast hCG and the hormone hCG all together control pregnancy implantation. Clin Chim Acta 2009 (in press).

[30] Cole LA. Menstrual cycle hCG. Am J Obstet Gynecol 2019 (in press).

My journey with human chorionic gonadotropin: development of a unique vaccine for control of fertility

3.7

G.P. Talwar

Introduction

Human chorionic gonadotropin (hCG) is not normally made by any organ of women (or men) and emerges only after fertilization of the egg and its development as an embryo. An in vitro fertilized egg, cultured till blastocyst stage, renders the medium positive for hCG as reported by Bob Edwards [1]. The presence of hCG in blood is a standard test for diagnosis of pregnancy implying that normal nonpregnant women do not make it. John Hearn et al. [2] observed that marmoset embryos exposed to anti-hCG antibodies fail to implant, whereas the same exposed to globulins from a nonimmunized animal implant perfectly. The fact that hCG is made only after fertilization of the egg and has presumably a crucial role in implantation of the embryo leading to pregnancy was the rationale for choice of hCG as a target for immunological intervention. It was also expected that inducing antibodies against hCG would not create cross-reaction with other organs of the body and would have no side effects.

Structure of hCG

hCG is composed of two subunits, α and β. α-Subunit of hCG is identical to the α-subunits of three other pituitary hormones, TSH, FSH, and LH. It is the β-subunit which imparts identity to these hormones and is presumably responsible for their diverse biological actions. The structures of α- and β-subunits of hCG and the way they are linked have been described [3]. Fig. 3.7.1 shows the structure of hCG and its subunits.

100 Years of Human Chorionic Gonadotropin. https://doi.org/10.1016/B978-0-12-820050-6.00019-9

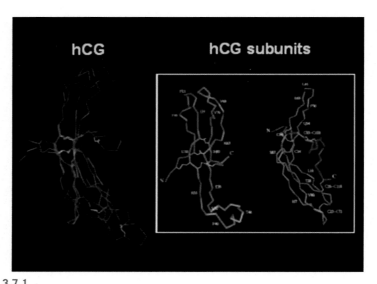

FIGURE 3.7.1

Structures of hCG and its α- and β-subunits [3].

The amino acid sequence of these hormones is known. The β-subunit of hCG is 145 amino acids long, the terminal 35 amino are additional to those present in β-hLH. Being given that the β subunit of hCG distinguishes hCG from three other pituitary hormones, it was logical to design the anti-hCG vaccine employing its β subunit. This was linked to a carrier to make it immunogenic. Originally tetanus toxoid was chosen as the carrier for two reasons. It was an approved vaccine made by industry and is available at low price. Furthermore, it provides protection against tetanus from which several deaths took place in rural parts of India in 1970s (at present government has introduced compulsory immunization of all children with DPT in schools). Linking β-hCG with TT (tetanus toxoid) was expected to induce antibodies against both hCG and TT. This was indeed the case. Four women volunteered to get immunized with β hCG- T vaccine initially made by us. All of them formed antibodies not only against tetanus but also against hCG [4]. Fig. 3.7.2 shows the typical response in a woman.

It was further necessary to see whether the antibodies induced against hCG by βhCG-TT recognized and bound the whole hormone, hCG. This was indeed the case. Injection of 2000 IU of hCG followed by 4000 IU as also a bulk dose of 5000 IU of hCG led to a drop of anti-hCG antibody titers, which returned in course of time to original antibody titers before these challenges (Fig. 3.7.3). The antitetanus titers remained unchanged indicating that the vaccine β-hCG-TT induces two independent sets of antibodies against both hCG and tetanus.

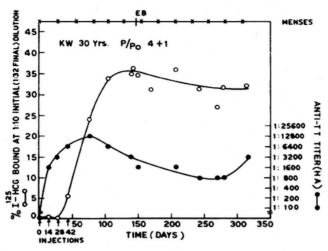

FIGURE 3.7.2

Kinetics of antibody titers against hCG and tetanus in a woman KW 30 years old with four children and one termination of pregnancy. ×× at the upper abscissa indicates the menstruation days, which remained regular postimmunization [4].

Safety

Extensive toxicology and safety studies were carried out in rodents and rhesus monkeys with the βhCG-TT vaccine indicating its safety and lack of any side effects in recipients. An entire issue of *Contraception* 1976 is devoted to these studies.

Vaccine employing carboxy terminal peptides of hCG

The β-subunit of hCG is composed of 145 amino acids with a unique carboxy terminal sequence (CTP) of 35 amino acids not present in β-hLH. It was logical to inquire whether the vaccine against CTP should not be used as a better and safer vaccine than the one employing the entire β subunit of hCG. The CTP vaccine had poor antigenicity and required the use of strong adjuvants, often adding to toxicity. What was amazing was that antibodies generated by the 35 amino acids CTP were no doubt non-cross-reactive with hLH, but had an unexpected cross-reaction with the human pancreatic cells and pituitary as observed by Noel Rose et al. at Johns Hopkins [6]. Furthermore, Louvet et al. [7] in Canfield's Laboratory reported that the sera against the unique structure region of β-hCG though totally devoid of cross-reaction with hLH had no neutralizing effect on hCG. We experimented also with the peptides comprising terminal 45 and 53 amino acids [8,9]. These peptides

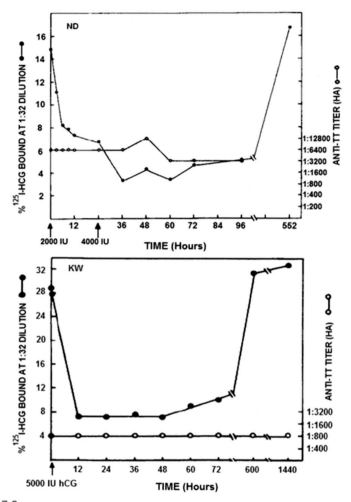

FIGURE 3.7.3

Injection of one or two lots of hCG caused a temporary drop in anti-hCG antibody titers, which return to original level in course of time, the antitetanus remained at the same level indicating that the vaccine generated independent antibodies against both hCG and tetanus [4,5].

induced non-hLH reactive antibodies. Their immunogenicity as compared with the vaccine employing the terminal 35 amino acids peptide was improved but still not attained enough immunogenicity, and the antibodies induced were not of as high affinity for hCG, as those induced by the entire β-subunit.

Are there any serious consequences of partial cross-reactivity with hLH?

Population Council Laboratory, Rockefeller University, carried out extensive toxicology studies on the long-term effects, if any, on pituitary of monkeys immunized with β-oLH along with Freund's complete adjuvant. In spite of the sustained LH-reactive high antibodies, no adverse effect was observed on pituitary functions and histology [10]. Noel Rose et al. also reported the complete safety of our anti-hCG vaccine in primates [6].

The International Committee on Contraception Research (ICCR) of Population Council carried out immunogenicity and safety studies on βhCG-TT vaccine in women in Finland, Sweden, Chile, and Brazil, confirming our observations [11] on the trials conducted in India [4]. Immunization against hCG with partially cross-reactive antibodies with hLH neither impaired ovulation nor induced any observable side effects on body functions. What was needed now was further improvement in immunogenicity of the vaccine without recourse to strong adjuvants.

Heterospecies dimer

The ability of β-subunit of hCG to associate with α-subunit of gonadotropins is preserved across species. β hCG can readily combine with α-subunit of ovine LH generating a dimer HSD. HSD coupled with TT generates higher titers of anti-hCG antibodies with improved bioneutralization capacity as shown by data in Table 3.7.1.

Linking of HSD to diphtheria toxoid

It was noticed that repeated immunization with β-hCG or HSD linked to tetanus toxoid as carrier led to a stage of nonresponsiveness for inducing anti-hCG antibodies [13]. This lack of responsiveness could be overcome by presenting β-hCG or HSD linked to an alternate carrier such as diphtheria toxoid (DT).

Back to clinical trials

After having confirmed by trials in women in India, Finland, Sweden, Chile, and Brazil, the ability of β hCG linked to a carrier to generate antibodies against hCG, as well as its safety and reversibility, it was time to evaluate whether HSD-TT/DT vaccine elicited higher antibody titers in women without compromising safety and reversibility. Approvals were obtained from Institutional Ethics Committees and the Drugs Controller General of India (DCGI) to conduct Phase I followed

Table 3.7.1 hCG binding and neutralization capacity of anti-βhCG-TT or β hCG-cholera toxin B subunit (CHB) vaccines and anti-HSD-TT antisera generated in bonnet monkeys and rats [12].

Immunogen	No. of animals	hCG binding capacity (pg/mL) (I) (mean ± standard error of mean)	hCG neutralization capacity (pg/mL) (B) (mean ± standard error of mean)	B/Ix100
Bonnet monkeys				
βhCG-TT/ CHB	5	22.2 + 2.3	10.1 + 1.8	44 + 3.7
HSD-TT/ CHB	5	21.4 + 1.9	14.0 + 1.4	65 + 1.9
Rats				
βhCG-TT/ CHB	6	27.1 + 1.7	17.1 + 1.2	63 + 1.5
HSD-TT/ CHB	6	32.5 + 1.4	26.1 + 0.8	80 + 2.3

by Phase II clinical trials. The Phase I studies are reported in two papers published in *Contraception* 1990 [14,15]. The vaccine indeed induced higher antibody response. It was reversible and fully safe.

Historical phase II efficacy trials

The crucial question now was whether this vaccine inducing antibodies against hCG was indeed competent to prevent pregnancy in sexually active women. 148 women of reproductive age, who had given birth to at least two children, were enrolled for trial at three institutions: the All India Institute of Medical Sciences, Safdarjung Hospital, New Delhi and the Post Graduate Institute of Medical Education and Research, Chandigarh. They were required to have an IUD fitted until their antibody titers were sufficiently high and remained above 50 ng/mL for at least 3 months. While all women generated antibodies, 110 of them had titers above the putative threshold of 50 ng/mL for 3 months or longer. IUDs were taken out in these women, and they were exposed to pregnancy. Fig. 3.7.4 shows the typical observation in four women [16].

Antibodies appeared after three primary injections. Boosters were given as and when required to keep the antibody titers well above the putative threshold of 50 ng/mL. All of them remained protected from becoming pregnant for periods ranging from 26 to 32 cycles. They continued to menstruate and their menstrual

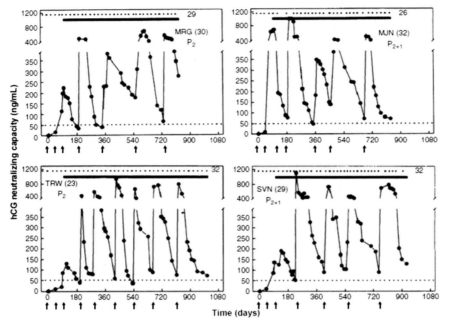

FIGURE 3.7.4

Anti-hCG response to the HSD vaccine in four sexually active women of proven fertility. MRG 30 year old and TRW 23 year old had two children each; MJN 32 year and SVN 29 year old had two children each and one elective termination of pregnancy. All of them remained protected from becoming pregnant over 26–32 cycles (……), at top edge represent the menstrual events which remained regular, solid lines denote the period over which they were exposed to pregnancy. Arrows indicate the day on which vaccine was given. Booster injections were given to keep antibody titers above 50 ng/mL [16].

cycles represented by dots …….. in the figure were regular. No one experienced extra bleeding. Their luteal phase progesterone was sufficiently high, indicating that they were ovulating normally and could conceive readily on decline of antibody titers in the absence of boosters.

The vaccine was highly effective. Only one pregnancy took place in 1224 cycles. The menstrual cycles of all immunized women remained regular, and the women kept on ovulating as gauged by luteal progesterone. Eight women completed 30 cycles without becoming pregnant, 9 were protected over 24–29 cycles, 12 for 18–23 cycles, 15 for 12–17 cycles, and 21 for 6–11 cycles. When we informed the women that we have to close the trial for analysis and report our findings, several women offered to pay for the vaccine to continue.

Reversibility and regain of fertility

During the trial, four women expressed the desire to have a child. No booster immunization was given to these women, and the antibody titers returned to near zero level in course of time. All of them became pregnant to bear another child.

Fig. 3.7.5 represents a woman who was protected for nearly a year after immunization with the vaccine. By not taking booster immunization, the titers came down, and in the immediate cycle when antibody titers came below 20 ng/mL, she conceived and gave birth to a normal infant.

Normalcy of children born to previously immunized women

Prof. Meharban Singh at the All India Institute of Medical Sciences, New Delhi, carried out an analysis of children born to the four women who were protected by the vaccine above 50 ng/mL titers, but on decline of antibody titers in absence of boosters, they conceived. Their progeny born was adjudged normal with respect to developmental landmarks and cognitive abilities of their siblings [17].

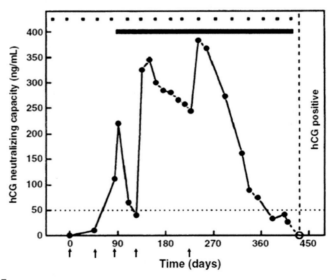

FIGURE 3.7.5

Regain of fertility on decline of antibodies. A 30-year-old subject (STS), with two gravidae and one elective abortion (P2+1), on immunization with the vaccine, remained protected from pregnancy for 12 cycles. In the absence of a booster injection, antibody titers declined and she became pregnant in the cycle starting on day 417. The extrapolated antibody titers at midcycle in the fertile month, shown by the dotted line, were <5 ng/mL. Arrows indicate the day on which vaccine was given [16].

Revival of the vaccine against hCG

I retired in 1994 from the Directorship of the National Institute of Immunology (NII), New Delhi, India. On request of my successor, the vaccine was left at NII. Nothing happened for 12 years. In 2006, at the initiative of the Indo-US Committee on Contraception Research, I got a grant to revive the vaccine. We thought of developing a genetically engineered recombinant vaccine so that it should be amenable to industrial production. The β-subunit of hCG was linked to B-subunit of heat-labile enterotoxin (LTB) of *Escherichia coli* as carrier (Fig. 3.7.6).

The carrier chosen this time does not evoke carrier-induced-immunosuppression which TT as carrier did on repeated use for long periods [18]. The fact that the suppression of immune response was carrier induced was confirmed by presenting hCGβ on an alternate carrier DT [13]. The B subunit of enterotoxin did not have these disadvantages. LTB has further adjuvant properties and evokes also mucosal response. Keeping all these properties in mind, the previous carriers TT and DT were abandoned and replaced by LTB.

hCGβ-LTB vaccine adsorbed on alhydrogel given along with autoclaved *Mycobacterium indicus pranii* (MIP formerly known as Mw), a vaccine which we had developed originally against leprosy [19] was found to be a potent potentiator of humoral and cell-mediated immune responses [20]. MiP is approved by the Drugs

TCC AAG GAC CCG CTT CGG CCA CGG TGC CGC CCC ATC AAT GCC ACC CTG GCT GTG GAG AAG
GAG GGC TGC CCC GTG TGC ATC ACC GTC AAC ACC ACC ATC TGT GCC GGC TAC TGC CCC ACC
ATG ACC CGC GTG CTG CAG GGG GTC CTG CCG GCC CTG CCT CAG GTG GTG TGC AAC TAC CGC
GAT GTG CGC TTC GAG TCC ATC CGG CTC CCT GGC TGC CCG CGC GGC GTG AAC CCC GTG GTC
TCC TAC GCC GTG GCT CTC AGC TGT CAA TGT GCA CTC TGC CGC CGC AGC ACC ACT GAC TGC
GGG GGT CCC AAG GAC CAC CCC TTG ACC TGT GAT GAC CCC CGC TTC CAG GAC TCC TCT TCC
TCA AAG GCC CCT CCC CCC AGC CTT CCA AGC CCA TCC CAA CTC CCG GGG CCC TCG GAC ACC
CCG ATC CTC CCA CAA **GTCTAGAA** GGA GCT CCT CAG TCT ATT ACA GAA CTA TGT TCG GAA TAT
CAC AAC ACA CAA ATA TAT ACG ATA AAT GAC AAG ATA CTA TCA TAT ACG GAA TCG ATG GCA
GGC AAA AGA GAA ATG GTT ATC ATT ACA TTT AAG AGC GGC GCA ACA TTT CAG GTC GAA GTC
CCG GGC AGT CAA CAT ATA GAC TCC CAA AAA AAA GCC ATT GAA AGG ATG AAG GAC ACA TTA
AGA ATC ACA TAT CTG ACC GAG ACC AAA ATT GAT AAA TTA TGT GTA TGG AAT AAA ACC CCC
AAT TCA ATT GCG GCA ATC AGT ATG GAA AAC TAG

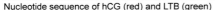
Nucleotide sequence of hCG (red) and LTB (green)

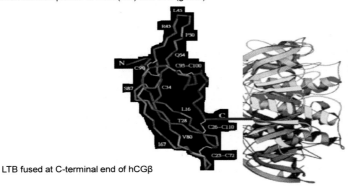
LTB fused at C-terminal end of hCGβ

FIGURE 3.7.6

Conceptualized structure of hCGβ-LTB vaccine. The carrier B chain of heat labile enterotoxin of *Escherichia coli* (LTB) is fused at C-terminal glutamine of hCGβ.

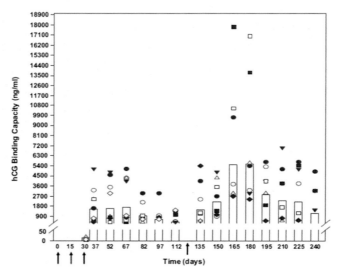

FIGURE 3.7.7

Antibody titers in Balb/C mice immunized with hCGβ-LTB. Titers in each mouse are represented by different symbols. Bar represents the geometric means at various times following immunization [21].

Controller General of India as well as by US FDA. It is licensed to a company and is available to public.

Fig. 3.7.7 shows antibody response to hCGβ-LTB vaccine in Balb/C mice [21]. Hundred percent of mice receiving the vaccine responded with formation of anti-hCG antibodies. The antibody titers went up to 5500 ng/mL in most of the mice and even higher up to 18,000 ng/mL in some mice. The titers remained well above 50 ng/mL for more than 3 months. Booster immunization resulted in high boosted response to the vaccine.

It is well established that immune response varies from individual to individual. Our initial studies were in Balb/C mice, in which the vaccine hCGβ-LTB was highly immunogenic. It was considered necessary to determine its immunogenicity in mice of other genetic strains. Thus studies were carried out in four other defined strains of mice namely FVB, C57Bl/6, SJL, and C3H. The vaccine-generated antibodies in all these strains of mice, although the titers varied [20].

Recombinant DNA and protein vaccines

Recombinant vaccines are expressed as both DNA and proteins. The DNA version is cheaper to make and is thermostable, thereby not requiring the "cold chain" for transportation and preservation. A large number of studies have been done on development of DNA vaccines [22–25]. However, a few DNA vaccines have succeeded in becoming DNA vaccines for human use [24–26].

We tried to determine whether priming of immune response with the DNA vaccine followed by protein version would be useful for immunization. It may be recalled that hCG vaccine demands on initial vaccination three primary immunizations to induce antibodies. On giving two of these primary injections with the DNA version of the vaccine followed by the protein version of the vaccine as third primary injection resulted in a distinctly elevated immune response to hCG [27]. Fig. 3.7.8A shows the antibody response to hCGβ-LTB vaccine along with MIP in Balb/C mice used for all three primary injections of the protein form of the vaccine, and Fig. 3.7.8B shows results where the first two injections were given with DNA vaccine followed by third primary injection with protein form of the vaccine. It would be observed that priming with DNA form of the vaccine followed by proteinic form elicits a higher antibody response in Balb/C mice than the one engendered by all three primary immunizations given with the protein form of the vaccine.

Approval of the recombinant vaccine by Review Committee on Genetic Manipulation (RCGM), is mandatory, as all products made by genetic engineering have to seek approval of this committee for further use. Accordingly, the entire data on the making of hCGβ-LTB as a recombinant vaccine, as also on its purification, physicochemical attributes, and immunogenicity were submitted to RCGM. After due deliberations, hCGβ-LTB received the approval of RCGM. RCGM asked us to carry out preclinical toxicology studies in two species of rodents on an international protocol conducted by a GLP Company. In addition, we considered it appropriate to conduct safety, immunogenicity, and efficacy studies in a primate subhuman species, the marmosets, which were carried out at the National Institute of Research in Reproductive Health, Mumbai.

Preclinical toxicology studies
In rodents

Preclinical toxicology studies in rodents were contracted to M/s Bioneeds at their GLP Facility in Bangalore, India. Studies were based on Schedule "Y" guidelines on Drugs and Cosmetics, guidelines of Institutional Animal Ethics Committee (IAEC), and biosafety issues related to genetically modified organisms.

Both DNA and protein forms of the vaccine were nonsensitizing to the skin of guinea pigs and manifested no clinical signs of toxicity, mortality, and changes in body weight. Both vaccines were nonmutagenic at the highest concentration tested by Bacterial Reverse Mutation and Mammalian Chromosome Aberration Tests. Similar observation on nonmutagenic property of the vaccines was made in vivo by Mammalian Erythrocyte Micronucleus Test in mice.

Single dose acute toxicity study was conducted in Sprague Dawley rats. Vaccinated rats were observed for mortality, clinical signs of toxicity, body weight, and

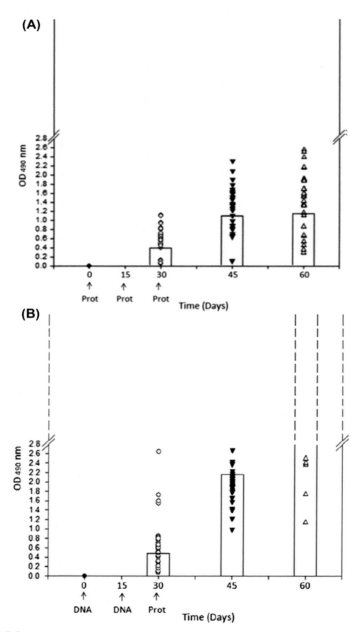

FIGURE 3.7.8

Effect of DNA priming on antibody titers in Balb/C mice. (A) Anti-hCG antibodies after three injections of protein form of the vaccine administered intramuscularly. (B) Anti-hCG antibodies titers in mice primed twice with DNA form of the recombinant hCGβ-LTB

gross pathological examination. No mortality, clinical signs of toxicity, and treatment-related changes in the body weight were observed. No changes in gross pathology (external and internal) were observed at even the highest dose tested. Repeat doses of the vaccines were also tested in rats, which were followed up to 90 days postimmunization. These studies showed no treatment-related changes in physical, physiological, clinical, hematological parameters, as also in histopathology profiles of the organs. Segment II studies conducted in rats showed that vaccines did not affect the embryo-fetal development. Body weight, food consumption, gross pathology remained normal, and no abnormal effect was observed in fetal sex ratio, fetal weight, external, visceral, and skeletal norms of fetuses.

In marmosets

Preclinical toxicology and safety studies in marmosets were carried out at the National Institute for Research in Reproductive Health, Mumbai, where alone marmoset colony is bred and maintained in India.

Studies were carried out in nine marmosets at three different doses. Two nonimmunized marmosets formed the control group. Active immunization of normal fertile females by the combination of DNA and protein vaccines did not show any adverse effect on the body weight or general activity. Profiles of steroid hormones, biochemical, and hematological parameters also remained similar to those of nonvaccinated animals. Vaccinated female marmosets did not become pregnant on cohabitation with normal male fertile marmosets, thus demonstrating the efficacy of hCGβ-LTB to prevent pregnancy in this primate.

Thus preclinical toxicology studies on the hCGβ-LTB vaccine in two species of rodents and a subhuman primate species, the marmosets, demonstrated the total safety of the recombinant hCGβ-LTB vaccine. RCGM reviewed and approved the preclinical toxicology data and forwarded its recommendation to the Drugs Controller General of India to grant permission for conduct of trials in women. A clinical trial protocol has been developed by an expert committee of the Indian Council of Medical Research. Permission has been granted by the DCGI for conducting the trials. Clinical studies will be carried out to determine the immunogenicity and safety of the recombinant vaccine in 50 women, 10 each at protein vaccine doses of 100, 200, 300, 400, and 500 µg after priming twice with the DNA version of the vaccine. From this part of the trial, the dose of the recombinant vaccine having the optimal immunogenicity will be chosen. This part of the trial

---

vaccine followed by the third injection with protein form of the vaccine. Symbols represent the individual values, while bar gives the geometric mean at various time points postimmunization. On day 60, the antibody titers in 35 out of 40 mice were higher than the scale [27].

would also confirm the safety of the recombinant vaccine. Part II of the trial would test the efficacy of the vaccine in 75 women.

During this time, the technology was been transferred to M/s Bharat Biotech, Hyderabad, India, for making the DNA and protein versions of the recombinant vaccine under GMP conditions, which will be employed for the clinical trials to be conducted under the auspices of the Indian Council of Medical Research.

Additional possible utility of anti-hCG vaccine

Our vaccine also gave interesting results in hCGβ expressing transgenic mice developed by Susana Rulli at the Instituto de Biologia y Medicina Experimental, Buenos Aires, Argentina (as discussed in Chapter 3.4). The female transgenic mice developed pituitary hypertrophy and mammary tumors over and above ovarian dysfunction [28]. Figs. 3.7.9 and 3.7.10 show that immunization of these transgenic hCGβ mice with our recombinant hCGβ-LTB vaccine prevented them from becoming obese. They do not develop insulin resistance and various other abnormalities [29]. Their life span became longer after immunization with hCGβ-LTB vaccine.

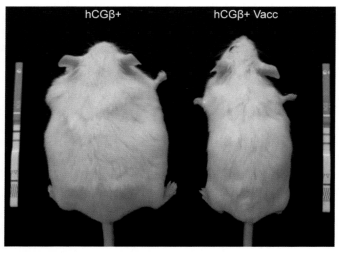

FIGURE 3.7.9

Physical appearance of a hCGβ transgenic mouse immunized with anti-hCG vaccine and control of the same age [29].

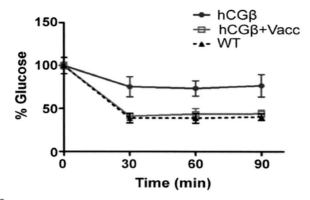

FIGURE 3.7.10

Insulin tolerance test in transgenic hCGβ mice and in those immunized with anti-hCG vaccine at 9 months of age ($P < .05$). Also given is the response in normal nontransgenic mice (WT) [29].

Summary

Briefly described herein is the long journey for devising a vaccine that is both safe and competent to prevent unwanted pregnancy in sexually active women. Starting from hCGβ-TT, we graduated to a heterospecies dimer consisting of hCGβ associated with α-subunit of ovine LH linked preferably to DT (Diphtheria toxoid). The historic Phase II trials on this vaccine showed not only safety and reversibility of the vaccine but also its ability to prevent pregnancy in sexually active women without derangement of regularity of menstrual cycles and hormonal profiles. Women continued to ovulate normally and remained protected at above 50 ng/mL antibody titers.

Women could conceive on antibody titers going below 20 ng/mL. Children born to such women were normal in their developmental landmarks and cognitive abilities with respect to their siblings.

In order to make this vaccine amenable to large-scale industrial production, it has been converted into a recombinant vaccine. Extensive preclinical safety studies were completed in two species of rodents and a subhuman primate species, the marmosets, which demonstrated total safety of the recombinant hCGβ-LTB vaccine. Approval of the recombinant vaccine has been obtained from the National Review Committee on Genetic Manipulations (RCGM). Also approval of the Drugs Controller General of India (DCGI) and Ethics Committees has been given for proceeding to clinical trial on a combined Phase I/II protocol.

Immunization of hCGβ transgenic mice with the recombinant hCGβ-LTB vaccine prevents obesity and their becoming insulin resistant.

References

[1] Fishel SB, Edwards RG, Evans CJ. Human chorionic gonadotropin secreted by preimplantation embryos cultured in vitro. Science 1984;223:816–8.

[2] Hearn JP, Gidley-Baird AA, Hodges JK, Summers PM, Webley GE. Embryonic signals during the peri-implantation period in primates. J Reprod Fertil Suppl 1988;36:49–58.

[3] Lapthorn AJ, Harris DC, Littlejohn A, Lustbader JW, Canfield RE, Machin KJ, et al. Crystal structure of human chorionic gonadotropin. Nature 1994;369:455–61.

[4] Talwar GP, Sharma NC, Dubey SK, Salahuddin M, Das C, Ramakrishnan S, et al. Isoimmunisation against human chorionic gonadotropin with conjugates of processed β-subunit of the hormone and tetanus toxoid. Proc Natl Acad Sci USA 1976;73:218–22.

[5] Talwar GP, Dubey SK, Salahuddin M, Das C. Antibody response to Pr-beta-HCG-TT vaccine in human subjects. Contraception 1976;13:237–43.

[6] Rose NR, Burek CL, Smith JP. Safety evaluation of hCG vaccine in primates: auto antibody production. In: Talwar GP, editor. Contraception Research for today and nineties. New York): Springer-Verlag; 1988. p. 231–9.

[7] Louvet JP, Ross GT, Birken S, Canfield RE. Absence of neutralizing effect of antisera to the unique structural region of human chorionic gonadotropin. J Clin Endocrinol Metab 1974;39:1155–8.

[8] Ramakrishnan S, Das C, Dubey SK, Salahuddin M, Talwar GP. Immunogenicity of three C-terminal synthetic peptides of beta subunit of human chorionic gonadotropin and properties of the antibodies raised against 45-amino acid C-terminal peptide. J Reprod Immunol 1979;1:249–61.

[9] Sahal D, Ramakrishnan S, Iyer KSN, Das C, Talwar GP. Immunological properties of a carboxy-terminal 53-amino acid peptide of the beta subunit of human chorionic gonadotropin. J Reprod Immunol 1982;4:145–56.

[10] Thau RB, Wilson CB, Sundaram K, Phillips D, Donelly T, Halmi NS, Bardin CW. Long-term immunization against beta subunit of ovine luteinizing hormone has no adverse effect on pituitary functions in rhesus monkeys. Am J Reprod Immunol Microbiol 1987;15:92–8.

[11] Nash H, Johansson ED, Talwar GP, Vasquez J, Segal S, Coutinho E, Luukkainen T, Sundaram K. Observations on the antigenicity and clinical effects of a candidate antipregnancy vaccine: beta-subunit of human chorionic gonadotropin linked to tetanus toxoid. Fertil Steril 1980;34:328–35.

[12] Talwar GP, Singh O, Rao LV. An improved immunogen for anti-human chorionic gonadotropin vaccine elicited antibodies reactive with a conformation native to the hormone without cross-reaction with human follicle stimulating hormone and human thyroid stimulating hormone. J Reprod Immunol 1988;14:203–12.

[13] Gaur A, Arunan K, Talwar GP. Bypass by an alternate carrier of acquired unresponsiveness to hCG upon repeated immunization with tetanus conjugated vaccine. Int Immunol 1990;2:151–5.

[14] Kharat I, Nair NS, Dhall K, Sawhney H, Krishna U, Krishna SM, Bannerjee AK, et al. Analysis of menstrual records of women immunized with anti-hCG vaccines inducing antibodies partially cross-reactive with hLH. Contraception 1990;41:293–9.

[15] Talwar GP, Hingorani V, Kumar S, Bannerjee AK, Shahani SM, Krishna U, et al. Phase I clinical trials with three formulations of anti-human gonadotropin vaccine. Contraception 1990;41:301−16.

[16] Talwar GP, Singh O, Pal R, Chatterjee N, Sahai P, Dhall K, et al. A vaccine that prevents pregnancy in women. Proc Natl Acad Sci USA 1994;91:8532−6.

[17] Singh M, Das SK, Suri S, Singh O, Talwar GP. Regain of fertility and normality of progeny born during below protective threshold antibody titres in women immunized with HSD-hCG vaccine. Am J Reprod Immunol 1998;39:195−8.

[18] Kaliyaperumal A, Chauhan VS, Talwar GP, Raghupathy R. Carrier-induced epitope-specific regulation and its bypass in a protein-protein conjugate. Eur J Immunol 1995;25:3375−80.

[19] Talwar GP. An immunotherapeutic vaccine for multibacillary leprosy. Int Rev Immunol 1999;18:229−49.

[20] Purswani S, Talwar GP, Vohra R, Pal R, Panda AK, Lohiya NK, Gupta JC. *Mycobacterium indicus pranii* is a potent immunomodulator for a recombinant vaccine against human chorionic gonadotropin. J Reprod Immunol 2011;91:24−30.

[21] Purswani S, Talwar GP. Development of a highly immunogenic recombinant candidate vaccine against human chorionic gonadotropin. Vaccine 2011;29:2341−8.

[22] Fioretti D, Lurescia S, Fazio VM, Monica RM. DNA vaccines: developing new strategies with cancer. J Biomed Biotechnol, Volume 2010: Article ID 174378.

[23] Pereira V, Turk MZ, Saraiva T, De Castro C, Souza B, Mancha Agresti P, Lima F, Pfeiffer V, Azevedo M, Rocha C, Pontes D, Azevedo V, Miyoshi A. DNA vaccines approach: from concepts to applications. World J Vaccines 2014;4:50−71.

[24] Wang S, Kennedy JS, West K, Montefiori DC, Coley S, Lawrence J, Shen S, Green S, Rothman AL, Ennis FA, Arthos J, Pal R, Markham P, Lu S. Cross-subtype antibody and cellular immune responses induced by a polyvalent DNA prime-protein boost HIV-1 vaccine in healthy human volunteers. Vaccine 2008;26:1098−110.

[25] Trimble CL, Peng S, Kos F, Gravitt P, Viscidi R, Sugar E, Pardoll D, Wu TC. A phase I trial of a human papillomavirus DNA vaccine for HPV16 + cervical intraepithelial neoplasia 2/3. Clin Cancer Res 2009;15:361−7.

[26] Okuda K, Wada Y, Shimada M. Recent developments in preclinical DNA vaccination. Vaccine 2014;2:89−106.

[27] Nand KN, Gupta J, Panda AK, Jain SK, Talwar GP. Priming with DNA enhances considerably the immunogenicity of hCGβ − LTB vaccine. Am J Reprod Immunol 2015;74:302−8.

[28] Rulli SB, Kuorelahti A, Karaer O, Pelliniemi LJ, Poutanen M. Reproductive disturbances, pituitary lactotrope adenomas, and mammary gland tumors in transgenic female mice producing high levels of human chorionic gonadotropin. Endocrinology 2002;143(10):4084−95.

[29] Talwar GP, Rulli SB, Vyas HK, Purswani S, Kabeer RS, Chopra P, Singh P, Atrey N, Nand KN, Gupta JC. Making of a unique Birth Control Vaccine against hCG with additional potential of therapy of advanced stage cancers and prevention of obesity and insulin resistance. J Cell Sci Ther 2014;5(2):1000159.

Evaluation of delivery systems for active immunization with synthetic peptides of hCG as a fertility control method: A collection of study data and discussion by the World Health Organization task force on the Regulation of Human Reproduction 1999–2007

3.8

Vernon C. Stevens, Stephen A. Butler

Preface by Dr. Stevens

Beginning in 1973, the Task Force on the Regulation of Human Reproduction began research to develop a vaccine against human chorionic gonadotropin (hCG) for the purpose of preventing pregnancy. The vaccine would principally be used in the least developed countries of the world where fewer contraceptives are available for use by poor women. In the pages that follow, some of the research studies conducted to find a safe, effective, and acceptable method of delivering the vaccine to women in rural and in crowded urban settings are shown. Studies were conducted in animals to test the production of antibodies and the reactions at the injection site elicited from vaccine formulations delivered by various vehicles. All vaccine immunogens used in these studies employed synthetic peptides representing sequences in the β-subunits of hCG that were specific to the hormone. The peptides were always linked to a foreign peptide or protein in order to allow antibodies to be formed to hCG since injecting hCG peptides alone would not cause the woman's immune system to react to the "self" peptides of hCG. Various hCG peptides were used throughout the several years of vaccine development up to the point of anticipated clinical trials at the Karolinska Institute in Stockholm, Sweden. At this time, a delivery system for the latest version of the vaccine was found that met the criteria for use in a safe and effective antifertility product. The details of the testing of numerous vaccine delivery systems between 1999 and 2007 are presented here.

Background

Human chorionic gonadotropin represents an ideal target for designing vaccines for fertility control for two main reasons: the molecule is only produced in significant quantities during pregnancy in humans and that to remove the molecule from the circulation results in pregnancy loss. There have been several attempts to design hCG vaccines for both pregnancy prevention and as a cancer therapy agent. During the period between 1973 and 2007, the World Health Organization (WHO) set up a task force on the use of vaccines for regulating fertility in collaboration with Vernon Steven's group at the Ohio State University (OSU) Research Foundation in the United States.

The vaccine was a hCGβ CTP/DT conjugate

This particular vaccine was developed in 1975 and during the next decade was evaluated using various delivery systems at the OSU as a potential method which could be applied to fertility control. Until now, these data have remained unpublished and are reproduced here with permission from Professor Vernon Stevens and sanctioned by the WHO.

Evaluation of a new vaccine delivery system

As previously reported, a new particle delivery system was developed which involved the incorporation of hCG immunogens with an inorganic biopolymer composite. This delivery system acted by releasing the vaccine contents from the matrix of components at the appropriate delivery site. Early, the delivery formulation manufactured by Buford Biomedical Inc. in Frederick, MD and the hCGβ CTP/DT conjugate, prepared at OSU, had been incorporated into this composite and provided for testing along with supplies of a nor MDP adjuvant were also made available.

Previous studies indicated that immunization with the conjugate biopolymer particles which were suspended in an emulsion of ISA719 (provided by Seppic) and PBS containing nor MDP elicited a high level of antibodies with a sustained duration of at least 6 months.

Unfortunately, these encouraging initial results were offset by the observation that injection sites in the immunized rabbits showed an unacceptable level of muscle reactivity. Because of this, significant efforts followed to identify an alternative vehicle for particle delivery that gave similar high level antibody profiles without the muscle damage.

Testing aqueous vehicles

Initial attempts to identify a more suitable vehicle for particle delivery focused on aqueous nonemulsion media which contained nor MDP, interleukin-2, CRL1005 (Vaxcel), or aluminum salts. Some of these studies are shown in Fig. 3.8.1. Calcium alginate, Alhydrogel, polyethylene glycol or a suspension of glycolipids were all used to construct liposomes. Adjuvants such as normal MDP, CRL1005, or interleukin-2 and conjugates incorporated in liposomes as immunization vehicles resulted in a significant level of antibodies. In all cases, maximum antibody levels were less than 100 nM/L and any levels which were attained declined after 8—10 weeks. Interestingly, tissue reactions for all of these vehicles were minimal.

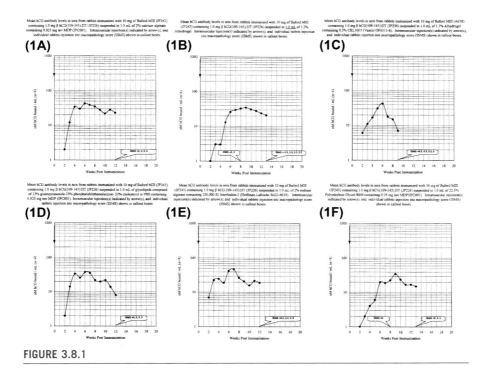

FIGURE 3.8.1

Testing coated particles

Earlier studies using a suspension of particles in the ISA719 emulsion produced excellent antibody levels but came with unacceptable muscle damage. In contrast, suspending particles in aqueous vehicles gave rise to minimal muscle damage but were inadequate for eliciting significant antibody levels. It was concluded that particles administered in the aqueous vehicle released the immunogen too rapidly to sustain a protracted immune response. A formulation with slower releasing properties was designed by coating the particles with polyethylene glycol.

These coated particles were compared with noncoated particles as well as the 719 emulsion and the aqueous vehicles. Adjuvant nor MDP was added to all vehicles. The results from these experiments are shown in Fig. 3.8.2.

As expected, the noncoated particles suspended in the 719 emulsion elicited an excellent antibody response profile which was comparable with those seen in the earlier studies shown in Fig. 3.8.2A. When the coated particles were mixed with the noncoated particles in the same vehicle, a slightly higher antibody response was seen and the levels were maintained for a longer duration (see Fig. 3.8.2B). In this experiment, muscle reactivity was elevated but only slightly as observed at the end of the study. It was suspected that if muscle damage had been evaluated during peak antibody levels, they would have been unacceptable, as seen previously, although there are no data to confirm this speculation.

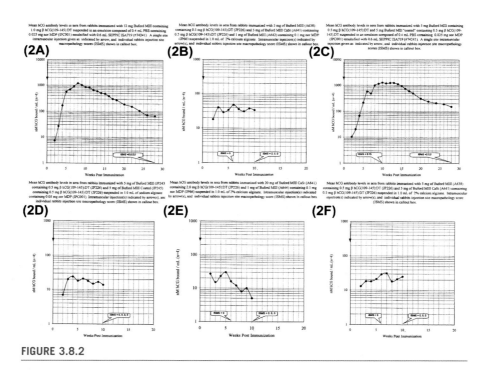

FIGURE 3.8.2

When the same particles when administered to rabbits in an aqueous vehicle, only very low levels of antibodies were attained in the animals as seen in Fig. 3.8.2C. Similar disappointing data were obtained when particles were coated in another material, calcium stearate, as shown in Fig. 3.8.2D–F. Thus, slowing down the rate of immunogen release, while improving the responses in 719 emulsion vehicle groups, did not improve the response to conjugate when the particles were given in aqueous vehicles.

The use of MDP particles as mixtures with conjugate particles

Another potential difference between the responses seen between 719 emulsion and the aqueous vehicle was that the adjuvant nor MDP was released slowly from the emulsion but free in the water of the aqueous vehicles. nor MDP is cleared very rapidly when administered in water, and if this could be slowed it was suggested that the responses to the immunogen may be improved. To test this hypothesis, nor MDP particles were prepared separately to conjugate particles, and together these two particles were coadministered in aqueous vehicles in various combinations. An alternative emulsion with no mannide monooleate was used instead of the 719 emulsifier to eliminate this as a potential cause of the unacceptable muscle reactions. The results of these combined studies are shown in Fig. 3.8.3.

As seen in Fig. 3.8.3A the response to the mixture of conjugate and nor MDP particles in a 719 emulsion (without adjuvant in the emulsion) elicited a typical profile of antibody levels, but even at the maximum, only about half of that found when the adjuvant was included in the emulsion, suggesting that the release rate of the nor MDP was not optimal. A very poor immune response resulted when the mixed particles were administered in 2% calcium alginate (Fig. 3.8.3B which was only slightly improved when spiking the vehicle with free conjugate and adjuvant (Fig. 3.8.3C). Furthermore, none of the emulsion formulations used to administer the mixture of adjuvant and conjugate particles, tested as potential alternatives to 719, elicited an improved antibody response over those of the aqueous vehicle formulations (Fig. 3.8.3D–G). In one of these experiments (Fig. 3.8.3E), a booster injection was given 3 months after the primary immunization to ascertain whether an additional depot of immunogen would result in a sustained elevation of antibodies. This was not the case. This observation further supported the conclusions that the particles released the immunogen too rapidly to elicit any significant immune response. One modification of the experiment used a 719 emulsion in which Tween 60 was added, but while responses were greater than those seen with other emulsions, this experiment still yielded a much lower response to that of the unmodified 719 emulsion (Fig. 3.8.3H).

Finally, the mixtures of adjuvant and conjugate particles were delivered using vehicles of a mixture of oils and surfactants without any aqueous components. These can be seen in Fig. 3.8.3I–M. None of these vehicles was more effective than an aqueous vehicle in eliciting antibody responses. A booster injection was given at 12 weeks in one of the oil formulations and the prompt elevation in antibody levels

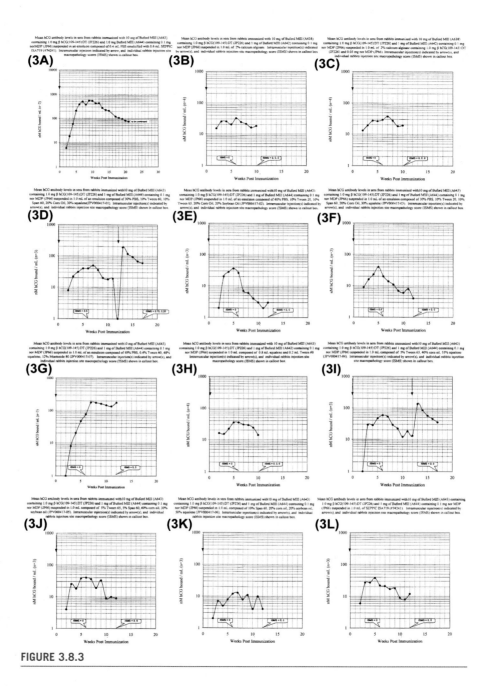

FIGURE 3.8.3

was observed. However, levels declined sharply shortly after the peak response (Fig. 3.8.3J). It is noteworthy that the oil phase of the 719 emulsion was ineffective in eliciting significant antibody levels when used alone as a vehicle (Fig. 3.8.3M).

Muscle reactions were minimal in animals from experiments using all of the formulations shown in Fig. 3.8.3.

Emulsions containing nor MDP

It was apparent from the initial experiments that the only effective vehicle tested to date was an emulsion containing nor MDP and that formulation (ISA 719/PBS) induced unacceptable muscle tissue damage. A series of other emulsions not containing mannide monooleate or, in most cases, no squalene, were tested as vehicles to deliver the particles containing the hCG immunogen. All new emulsions which were tested during these experiments contained nor MDP within the emulsion and also a control 719 emulsion with or without nor MDP. The data from these studies can be seen in Fig. 3.8.4.

Fig. 3.8.4A demonstrates the reproducibility of the excellent antibody profile elicited by delivering the immunogen and particles in a 719 emulsion containing nor MDP. In Fig. 3.8.4B, it can be seen that eliminating the nor MDP from the emulsion markedly reduces the immune response to the same dose of immunogen indicating its importance to the effective formulation. The importance of mannide monooleate to the response was tested by making and emulsion of it, called Montanide 80, with PBS containing either nor MDP or CRL1005 adjuvants (Fig. 3.8.4C and D). Only weak immune responses were induced from these immunizations, suggesting that the emulsifier in the 719 emulsion, by itself, is not capable of eliciting the desired antibody levels even when coadministered with potent adjuvant. Other emulsions containing monophosphate lipid A (MPL) (Ribi), squalene, corn oil, and various surfactants were also ineffective in inducing significant antibody levels when used at delivery vehicles (Fig. 3.8.4E–H). Interestingly, the stability of one of these emulsions was very good for more than 3 months at 25°in vitro and should an emulsion delivery be necessary for slowing immunogen release, this would provide a useful formulation. However, this was never the case and without further testing of the emulsion stability at 37 degrees, we could not conclude that the release of immunogen in vivo was slower than the ineffective aqueous vehicles. Within this series of experiments, oil-in-water vehicles were also tested. As with others tested here, the oil-in-water preparations, as expected, were not useful.

Testing reduced particle size

At the time of these studies, literature reports showed that the use of immunogens entrapped in nanospheres of polylactic and polyglycolic acids were very effective delivery systems for vaccines when administered in only PBS. A combination of these nanospheres with microspheres has been effective in stimulating antibody profiles lasting 1 year or more. While the release rates from these polymers were more controlled

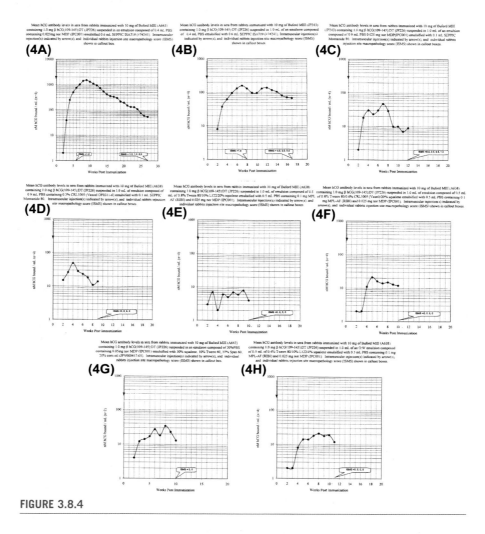

FIGURE 3.8.4

and possibly slower than the Buford composite used previously, it seemed worthwhile to attempt making a preparation of microparticles of the immunogen for testing.

The Gilson Company prepared particles for this study using one of their milling machines which would yield particles of 1−5 nm, as opposed to the 45−150 nM particles previously supplied by Buford. These particles were produced using a dry milling operation which caused particle clumping and potentially much larger particles in a batch. In addition, this dry process generated a lot of heat and the conjugate was exposed to temperatures exceeding 100°C. Despite these two potential problems, the conjugates produced into the smaller milled particles were tested in our model, and the results are shown in Fig. 3.8.5.

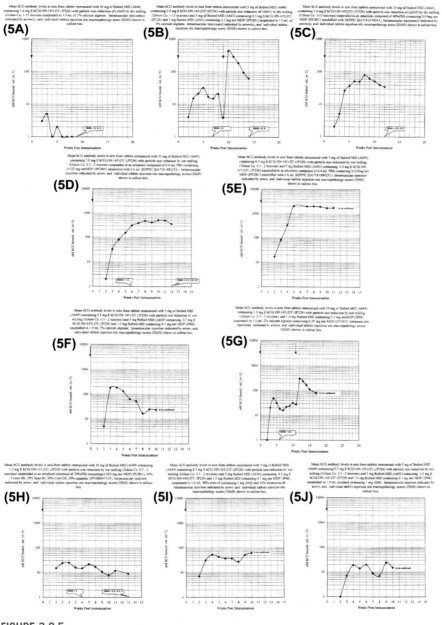

FIGURE 3.8.5

Fig. 3.8.5A shows the antibody levels elicited when the reduced size particles were given in an aqueous vehicle. A very weak response was observed. Fig. 3.8.5B shows the data from an experiment where the milled particles were mixed with unmilled particles in an aqueous vehicle. A slightly higher response was elicited but was far from useful. A booster injection was given at 9 weeks, which resulted in a significant rise in antibody levels. Unfortunately, this rise was followed by a rapid decline. These findings strongly suggest that the particles adequately prime the B-cell lymphocytes with the first immunization, but failed to sustain a supply of immunogen to expand the clones and maintain antibody production.

The controlled experiment for the study is shown in Fig. 3.8.5C. Using the standard 719 emulsion containing nor MDP as a vehicle, the dry milled particles were administered to rabbits. While a much better antibody profile was found, the levels of antibodies produced were much lower than expected. This indicated that the immunogen was partially damaged by the milling process, most probably by the heat.

Considering the drawbacks of the milling process and the size of the particles made possible, we turned to a reduced particle size in a liquid suspension. Isobutanol was selected as the liquid since it could be evaporated from the particles after the milling process. Dry particles estimated to be 0.5—2.0 nM in size were achieved. Results for the control are seen in Fig. 3.8.5D. Following immunization with these, very good antibody profiles were observed although the levels were about half that normally found with unmilled particles. In addition, the rate of rise in antibody levels with time appeared to be slower during the first few weeks following immunization. The interpretation of this result is difficult but it would seem to indicate that the weaker response was due to partial immunogen damage by the milling process.

A further study using the 719 emulsion vehicle was conducted in which the milled particles were mixed with unmilled particles. The total immunogen dose was the same as the previous experiment. Here, the antibody levels were twice as high as with the unmilled particles (Fig. 3.8.5E). Despite this encouraging finding, the goal was to avoid using 719 emulsion for vaccine delivery. Accordingly, other vehicles were tested using mixtures of milled and unmilled particles and are shown in Figs. 3.8.5F and G. The responses in these cases were better than most found to date but were still lower than required. As the priming of immune cells was apparent, a boosted injection was given at 11 weeks following the first immunization, and as seen before, a significant rise in antibody levels was followed by a rapid decline (Fig. 3.8.5F). Figs. 3.8.5H—J show the poor responses seen using mixtures of particles in experimental emulsions such as corn oil and squalene combined with aluminum monostearate (AMS).

To summarize, the use of reduced particle size of the Buford composite indicate that the process employed for particle size reduction is not suitable for product manufacture and a more suitable processes should be identified.

In vitro release rate studies

Studies were next conducted on the release rates of immunogen from regular, non-milled particles and regular particles coated with calcium stearate suspended in PBS. The release rate of regular particles, contained in an ISA/PBS emulsion, released into PBS through a permeable membrane was tested. All studies were carried out at 37°C with rotation. PBS was replaced daily for 30 days and each time, the tube was centrifuged to eliminate any particles before assay. The amount of immunogen released was estimated by BCA protein essay, and results are shown in Fig. 3.8.6A and B. It is apparent that calcium stearate-coated particles released immunogen into the buffer slower than uncoated particles. However, when compared with those released from 719 emulsion, an even greater difference in rates is shown. Immunogen was still being released from the emulsion at 30 days while release was complete in the regular particles directly to PBS after 11 days. These differences in release rates undoubtedly account for the major differences in immune responses observed using these vehicles for immunizations. These findings are related to Buford particles and indicate slower releasing particles could be prepared. Perhaps a mixture of particles could be employed to yield a product administered in aqueous vehicles that would provide the desired antibody profile without unacceptable muscle tissue damage.

The following studies were carried out using an existing laboratory made hCGβ-CTP conjugate. Further studies would contain newly available GMP lots of CTP/DT and loop/DT conjugates. It should also be noted that Buford Biomedical changed its name to Royer Biomedical and the preparation used in studies here was known as Royer MIII.

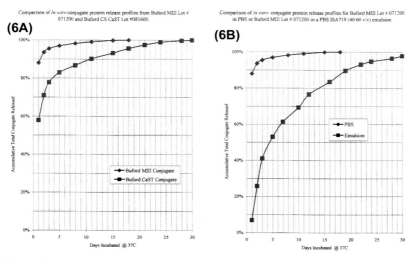

FIGURE 3.8.6

Evaluation of modified inorganic biopolimer formulations in various vehicles

The new Royer particles were prepared with the following agents added to PBS in order to slow the conjugate release.

- Chitosan added to emulsion vehicles (were included in the composition of the particles cross-linked to the biopolymer with glutaraldehyde)
- Biopolymer cross-linked with glutaraldehyde
- Butyl stearate added to particles
- Gelatin cross-linked to biopolymer with glutaraldehyde
- BSA cross-linked to biopolymer with glutaraldehyde

As before, the release rates were demonstrated using BCA protein essay in aliquots removed from the suspensions at time points up to 35 days and are shown in Fig. 3.8.7.

These modified particles were employed in in vivo studies using rabbits as previously described. As a positive control and to assess Chitosan as an adjuvant, standard MIII particles were suspended in emulsions together with Chitosan mixed in

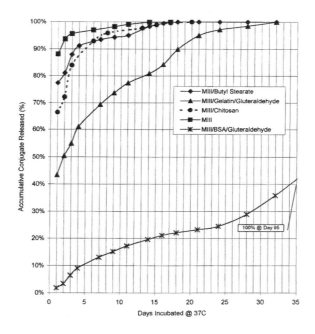

FIGURE 3.8.7

Comparison of in vitro conjugate protein release profiles from Buford (Royer) Biomedical MIII formulations containing βhCG(109−145):DT conjugate incorporated in MIII alone, MIII + butyl stearate, MIII + gelatin/glutaraldehyde, MIII + BSA/glutaraldehyde, or MIII + chitosan.

PBS and in an emulsion (Fig. 3.8.8A and B). Both formulations elicited an excellent level of antibodies following a single injection; however, examination of muscle tissue at 6 weeks revealed an unacceptable level of tissue damage. No further studies of Chitosan added to emulsions were performed.

Fig. 3.8.8C and D show results of immunizations when conjugates were incorporated into MIII particles and then suspended in either water or aqueous vehicles. Neither of these preparations elicited good responses, and similar results were seen with gelatin or BSA (Fig. 3.8.8E and F). However, after booster injections of some of these preparations, a rapid and significant elevation in antibodies was seen indicating that the rabbits were sensitized to the immunogen but a sustained antigen release was absent (Fig. 3.8.8G and H). These findings were inconsistent with the in vitro studies, perhaps explaining other protein assays measuring release of biopolymer, gelatin, or BSA but not that of the hCG peptide conjugate.

The conclusion here is that the particles are released too much rapidly to sustain antibody production at the levels required except when they are suspended in a stable water-in-oil emulsion such as our standard PBS/ISA 719 formulation.

Evaluation of compounds for the reduction of local reactions

Reports in the literature at the time suggested that certain molecules are available that would inhibit inflammation. It was decided that these would be tested in the aqueous phase of an ISA719 emulsion with a dose of conjugate known to cause excessive tissue reactions. The rabbits used in the studies were sacrificed after 5 weeks following immunization and muscle tissue examined in accordance with our earlier studies (and 0−3 scale where 0 was no muscle damage and three was severe muscle damage). The first two experiments using clarithromycin (Biaxin), a superoxide inhibitor, and pentoxifylline, a TNFα inhibitor, gave rise to unacceptable tissue reaction scores as seen previously (Fig. 3.8.9A and B). A compliment inhibitor, FUT-175, gave rise to a slightly reduced tissue score, suggesting a modest reduction in inflammation may have occurred which would warrant possible further investigation (Fig. 3.8.9C).

Immunogenicity testing of new hCG Peptide/DT conjugates

Ahead of Phase I Clinical Trials, new hCGβ (109−145)/DT called (CTP/DT) and hCGβ (38−57)[39Hyp]/DT called (LOOP/DT) conjugates were tested using the standard PBS/nor MDP/ISA719 emulsion. First, at 0, 2, and 4 weeks (Fig. 3.8.10A) and then at 3 and 6 weeks (Fig. 3.8.10B). Tissue scores were low, and antibody levels were high, at least twice that seen with previous conjugates. Subsequently, lower doses were tested to precede the Phase I trial, and these are seen in Fig. 3.8.10C−E. Both lower doses and low volumes elicited antibody levels equal to those used previously with higher doses and volumes. However, tissue scores were also unexpectedly and unacceptably high. Based on these data and in consideration of an additional local tolerance study of these conjugates, it was decided to abandon plans for the Phase I study using these systems. Research returned to identify a system which would be both immunogenic and tolerated by the muscle tissue.

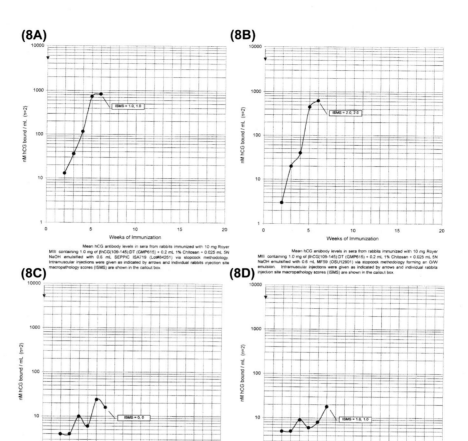

(8A)

Mean hCG antibody levels in sera from rabbits immunized with 10 mg Royer MIII containing 1.0 mg of βhCG(109-145):DT (GMP615) + 0.2 mL 1% Chitosan + 0.025 mL 5N NaOH emulsified with 0.6 mL SEPPIC ISA719 (Lot#84251) via stopcock methodology. Intramuscular injections were given as indicated by arrows and individual rabbits injection site macropathology scores (ISMS) are shown in the callout box.

(8B)

Mean hCG antibody levels in sera from rabbits immunized with 10 mg Royer MIII containing 1.0 mg of βhCG(109-145):DT (GMP615) + 0.2 mL 1% Chitosan + 0.025 mL 5N NaOH emulsified with 0.6 mL MF59 (OSU12901) via stopcock methodology forming an O/W emulsion. Intramuscular injections were given as indicated by arrows and individual rabbits injection site macropathology scores (ISMS) are shown in the callout box.

(8C)

Mean hCG antibody levels in sera from rabbits immunized with 10 mg Royer MIII w/chitosan-gluteraldehyde (A662) containing 1.0 mg of βhCG(109-145):DT (GMP615) + 1 mg Royer MIII (A644) containing 0.1 mg norMDP (IPC001) + 1.0 mg Royer MIII w/calcium stearate (A645) containing 0.1 mg norMDP (IPC001) 0.9 mL PBS emulsified with 0.1 mL MF59 (OSU12901) via stopcock methodology forming an O/W emulsion. Intramuscular injections were given as indicated by arrows and individual rabbits injection site macropathology scores (ISMS) are shown in the callout box.

(8D)

Mean hCG antibody levels in sera from rabbits immunized with 10 mg Royer MIII w/chitosan-gluteraldehyde (A662) containing 1.0 mg of βhCG(109-145):DT (GMP615) + 1 mg Royer MIII (A644) containing 0.1 mg norMDP (IPC001) + 1.0 mg Royer MIII w/calcium stearate (A645) containing 0.1 mg norMDP (IPC001) suspended in 1.0 mL 2% calcium alginate. Intramuscular injections were given as indicated by arrows and individual rabbits injection site macropathology scores (ISMS) are shown in the callout box.

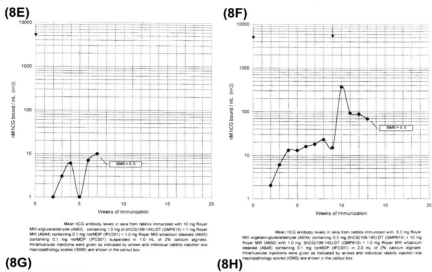

(8E)

Mean hCG antibody levels in sera from rabbits immunized with 10 mg Royer MIII w/gluteraldehyde (A663) containing 1.0 mg of [hCG(109-145):DT (GMP615) + 1 mg Royer MIII (A644) containing 0.1 mg norMDP (IPC001) + 1.0 mg Royer MIII w/calcium stearate (A645) containing 0.1 mg norMDP (IPC001) suspended in 1.0 mL of 2% calcium alginate. Intramuscular injections were given as indicated by arrows and individual rabbits injection site macropathology scores (ISMS) are shown in the callout box.

(8F)

Mean hCG antibody levels in sera from rabbits immunized with 5.0 mg Royer MIII w/gelatin-gluteraldehyde (A654) containing 0.5 mg βhCG(109-145):DT (GMP615) + 10 mg Royer MIII (A650) with 1.0 mg βhCG(109-145):DT (GMP615) + 1.0 mg Royer MIII w/calcium stearate (A645) containing 0.1 mg norMDP (IPC001) in 2.0 mL of 2% calcium alginate. Intramuscular injections were given as indicated by arrows and individual rabbits injection site macropathology scores (ISMS) are shown in the callout box.

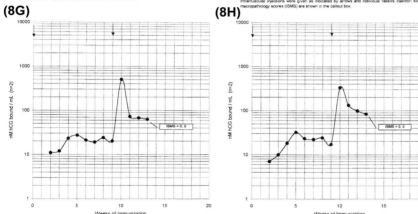

(8G)

Mean hCG antibody levels in sera from rabbits immunized with 5.0 mg Royer MIII w/butyl stearate (A652) containing 0.5 mg βhCG(109-145):DT (GMP615) + 5.0 mg Royer MIII w/BSA-gluteraldehyde (A653) containing 0.5 mg βhCG(109-145):DT (GMP615) + 5.0 mg Royer MIII w/gelatin-gluteraldehyde (A654) containing 0.5 mg βhCG(109-145):DT (GMP615) + 10 mg Royer MIII (A650) with 1.0 mg βhCG(109-145):DT (GMP615) + 1.0 mg Royer MIII w/calcium stearate (A645) containing 0.1 mg norMDP (IPC001) in 2.0 mL of 2% calcium alginate. Intramuscular injections were given as indicated by arrows and individual rabbits injection site macropathology scores (ISMS) are shown in the callout box.

(8H)

Mean hCG antibody levels in sera from rabbits immunized with 5.0 mg Royer MIII w/butyl stearate (A652) containing 0.5 mg βhCG(109-145):DT (GMP615) + 5.0 mg Royer MIII w/BSA-gluteraldehyde (A653) containing 0.5 mg βhCG(109-145):DT (GMP615) +10 mg Royer MIII (A650) with 1.0 mg βhCG(109-145):DT (GMP615) + 1.0 mg Royer MIII w/calcium stearate (A645) containing 0.1 mg norMDP (IPC001) in 2.0 mL of 2% calcium alginate. Intramuscular injections were given as indicated by arrows and individual rabbits injection site macropathology scores (ISMS) are shown in the callout box.

FIGURE 3.8.8

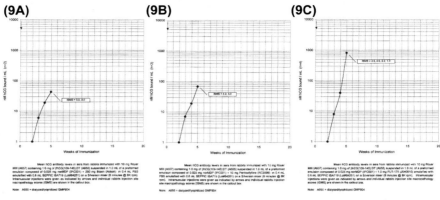

FIGURE 3.8.9

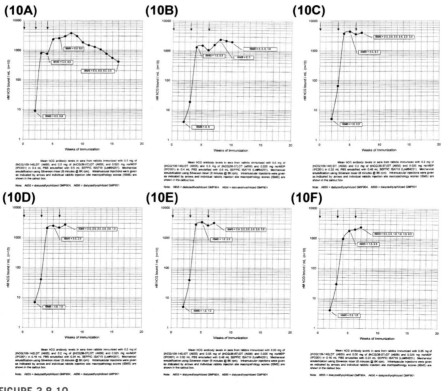

FIGURE 3.8.10

Testing varying doses of immunogens contained in Royer biomedical particles and delivered in emulsion

In view of the recent findings, it was decided to study lower doses of the conjugate using the Royer MIII particles delivered in the ISA/719 emulsion. It was suggested that lower doses of the new conjugate would give adequate antibody levels without muscle damage. The results of these studies are shown in Fig. 3.8.11 (Fig. 3.8.11A and B using CTP and LOOP conjugates, respectively). These experiments confirmed the excellent responses seen previously at 1.0 mg of the CTP conjugate as did a combination of half CTP (0.5 mg) and half LOOP conjugate (0.5 mg) (Fig. 3.8.11C) total 1.0 mg. Considerably lower doses were also tested with very similar responses: 0.195 mg (Fig. 3.8.11D) and 0.039 mg (Fig. 3.8.11E). As can be seen, adequate levels of antibodies were elicited with tissue scores well below the maximum anticipated to be clinically acceptable. The duration of the elevated levels of antibodies, above speculated levels necessary for efficacy, was at least 6 months. In Fig. 3.8.11E, a booster injection was given to three animals to see further effects on antibody levels and tissue tolerance. As shown, a subsequent elevation in

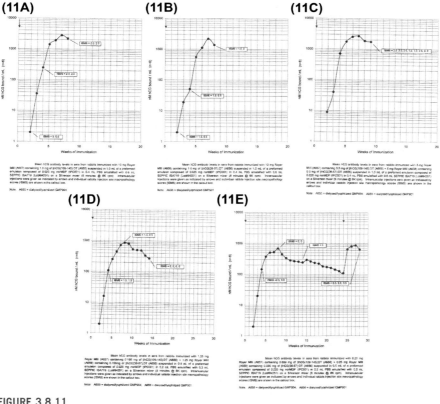

FIGURE 3.8.11

antibodies followed the boost without any increase in tissue damage scores. An expanded study was initiated using 10 rabbits in each group receiving 0.04, 0.08, and 0.12 mg which confirmed the earlier smaller study and a comparison of mean antibody levels for each group can be seen in Fig. 3.8.12. These findings provided promise that this particular formulation should be investigated further for possible use in a clinical trial.

Evaluation of the effect of Cyclofem on antibody production

Given that the immune response during the first month of the advanced prototype vaccine (APV) would not provide sufficient contraceptive protection, it was proposed that an injectable steroid contraceptive would be administered at the same time as APV immunization. The medroxyprogesterone acetate plus ethinyl estradiol product Cyclofem was suggested as a possible candidate and as such should be tested with the simultaneous administration of APV. The data for this study can be seen in Fig. 3.8.13 and indicates that Cyclofem can be administered at the same time as APV offering protection against pregnancy for the first month after immunization without affecting the antibody response.

Immunogenicity and safety of the inorganic biopolimer composite vaccine formulation in rabbits

As described above and as shown in Fig. 3.8.12, a single injection of the composite particles suspended in an emulsion vehicle was capable of eliciting high levels of

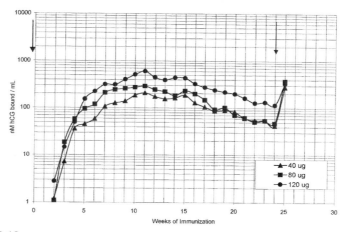

FIGURE 3.8.12

Comparison of mean hCG antibody levels in sera from rabbits immunized using three dose levels of Royer Biomedical MIII each comprising equal portions of (A657) βhCG(109−145):DT and (A658) βhCG(38 57):DT suspended in an ISA719 emulsion (40: 60, w/o) containing nor MDP (0.05 mg/mL emulsion). Doses of 40, 80, or 120 ug of conjugate equivalent suspended in 0.5 mL emulsion for injection.

Mean hCG antibody levels in sera from rabbits immunized with 1.33 mg of MIII (UPM- Lot#1139A-003-078) containing 0.1 mg βhCG(109-145):DT + 0.1 mg βhCG (38-57):DT suspended in an emulsion of 0.2 mL PBS containing 0.025 mg nor-MDP and 0.3 mL mannide monooleate (SEPPIC ISA719, Lot# 84251). MIII stored at 4° C for 3 months prior to injection. Injection given at day 0.

(18A)

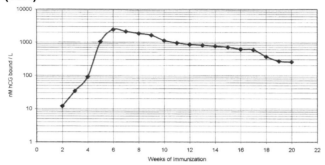

Mean hCG antibody levels in sera from rabbits immunized with 1.28 mg of MIII (UPM- Lot#1139A-003-078) containing 0.1 mg βhCG(109-145):DT + 0.1 mg βhCG (38-57):DT suspended in an emulsion of 0.2 mL PBS containing 0.025 mg nor-MDP and 0.3 mL mannide monooleate (SEPPIC ISA719, Lot# 84251). MIII stored at 4° C for 6 months prior to injection. Injection given at day 0.

(18B)

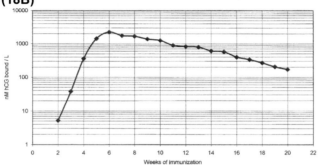

Mean hCG antibody levels in sera from rabbits immunized with 1.28 mg of MIII (UPM- Lot#1139A-003-078) containing 0.1 mg βhCG(109-145):DT + 0.1 mg βhCG (38-57):DT suspended in an emulsion of 0.2 mL PBS containing 0.025 mg nor-MDP and 0.3 mL mannide monooleate (SEPPIC ISA719, Lot# 84251). MIII stored at 4° C for 30 months prior to injection. Injection given at day 0.

(18C)

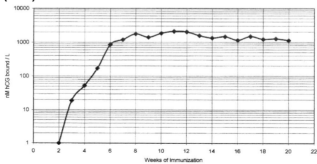

FIGURE 3.8.18

shown that the use of totally synthetic peptide immunogens, delivered in biodegradable microspheres of polylactic/polyglycolide, offer promise for vaccines that are safer, more predictable, and more economical to manufacture.

Later studies with collaborating partners, CG Therapeutics, involved testing a preformed vaccine formulation in ready-to-use syringes which were stored at 4°C for up to 8 months without seeing any decrease in antibody responses. These latest studies indicated that this product would be suitable for widespread use as a commercial pharmaceutical.

Final conclusions by Dr. Stevens

Numerous attempts to deliver a vaccine containing a diphtheria toxoid/peptide of the C-terminal 35 amino acids of the β-subunit of hCG (CTP) conjugate in several aqueous vehicles were unsuccessful. I wish to express my sincere thanks to Mr. John E. Powell for conducting assisting with all of the experiments described in the figures. While all of these vehicles were found safe as no inflammation was seen at the injection site, none were able to elicit antibody levels considered adequate to prevent pregnancy if used in women. Several peptide immunogens were tested in a large number of formulations and only those delivered with some oil content in the vehicle produced high antibody levels in rabbits. However, the incorporation of immunogens into particles of an inorganic salt allowed the use of a smaller volume of an oil-containing vehicle that caused only minor damage to tissues at the site of vaccine administration. Also, the shelf life of peptide conjugates which were a combination of CTP and a peptide representing the 38−57 sequence of the β-subunit, were evaluated. The production and storage of manufactured products in bulk quantities were also established. Thus, the latest studies showed that the hCG vaccine, developed by WHO, met all criteria necessary to be a commercial product. Nonetheless, only one pharmaceutical company licensed the vaccine, but only after a short time, it returned the license. The reasons given were fear of negative publicity from religious groups and low profits from sales in developing countries. Despite the rejection of such a unique and desirable contraceptive, the need for such a method persists.

Cancer and therapy

Negative control—how hCG, and a failed experiment, changed my life

Ray K. Iles

After graduating, my scientific career was going to be in cancer immunology and modulation of MHC antigen expression in urogenital tumors, working on a grant from the Imperial Cancer Research Fund (forerunner of Cancer Research UK) under the medical oncologist Tim Oliver and urologist John Blandy, at the London Hospital Medical School. This involved attending operations, collecting fresh tissue samples, and establishing primary cultures of the tumor cells. The tumors I attempted to culture included testicular germ cell tumors. These were a mixture of seminomas and nonseminomas with trophoblast differentiation. I was successful in propagating several testicular germ cell cultures through multiple passages.

Knowing that the male patients, from which the tumors had been taken, had been serum positive for "hCG," I harvested spent culture media from these testicular germ cell cultures and sent them to our partner laboratory at St Bartholomew's Hospital Medical College for hCG immunoassay. Being a vigilante and well-trained young scientist, I also took spent culture media from bladder cancers I was growing at the same time to act as a negative control. The results came back from the clinical immunoassay laboratory as negative for any hCG in my testicular germ cell tumors. However, my controls were positive with significant amounts of hCG! [1,2].

This observation changed my entire life. Professor Tim Chard, head of the laboratory at Barts and Department of Reproductive Physiology, asked me to join him, and we wrote our first grant together to investigate this surprising finding. I repeated the immunoassay experiments and conducted protein chemistry and molecular characterized that showed that in fact these bladder cancers were only producing the free β-subunit of hCG [3—5]. Clinical studies showed ectopic free hCGβ expression can be detected in 30%—50% of all patients with common epithelial cancers. Furthermore, such expression is associated with highly aggressive tumors that rapidly metastasize [6—8]. Although we have hypothesized that cellular mechanism by which expression of the β-subunit of hCG may act as an auto or paracrine growth factor inhibiting apoptosis [9—11], the molecular genetics of β-subunit gene expression requires much more investigation [12].

100 Years of Human Chorionic Gonadotropin. https://doi.org/10.1016/B978-0-12-820050-6.00021-7

As an aside note, it transpires that testicular germ cell tumors do not express hCG genes when in culture. Thus, trophoblast differentiation of the germ cell tumors is dependent on multiple differentiation factors present "in vivo" rather than an innate program to do so.

References

[1] Iles RK, Oliver RTD, Kitau M, Walker C, Chard T. *In vitro* secretion of human chorionic gonadotrophin by bladder tumour cells. Br J Cancer 1987;55:623−6.

[2] Iles RK, Purkis PE, Whitehead PC, Oliver RTD, Leigh I, Chard T. Expression of β human chorionic gonadotrophin by non − trophoblastic non-endocrine "normal" and malignant epithelial cells. Br J Cancer 1990;61:663−6.

[3] Iles RK, Chard T. Immunochemical analysis of the human chorionic gonadotrophin-like material secreted by "normal" and neoplastic urothelial cells. J Mol Endocrinol 1989;2:107−12.

[4] Iles RK, Czepulkowski BH, Young BD, Chard T. Amplification or rearrangement of the β − hCG-hLH gene cluster is not responsible for the ectopic production of βhCG by bladder tumour cells. J Mol Endocrinol 1989;2:113−7.

[5] Iles RK, Lee CL, Oliver RTD, Chard T. Composition of intact hormone and free subunit in the human chorionic gonadotrophin-like material found in serum and urine of patients with carcinoma of the bladder. Clin Endocrinol 1990;32:355−64.

[6] Iles RK, Jenkins BJ, Oliver RTD, Blandy JP, Chard T. βhCG in serum and urine: a marker for metastatic urothelial cancer. Br J Urol 1989;64:241−4.

[7] Iles RK, Chard T. Review: human chorionic gonadotrophin expression by bladder cancers: biology & clinical potential as an indicator of poor prognosis. J Urol 1991;145: 453−8.

[8] Iles RK, Persad R, Sharma KB, Dickinson A, Smith P, Chard T. Urinary concentration of human chorionic gonadotrophin and its fragments as a prognostic marker in bladder cancer. Br J Urol 1996;77:61−9.

[9] Gillott DJ, Iles RK, Chard T. The effects of β human chorionic gonadotrophin (βhCG) on the in vitro growth of bladder cancer cell lines. Br J Cancer 1996;73:323−6.

[10] Butler SA, Laidler P, Porter JR, Kicman AT, Chard T, Cowen DA, Iles RK. The β subunit of human chorionic gonadotrophin exists as a homodimer. J Mol Endocrinol 1999; 22:185−92.

[11] Butler SA, Ikram MK, Mathieu S, Iles RK. The increase in carcinoma cell population induced by the free beta subunit of human chorionic gonadotrophin is a result of an anti-apoptotic effect and not cell proliferation. Br J Cancer 2000;82:1553−6.

[12] Burczynska BB, Kobrouly L, Butler SA, Naase M, Iles RK. Novel insights into the expression of *CGB1 & 2* genes by epithelial cancer cell lines secreting ectopic free hCGβ. Anticancer Res 2014;34:2239−48.

Human chorionic gonadotropin in cancer—where are we?

4.2

Anna Jankowska, Anna Szczerba

Similarities between embryogenesis and carcinogenesis have been postulated since the beginning of the last century. The discovery of carcinoembryonic antigens allowed to hypothesize that tumor cells mimic the development of embryonic cells [1]. Both during embryonic development and oncogenesis, specific antigens such as α fetoprotein (AFP), carcinoembryonic antigen (CEA), growth hormone (GH), insulin growth factor (IGF), fibroblast growth factor (FGF), tumor growth factor (TGF), and epidermal growth factor (EGF) are expressed [2]. One of these antigens, considered a key factor regulating both fetal development and tumor growth, is human chorionic gonadotropin (hCG) [3,4].

The expression of hCG, especially its free β-subunit (hCGβ) by many cancers of different origin, is well documented [5,6].

Despite numerous studies, the exact role and mechanisms of hCGβ action in cancer remain unexplained. This is probably due to the fact that hCGβ is encoded by eight different genes (*CGBs*) which are not equally active. Translation of their transcripts gives rise to several protein isoforms, which additionally differ in terms of posttranslational modifications and biological activity. What is more, it has been showed that hCGβ action is mediated through various receptors and mechanisms [4,6–8]. Nevertheless, no matter which gene is active and what form of the hormone is produced, the fact remains that hCGβ seems to be a crucial agent driving tumor growth, cancer progression, and metastasis, and it determines response to treatment and survival of cancer patients [9–14].

The basic biological effect of hCGβ in cancer is linked with its ability to block apoptotic processes, promote cell proliferation, and promote tumor growth. This effect was demonstrated in studies conducted both in vitro on cell lines and ex vivo on tumor tissues, as well as using mouse models [5,15,16].

In pregnancy, hCG promotes angiogenesis and determines immune tolerance to the fetus. It has been postulated that the hormone may contribute to neovascularization and lead to the desensitization of the patient's immune system also in oncogenesis [17,18].

We have previously demonstrated that hCGβ is a useful marker of cervical, ovarian, and endometrial cancers [16,19,20]. The results of our experiments document the expression of genes encoding hCGβ also in blood of cancer patients (with gynecological as well as head and neck, breast, digestive system, lung, prostate, pancreas tumors), where it might indicate the presence of circulating tumor cells (CTCs) [21,22]. The critical role of these cells in metastasis is very well recognized [23,24]. CTCs' presence in peripheral blood of cancer patients may allow for assessment of cancer recurrence risk, response to treatment monitoring, follow-up studies as well as development of novel therapeutic agents [24−26]. Therefore, early detection of CTCs using *CGBs* as their marker is a promising diagnostic and prognostic tool for cancer patients.

According to the theory of tumor heterogeneity and its genetic instability, once CTCs detach from the primary tumor, they may change their expression profile, adapting to a new microenvironment [27]. Thus, CTC populations may consist of many subpopulations with different genotypes and phenotypes. This diversity is mainly acquired in the process known as the epithelial-mesenchymal transition (EMT), in which epithelial cells change their size and shape and lose the ability of cell adhesion to acquire migration properties typical for mesenchymal cells [28,29].

It has recently been proved that hCGβ expression in human ovarian, lung, and colorectal cancers regulates the EMT process [30−32], and we believe that hCGβ production may characterize tumor cells at different stages of tumor development including cancer progression and metastasis.

In ovarian cancer, it has been shown that hCGβ induced morphological changes in and increased cell adherence. These changes were accompanied by upregulation of EMT-associated proteins (vimentin, N-cadherin, β-catenin, Slug, Snail) and downregulation of epithelial markers expression (E-cadherin and claudin). Moreover, the presence of the hCG β-subunit promoted migration and invasion of cancer cells as well as facilitated metastasis. In contrast, knocking down hCGβ expression had the opposite effect [30].

The clinical significance of hCGβ was documented also for colorectal cancer (CRC). It has been showed that hCGβ expression increased invasiveness, migration ability, and metastatic potential in both cell lines and mouse models. The study confirmed that, similarly to ovarian cancer, hCGβ altered the expression of EMT-related genes encoding: E-cadherin, phospho-SMAD2, SNAIL, and TWIST. Additionally, analysis of CRC specimens and preoperative serum samples demonstrated a correlation of hCGβ expression with clinical data and unfavorable patient outcomes [31].

The enhanced invasiveness of tumor cells in human colorectal and lung cancers upon exogenous hCG treatment was showed to be associated also with an increase in expression of MMP-2, MMP-9, VEGF, and IL-8. Additionally, the authors of the studies proved that anti-hCG antibodies restricted the growth of implanted tumors in nude mice [32].

The antitumor efficacy and the immunogenicity of anti-hCG vaccination in cell lines and mice models have been described previously [33−35]. A vaccine based on the carboxy-terminal peptide (CTP) of hCGβ demonstrated clinical benefits in patients with colorectal cancer. The average survival of patients with optimal antibody response was two times greater compared with those without optimal response [36]. The results of these studies provide further rationale for anti-hCGβ vaccination as a treatment approach toward gonadotropin-sensitive tumors.

Anti-hCGβ antibodies have been observed to remain at detectable levels in the human body for more than 1 year [37]. It is also known that CTCs, responsible for the development of metastasis, may be present not only in preoperative state but also in patients who underwent complete removal of the primary tumor [38,39]. Therefore, immunodepletion of hCGβ expressed by primary tumor cells or by CTCs, whether by active or passive immunization may become an attractive therapeutic approach for patients at different stages of the disease.

While most existing anti-hCGβ therapeutic strategies are based on the use of antibodies which block ectopically expressed hCGβ, it has to be pointed out that the same results may be achieved with the potential of gene silencing. This technology was successfully used in vitro to inhibit proliferation and induce apoptosis of cancer cells [16,40,41]. What is more blocking of genes coding hCGβ as well as hCGα has been shown to reduce not only free hormone subunits but also heterodimeric hCG [42−44].

In fact, in case of cancers synthesizing human chorionic gonadotropin, gene silencing seems a more adequate approach. It has been demonstrated that malignancies produce a variety of hCG-related molecules, namely regular hCG, hyperglycosylated hCG, and hyperglycosylated hCG free β-subunit of hormone [5]. Therefore, anti-hCGβ vaccinations alone may not eliminate all of these peptide forms and fail in tumor growth and malignancy suppression.

In this context, gene therapy and silencing of particular genes encoding hCGβ may be more effective and become an alternative or a part of combination therapy with vaccines.

References

[1] Beard J. Embryological aspects and etiology of carcinoma. Lancet 1902;1:1758−61.
[2] Knöchel W, Tiedemann H. Embryonic inducers, growth factors, transcription factors and oncogenes. Cell Differ Dev 1989;26(3):163−71.
[3] Srisuparp S, Strakova ZFA. The role of chorionic gonadotropin (CG) in blastocyst implantation. Arch Med Res 2001;32:627−34.
[4] Rull K, Hallast P, Uusküla L, Jackson J, Punab M, Salumets A, et al. Fine-scale quantification of HCG beta gene transcription in human trophoblastic and non-malignant non-trophoblastic tissues. Mol Hum Reprod 2008;14(1):23−31.
[5] Cole LA. HCG variants, the growth factors which drive human malignancies. Am J Cancer Res 2012;2(1):22−35.
[6] Iles RK, Butler SA. Gonadotropins and gonadotropin receptors—evolutional genetics, signalling mechanisms, extra gonadal function and roles in oncogenesis. Mol Cell Endocrinol 2010;329(1−2):1−2.

[7] Fournier T. Human chorionic gonadotropin: different glycoforms and biological activity depending on its source of production. Ann Endocrinol 2016;77(2):75−81.

[8] Stenman U. Biomarker development, from bench to bedside. Crit Rev Clin Lab Sci 2016;53(2):69−86.

[9] Acevedo HF, Hartsock RJ. Metastatic phenotype correlates with high expression of membrane-associated complete beta-human chorionic gonadotropin in vivo. Cancer 1996;78(11):2388−99.

[10] Crawford RA, Iles RK, Carter PG, Caldwell CJ, Shepherd JH, Chard T. The prognostic significance of beta human chorionic gonadotrophin and its metabolites in women with cervical carcinoma. J Clin Pathol 1998;51(9):685−8.

[11] Vartiainen J, Lehtovirta P, Finne P, Stenman UH, Alfthan H. Preoperative serum concentration of hCGbeta as a prognostic factor in ovarian cancer. Int J Cancer 2001;20; 95(5):313−6.

[12] Hotakainen K, Ljungberg B, Haglund C, Nordling S, Paju A, Stenman U-H. Expression of the free beta-subunit of human chorionic gonadotropin in renal cell carcinoma: prognostic study on tissue and serum. Int J Cancer 2003;104(5):631−5.

[13] Fukuoka K, Yanagisawa T, Suzuki T, Shirahata M, Adachi J, Mishima K, et al. Human chorionic gonadotropin detection in cerebrospinal fluid of patients with a germinoma and its prognostic significance: assessment by using a highly sensitive enzyme immunoassay. J Neurosurg Pediatr 2016;18(5):573−7.

[14] Morris CD, Hameed MR, Agaram NP, Hwang S. Elevated β-hCG associated with aggressive Osteoblastoma. Skeletal Radiol 2017;46(9):1187−92.

[15] Butler SA, Ikram MS, Mathieu S, Iles RK. The increase in bladder carcinoma cell population induced by the free beta subunit of human chorionic gonadotrophin is a result of an anti-apoptosis effect and not cell proliferation. Br J Canc 2000;82(9):1553−6.

[16] Jankowska A, Gunderson SI, Andrusiewicz M, Burczynska B, Szczerba A, Jarmolowski A, et al. Reduction of human chorionic gonadotropin beta subunit expression by modified U1 snRNA caused apoptosis in cervical cancer cells. Mol Cancer 2008;7:26.

[17] Bansal AS, Bora SA, Saso S, Smith JR, Johnson MR, Thum M-Y. Mechanism of human chorionic gonadotrophin-mediated immunomodulation in pregnancy. Expert Rev Clin Immunol 2012;8(8):747−53.

[18] Tsampalas M, Gridelet V, Berndt S, Foidart J-M, Geenen V, d'Hauterive SP. Human chorionic gonadotropin: a hormone with immunological and angiogenic properties. J Reprod Immunol 2010;85(1):93−8.

[19] Nowak-Markwitz E, Jankowska A, Andrusiewicz M, Szczerba A. Expression of beta-human chorionic gonadotropin in ovarian cancer tissue. Eur J Gynaecol Oncol 2004; 25(4):465−9.

[20] Jankowska AG, Andrusiewicz M, Fischer N, Warchol PJB. Expression of hCG and GnRHs and their receptors in endometrial carcinoma and hyperplasia. Int J Gynecol Cancer 2010;20(1):92−101.

[21] Andrusiewicz M, Szczerba A, Wołuń-Cholewa M, Warchoł W, Nowak-Markwitz E, Gąsiorowska E, et al. CGB and GNRH1 expression analysis as a method of tumor cells metastatic spread detection in patients with gynecological malignances. J Transl Med 2011;9:130.

[22] Szczerba A, Adamska K, Warchol W, Andrusiewicz M, Nowak-Markwitz E, Jankowska A. Evaluation of CGB, GNRH1, MET and KRT19 genes expression profile

as a circulating tumor cells marker in blood of cancer patients. J Mol Biomark Diagn 2015;s6(4):1−8.

[23] Zhou L, Dicker DT, Matthew E, El-Deiry WS, Alpaugh RK. Circulating tumor cells: silent predictors of metastasis. F1000Res 2017;6:1445.

[24] Masuda T, Hayashi N, Iguchi T, Ito S, Eguchi H, Mimori K. Clinical and biological significance of circulating tumor cells in cancer. Mol Oncol 2016;10(3):408−17.

[25] Micalizzi DS, Maheswaran S, Haber DA. A conduit to metastasis: circulating tumor cell biology. Genes Dev 2017;31(18):1827−40.

[26] Millner LM, Linder MW, Valdes R. Circulating tumor cells: a review of present methods and the need to identify heterogeneous phenotypes. Ann Clin Lab Sci 2013; 43(3):295−304.

[27] Gerlinger M, Swanton C. How Darwinian models inform therapeutic failure initiated by clonal heterogeneity in cancer medicine. Br J Canc 2010;103(8):1139−43.

[28] Heerboth S, Housman G, Leary M, Longacre M, Byler S, Lapinska K, et al. EMT and tumor metastasis. Clin Transl Med 2015;4(1):6.

[29] Jie X-X, Zhang X-Y, Xu C-J. Epithelial-to-mesenchymal transition, circulating tumor cells and cancer metastasis: mechanisms and clinical applications. Oncotarget 2017; 8(46):81558−71.

[30] Liu N, Peng S-M, Zhan G-X, Yu J, Wu W-M, Gao H, et al. Human chorionic gonadotropinï β regulates epithelial-mesenchymal transition and metastasis in human ovarian cancer. Oncol Rep 2017;38(3):1464−72.

[31] Kawamata F, Nishihara H, Homma S, Kato Y, Tsuda M, Konishi Y, et al. Chorionic gonadotropin-β modulates epithelial-mesenchymal transition in colorectal carcinoma metastasis. Am J Pathol 2018;188(1):204−15.

[32] Khare P, Bose A, Singh P, Singh S, Javed S, Jain SK, et al. Gonadotropin and tumorigenesis: direct and indirect effects on inflammatory and immunosuppressive mediators and invasion. Mol Carcinog 2017;56(2):359−70.

[33] Acevedo HF, Raikow RB, Powell JE, Stevens VC. Effects of immunization against human choriogonadotropin on the growth of transplanted Lewis lung carcinoma and spontaneous mammary adenocarcinoma in mice. Cancer Detect Prev Suppl 1987;1:477−86.

[34] Cole LA, Butler SA. B152 anti-hyperglycosylated human chorionic gonadotropin free β-Subunit. A new, possible treatment for cancer. J Reprod Med 2015;60(1−2):13−20.

[35] Morse MA, Chapman R, Powderly J, Blackwell K, Keler T, Green J, et al. Phase I study utilizing a novel antigen-presenting cell-targeted vaccine with toll-like receptor stimulation to induce immunity to self-antigens in cancer patients. Clin Cancer Res 2011; 17(14):4844−53.

[36] Moulton HM, Yoshihara PH, Mason DH, Iversen PL, Triozzi PL. Active specific immunotherapy with a beta-human chorionic gonadotropin peptide vaccine in patients with metastatic colorectal cancer: antibody response is associated with improved survival. Clin Cancer Res 2002;8(7):2044−51.

[37] Triozzi PL, Stevens VC. Human chorionic gonadotropin as a target for cancer vaccines. Oncol Rep 1999;6(1):7−17.

[38] Müller V, Alix-Panabières C, Pantel K. Insights into minimal residual disease in cancer patients: implications for anti-cancer therapies. Eur J Cancer 2010;46(7):1189−97.

[39] Cohen SJ, Punt CJA, Iannotti N, Saidman BH, Sabbath KD, Gabrail NY, et al. Prognostic significance of circulating tumor cells in patients with metastatic colorectal cancer. Ann Oncol 2009;20(7):1223−9.

[40] Hamada AL, Nakabayashi K, Sato A, Kiyoshi K, Takamatsu Y, Laoag-Fernandez JB, et al. Transfection of antisense chorionic gonadotropin β gene into choriocarcinoma cells suppresses the cell proliferation and induces apoptosis. J Clin Endocrinol Metab 2005;90(8):4873−9.

[41] Burczynska B, Booth MJ, Iles RK, Shah A, Shiled A, Butler SA. Stable knockdown of hCGβ mRNA expression in bladder cancer cells results in significant growth inhibition. Anticancer Res 2013;33(9):3611−4.

[42] Ghosh NK, Cox RP. Production of human chorionic gonadotropin in HeLa cell cultures. Nature 1976;259(5542):416−7.

[43] Lieblich JM, Weintraub BD, Rosen SW, Chou JY, Robinson JC. HeLa cells secrete α subunit of glycoprotein tropic hormones. Nature 1976;260(5551):530−2.

[44] Cox GS. Glycosylation of the chorionic gonadotropin a subunit synthesized by HeLa cells. Cancer Res 1981;41(8):3087−94.

LH/hCG receptor–independent activities of hCG and hCGβ

4.3

Hannu K. Koistinen, Ulf-Håkan Stenman

Human chorionic gonadotropin (hCG) is a heterodimer consisting of an α- and a β-subunit (hCGα and hCGβ) that are noncovalently linked. The α-subunit is identical to those in other glycoprotein hormones, i.e., LH, FSH, and TSH. While intact hCG heterodimer binds to the LH/hCG receptor (LHCGR) in the corpus luteum, stimulating progesterone production essential for successful pregnancy [1], the free β-subunit does not activate the LHCGR [2–4]. However, free hCGβ is present in several tissues, including many nontrophoblastic tumors, which may produce free hCGβ, but very rarely intact hCG [5]. Therefore, it is plausible that hCGβ and hCG have functions, which are independent of the LHCGR. Indeed, several LHCGR-independent activities for hCG and hCGβ have been described. Here we review some of these proposed activities in relation to pregnancy and cancer, and at the same time, emphasize the need to use highly purified and well characterized hCG preparations and careful study design for characterizing such activities.

Trophoblast invasion and pregnancy

Placental trophoblast cell invasion into the decidualized endometrium is necessary for successful pregnancy [6]. This process is tightly regulated, and several paracrine and autocrine factors that regulate trophoblast invasion, at least in *in vitro* models, are known [7]. One of these factors is hCG, which stimulates trophoblast invasion [8–11] and is the first trophoblast marker detected in the maternal blood. We have found that, contrary to hCG, the endometrial glycoprotein glycodelin inhibits trophoblast invasion, which is specifically modulated by glycosylation [12,13]. Whether glycosylation modulates the activity of trophoblast-derived hCG is controversial. So-called hyperglycosylated hCG (hCG-h) [14] has been proposed to be more active in stimulating trophoblast invasion than nonhyperglycosylated hCG [15,16]. hCG-h is produced by invasive cytotrophoblasts and is secreted into maternal blood, where it is the major form of hCG during the first 4–5 weeks of pregnancy, declining thereafter [17,18]. We have not found large differences between various highly purified and well-characterized hCG isoforms, including hCG and hCG-h, in their ability to stimulate invasion of primary trophoblast cells and JEG-3 choriocarcinoma cells, often used for studying trophoblasts invasion [11].

100 Years of Human Chorionic Gonadotropin. https://doi.org/10.1016/B978-0-12-820050-6.00023-0

Importantly, we found that free hCGβ is also able to stimulate trophoblast invasion [11]. It is likely that both hCG and hCGβ act through the same receptor, as their effect on invasion was very similar and the binding of labeled hCGβ on JEG-3 cells was blocked with excess of hCG. Since LHCGR is not stimulated by hCGβ [2–4], this receptor is probably not LHCGR. Furthermore, LHCGR antibody did not have any effect on the binding of hCGβ to JEG-3 cells, while it inhibited the binding of LH, and knockdown of LHCGR by RNAi did not affect the stimulatory effect of hCG or hCGβ on trophoblast invasion. Together these findings strongly suggest that the effect of hCG and hCGβ on trophoblast invasion is independent of LHCGR [11].

It has been hypothesized that hCG-h stimulates trophoblast invasion via the TGF-β receptor (TGFβR) [14]. However, we have not found significant differences between the ability of hCG and hCG-h, isolated form pregnancy urine, to stimulate trophoblast invasion, thus, the hCG-h specific activation of the TGFβR may not mediate the stimulation. Furthermore, TGFβ has been found to inhibit, rather than stimulate, the invasion of normal trophoblast cells, while it has not been found to have any effect on invasion of JEG-3 cells [19,20]. Further still, we have shown that highly purified hCG, hCGβ, or their hyperglycosylated forms do not activate TGFβR in cells transfected with a reporter gene for TGFβRI/II activation [21].

It appears that downstream of the primary stimulus by hCG and hCGβ, extracellular matrix degrading enzymes, matrix metalloproteinases (MMPs), and urokinase-type plasminogen activator (uPA) are involved in trophoblast invasion [7,8,10,11,22,23]. It has also been suggested that hCG-stimulated trophoblast invasion is mediated by recycling of the IGF-II/mannose-6 phosphate receptor [9]. Interestingly, hCGβ has been found to increase the invasion of cancer cells concomitantly with decreased expression of cell adhesion molecule E-cadherin (see below). This may mediate the proinvasive activity of hCG and hCGβ in trophoblast cells, as E-cadherin is known to be downregulated during trophoblast invasion [7].

hCG may have an additional LHCGR-independent role in modulating the uterine natural killer cells, which are a phenotypically distinct population of natural killer cells and may further regulate the trophoblast cells and pregnancy outcome [24]. hCG has been found to increase the proliferation of these cells [25]. Curiously, this is mediated via the mannose receptor (CD206), rather than via the classical LHCGR, which is not expressed in these cells. Deglycosylated hCG did not have such an effect and the effect could be blocked with excess of mannose.

Cancer

Since the expression of hCGβ has been observed in several nontrophoblastic cancers, including bladder, renal, gastrointestinal, ovarian, prostate, and breast cancers [5,26], and in cancer patients elevated serum levels of hCGβ are associated with adverse prognosis, it is plausible that hCGβ has a functional role(s) in cancer.

Although trophoblast invasion is more controlled, with respect to timing and extent of invasion, than cancer cell invasion, hCGβ has been found to facilitate metastasis of ovarian cancer xenograft cells [27] and increase the invasion and migration in several cancer cell models, including those of prostate, ovarian and breast cancer, and glioblastoma [26–30]. In several models, this was associated with epithelial-to-mesenchymal transition-like changes in cells, including downregulation of E-cadherin, and other changes, like upregulation of MMP-2 and activation of mitogen-activated protein kinase (MAPK)-signaling, as detected by extracellular-signal-regulated kinase (ERK) 1/2 phosphorylation [26–28,31]. Several studies have also described LHCGR-mediated stimulation of ERK1/2 phosphorylation in various cell types, including placental cells, by different hCG preparations [10,32,33]. Furthermore, other gonadotropins have been shown to have similar effects as hCG on ovarian cancer cells in promoting migration and by activation of ERK1/2 signaling [34]. However, we have not observed any increase in phosphorylation of ERK1/2 in JEG-3 cells treated with different highly purified hCG preparations [21].

In these studies, various hCGβ preparations, gene knockdown [26,27], and transgenic expression approaches have been used [27–31]. All these approaches have their limitations, especially when LHCGR-independent hCGβ actions are considered. hCG and hCGβ preparations may be contaminated with growth factors (see below), hCGβ (purified preparation or expressed in the cells) may form complexes with hCGα, if it is endogenously produced by the cells, and knockdown of hCGβ would affect also the levels of hCG dimer. Therefore, it would be important to control the presence of free hCGβ and hCG dimer. In some of the studies, the effect of transfected hCGβ on ERK phosphorylation has been transient and, unfortunately, not compared with the potential effect caused by transfection alone [31]. Similar response of hCGβ transfection has been observed both using OVCAR-3 and SKOV-3 ovarian cancer cells [31], of which the latter was not found to express LHCGR as studied by quantitative RT-PCR, suggesting an LHCGR-independent regulation. It should be noted that regarding the LHCGR expression in these cells, the opposite has also been reported, i.e., that LHCGR is expressed in SKOV-3, but not in OVCAR-3 cells [35]. This highlights the importance to use properly authenticated cells and also the phenotypic drift that may arise during multiple passaging of the cells [36,37].

In breast cancer cells, BRCA1 mutation (or knockdown of wild-type BRCA1 by RNA interference) has been found to promote hCGβ expression [26]. In these cells, hCGβ promoted migration and invasion, and this was suggested to be mediated through TGFβRII signaling [26]. hCGβ and hyperglycosylated hCG have been found to stimulate cell proliferation, which also has been proposed to be mediated by TGFβR [38–40]. The cell growth-stimulatory effect has been proposed to be related to the ability of hCG to prevent apoptosis [41–43], which may be LHCGR-dependent [43]. TGFβR has been proposed to also mediate angiogenic activity of hCG-h [44], while nonhyperglycosylated hCG has been suggested to promote angiogenesis via LHCGR [45]. However, while both hCG-h and hCG are able to stimulate LHCGR [4], it is controversial whether different hCG isoforms are able to stimulate TGFβR or not. Nonspecific effects may be caused by growth factor contamination present in several hCG preparations (see below). Furthermore, as discussed above, we have not detected TGFβRI/II activation by highly purified hCG, hCGβ, or their hyperglycosylated forms. To note, in TGFβR receptor studies, cell type—specific differences in responses, due to different expression of different TGFβRs and downstream signaling molecules, are possible.

Word of caution for interpreting results obtained with impure hCG and hCGβ preparations

hCG concentrations used in cell culture studies are often high, reflecting physiological hCG levels found in pregnancy [46] and, thus, even a relatively minor contamination with potent growth factors may be significant and affect the results. Indeed, several hCG preparations have been found to contain significant amounts of impurities, including EGF [47,48]. We have found EGF and TGF-β1 contaminations even in some immunoaffinity-purified hCG preparations [21]. These growth factors have been present at levels high enough to induce ERK1/2 phosphorylation and activation of TGFβR, respectively. Based on these findings, it is of utmost importance that the purity of hCG and hCGβ preparations is controlled. Furthermore, for studies aiming to elucidate the effect of glycosylation (like those addressing the functions of hCG-h), it is important to properly characterize the hCG isoforms present in the preparations. It is, however, noteworthy, that the observed contaminants, including TGF-β1, EGF [21,47,48] and other factors [49,50], do not explain all the suggested LHCGR-independent activities of hCG and hCGβ, like stimulation of trophoblast and cancer cell invasion.

Conclusions and future directions

It has become evident that hCG and hCGβ have activities, like stimulation of trophoblast and cancer cell invasion, which are independent of LHCGR. However, the detailed mechanism of these and the impact of the glycosylation of hCG and hCGβ in mediating those is controversial and warrant further studies with careful experimental design and rigorous controls. Special caution should be devoted to the purity of hCG preparations and proper model systems (not discussed here, but likely to have a huge impact on the results). In addition to purity, characterization of the hCG preparations used and the hCG-forms expressed in the cells, with respect to hCG isoforms, including potential internal cleavages (nicked hCG) and glycosylation, is important. Hyperglycosylated hCG-h, which has been proposed to functionally differ from nonhyperglycosylated hCG, is defined by its reaction with monoclonal antibody B152 [51]. The antibody, however, recognizes variety of differentially glycosylated hCG-h forms, including the one present in early pregnancy and differentially glycosylated cancer-associated hCG-h forms [52]. In addition to using purified hCG preparations, gene knockdown/knockout techniques and transgenic expression (providing that the used cells can produce properly glycosylated hCG) are important and have already been used in several studies referred to above. With these and other techniques, it is likely that LHCGR-independent mechanisms of hCG action will be uncovered in the future.

Acknowledgments

Our original studies referred to here have been supported by the Sigrid Jusélius Foundation and Finnish Cancer Foundation.

References

[1] Yoshimi T, Strott CA, Marshall JR, Lipsett MB. Corpus luteum function in early pregnancy. J Clin Endocrinol Metab 1969;29:225—30.

[2] Catt KJ, Dufau ML, Tsuruhara T. Absence of intrinsic biological activity in LH and hCG subunits. J Clin Endocrinol Metab 1973;36:73—80.

[3] Ryan RJ, Charlesworth MC, McCormick DJ, Milius RP, Keutmann HT. The glycoprotein hormones: recent studies of structure-function relationships. FASEB J 1988;2:2661—9.

[4] Koistinen H, Koel M, Peters M, Rinken A, Lundin K, Tuuri T, Tapanainen JS, Alfthan H, Salumets A, Stenman UH, Lavogina D. Hyperglycosylated hCG activates LH/hCG-receptor with lower activity than hCG. Mol Cell Endocrinol 2019;479:103—9.

[5] Stenman UH, Alfthan H, Hotakainen K. Human chorionic gonadotropin in cancer. Clin Biochem 2004;37:549—61.

[6] Lunghi L, Ferretti ME, Medici S, Biondi C, Vesce F. Control of human trophoblast function. Reprod Biol Endocrinol 2007;5:6.

[7] Knöfler M. Critical growth factors and signalling pathways controlling human trophoblast invasion. Int J Dev Biol 2010;54:269—80.

[8] Zygmunt M, Hahn D, Munstedt K, Bischof P, Lang U. Invasion of cytotrophoblastic JEG-3 cells is stimulated by hCG in vitro. Placenta 1998;19:587—93.

[9] Zygmunt M, McKinnon T, Herr F, Lala PK, Han VK. HCG increases trophoblast migration in vitro via the insulin-like growth factor-II/mannose-6 phosphate receptor. Mol Hum Reprod 2005;11:261—7.

[10] Prast J, Saleh L, Husslein H, Sonderegger S, Helmer H, Knöfler M. Human chorionic gonadotropin stimulates trophoblast invasion through extracellularly regulated kinase and AKT signaling. Endocrinology 2008;149:979—87.

[11] Lee CL, Chiu PCN, Hautala L, Salo T, Yeung WSB, Stenman UH, Koistinen H. Human chorionic gonadotropin and its free beta-subunit stimulate trophoblast invasion independent of LH/hCG receptor. Mol Cell Endocrinol 2013;375:43—52.

[12] Lam KK, Chiu PC, Chung MK, Lee CL, Lee KF, Koistinen R, Koistinen H, Seppälä M, Ho PC, Yeung WS. Glycodelin-A as a modulator of trophoblast invasion. Hum Reprod 2009;24:2093—103.

[13] Lam KKW, Chiu PCN, Lee C-L, Pang RTK, Leung CON, Koistinen H, Seppälä M, Ho P-C, Yeung WSB. Glycodelin-A interacts with siglec-6 to suppress trophoblast invasiveness by down-regulating ERK/c-Jun signaling pathway. J Biol Chem 2011;286: 37118—27.

[14] Cole LA. hCG, the wonder of today's science. Reprod Biol Endocrinol 2012;10:24.

[15] Handschuh K, Guibourdenche J, Tsatsaris V, Guesnon M, Laurendeau I, Evain-Brion D, Fournier T. Human chorionic gonadotropin produced by the invasive trophoblast but not the villous trophoblast promotes cell invasion and is down-regulated by peroxisome proliferator-activated receptor-gamma. Endocrinology 2007;148:5011—9.

[16] Evans J, Salamonsen LA, Menkhorst E, Dimitriadis E. Dynamic changes in hyperglycosylated human chorionic gonadotrophin throughout the first trimester of pregnancy and its role in early placentation. Hum Reprod 2015;30:1029—38.

[17] Kovalevskaya G, Birken S, Kakuma T, O'Connor JF. Early pregnancy human chorionic gonadotropin (hCG) isoforms measured by an immunometric assay for choriocarcinoma-like hCG. J Endocrinol 1999;161:99—106.

[18] Stenman UH, Birken S, Lempiäinen A, Hotakainen K, Alfthan H. Elimination of complement interference in immunoassay of hyperglycosylated human chorionic gonadotropin. Clin Chem 2011;57:1075—7.

[19] Lash GE, Otun HA, Innes BA, Bulmer JN, Searle RF, Robson SC. Inhibition of trophoblast cell invasion by TGFB1, 2, and 3 is associated with a decrease in active proteases. Biol Reprod 2005;73:374—81.

[20] Graham CH, Connelly I, MacDougall JR, Kerbel RS, Stetler-Stevenson WG, Lala PK. Resistance of malignant trophoblast cells to both the antiproliferative and anti-invasive effects of transforming growth factor-beta. Exp Cell Res 1994;214:93—9.

[21] Koistinen H, Hautala L, Koli K, Stenman UH. Absence of TGF-β receptor activation by highly purified hCG preparations. Mol Endocrinol 2015;29:1787—91.

[22] Ferretti C, Bruni L, Dangles-Marie V, Pecking AP, Bellet D. Molecular circuits shared by placental and cancer cells, and their implications in the proliferative, invasive and migratory capacities of trophoblasts. Hum Reprod Update 2007;13:121—41.

[23] Fluhr H, Bischof-Islami D, Krenzer S, Licht P, Bischof P, Zygmunt M. Human chorionic gonadotropin stimulates matrix metalloproteinases-2 and -9 in cytotrophoblastic cells and decreases tissue inhibitor of metalloproteinases-1,-2, and -3 in decidualized endometrial stromal cells. Fertil Steril 2008;90:1390—5.

[24] Gaynor LM, Colucci F. Uterine natural killer cells: functional distinctions and influence on pregnancy in humans and mice. Front Immunol 2017;8:467.

[25] Kane N, Kelly R, Saunders PT, Critchley HO. Proliferation of uterine natural killer cells is induced by human chorionic gonadotropin and mediated via the mannose receptor. Endocrinology 2009;150:2882—8.

[26] Sengodan SK, Nadhan R, Nair RS, Hemalatha SK, Somasundaram V, Sushama RR, Rajan A, Latha NR, Varghese GR, Thankappan RK, Kumar JM, Chil A, Anilkumar TV, Srinivas P. BRCA1 regulation on β-hCG: a mechanism for tumorigenicity in BRCA1 defective breast cancer. Oncogenesis 2017;6:e376.

[27] Liu N, Peng SM, Zhan GX, Yu J, Wu WM, Gao H, Li XF, Guo XQ. Human chorionic gonadotropin β regulates epithelial-mesenchymal transition and metastasis in human ovarian cancer. Oncol Rep 2017;38:1464—72.

[28] Wu W, Walker AM. Human chorionic gonadotropin beta (HCGbeta) downregulates E-cadherin and promotes human prostate carcinoma cell migration and invasion. Cancer 2006;106:68—78.

[29] Li Z, Li C, Du L, Zhou Y, Wu W. Human chorionic gonadotropin β induces migration and invasion via activating ERK1/2 and MMP-2 in human prostate cancer DU145 cells. PLoS One 2013a;8(2):e54592.

[30] Li Z, Du L, Li C, Wu W. Human chorionic gonadotropin β induces cell motility via ERK1/2 and MMP-2 activation in human glioblastoma U87MG cells. J Neuro Oncol 2013b;111:237–44.

[31] Głodek A, Jankowska A. CGB activates ERK and AKT kinases in cancer cells via LHCGR-independent mechanism. Tumour Biol 2014;35:5467–79.

[32] Shiraishi K, Ascoli M. Lutropin/choriogonadotropin stimulate the proliferation of primary cultures of rat leydig cells through a pathway that involves activation of the extracellularly regulated kinase 1/2 cascade. Endocrinology 2007;148:3214–25.

[33] Casarini L, Lispi M, Longobardi S, Milosa F, La Marca A, Tagliasacchi D, Pignatti E, Simoni M. LH and hCG action on the same receptor results in quantitatively and qualitatively different intracellular signalling. PLoS One 2012;7:e46682.

[34] Mertens-Walker I, Bolitho C, Baxter RC, Marsh DJ. Gonadotropin-induced ovarian cancer cell migration and proliferation require extracellular signal-regulated kinase 1/2 activation regulated by calcium and protein kinase Cδ. Endocr Relat Cancer 2010;17:335–49.

[35] Heublein S, Mayr D, Vrekoussis T, Friese K, Hofmann SS, Jeschke U, Lenhard M. The G-protein coupled estrogen receptor (GPER/GPR30) is a gonadotropin receptor dependent positive prognosticator in ovarian carcinoma patients. PLoS One 2013;8:e71791.

[36] Hughes P, Marshall D, Reid Y, Parkes H, Gelber C. The costs of using unauthenticated, over-passaged cell lines: how much more data do we need? Biotechniques 2007; 43(575):577–8.

[37] Fusenig NE, Capes-Davis A, Bianchini F, Sundell S, Lichter P. The need for a worldwide consensus for cell line authentication: experience implementing a mandatory requirement at the International Journal of Cancer. PLoS Biol 2017;15:e2001438.

[38] Gillott DJ, Iles RK, Chard T. The effects of β-human chorionic gonadotrophin on the in vitro growth of bladder cancer cell lines. Br J Cancer 1996;73:323–6.

[39] Cole LA, Butler S. Hyperglycosylated hCG, hCGβ and hyperglycosylated hCGβ: interchangeable cancer promoters. Mol Cell Endocrinol 2012;349:232–8.

[40] Burczynska B, Booth MJ, Iles RK, Shah A, Shiled A, Butler SA. Stable knockdown of hCGβ mRNA expression in bladder cancer cells results in significant growth inhibition. Anticancer Res 2013;33:3611–4.

[41] Butler SA, Ikram MS, Mathieu S, Iles RK. The increase in bladder carcinoma cell population induced by the free beta subunit of human chorionic gonadotrophin is a result of an anti-apoptosis effect and not cell proliferation. Br J Cancer 2000;82:1553–6.

[42] Szczerba A, Śliwa A, Kubiczak M, Nowak-Markwitz E, Jankowska A. Human chorionic gonadotropin β subunit affects the expression of apoptosis-regulating factors in ovarian cancer. Oncol Rep 2016;35:538–45.

[43] Hamada AL, Nakabayashi K, Sato A, Kiyoshi K, Takamatsu Y, Laoag-Fernandez JB, Ohara N, Maruo T. Transfection of antisense chorionic gonadotropin beta gene into choriocarcinoma cells suppresses the cell proliferation and induces apoptosis. J Clin Endocrinol Metab 2005;90:4873–9.

[44] Berndt S, Blacher S, Munaut C, Detilleux J, Perrier d'Hauterive S, Huhtaniemi I, Evain-Brion D, Noël A, Fournier T, Foidart JM. Hyperglycosylated human chorionic gonadotropin stimulates angiogenesis through TGF-β receptor activation. FASEB J 2013;27: 1309–21.

[45] Berndt S, Blacher S, Perrier d'Hauterive S, Thiry M, Tsampalas M, Cruz A, Péqueux C, Lorquet S, Munaut C, Noël A, Foidart JM. Chorionic gonadotropin stimulation of angiogenesis and pericyte recruitment. J Clin Endocrinol Metab 2009;94:4567—74.

[46] Jauniaux E, Bao S, Eblen A, Li X, Lei ZM, Meuris S, Rao CV. HCG concentration and receptor gene expression in placental tissue from trisomy 18 and 21. Mol Hum Reprod 2000;6:5—10.

[47] Saleh L, Prast J, Haslinger P, Husslein P, Helmer H, Knöfler M. Effects of different human chorionic gonadotrophin preparations on trophoblast differentiation. Placenta 2007;28:199—203.

[48] Yarram SJ, Jenkins J, Cole LA, Brown NL, Sandy JR, Mansell JP. Epidermal growth factor contamination and concentrations of intact human chorionic gonadotropin in commercial preparations. Fertil Steril 2004;82:232—3.

[49] Van Dorsselaer A, Carapito C, Delalande F, Schaeffer-Reiss C, Thierse D, Diemer H, McNair DS, Krewski D, Cashman NR. Detection of prion protein in urine-derived injectable fertility products by a targeted proteomic approach. PLoS One 2011;6: e17815.

[50] Kauffman HF, Hovenga H, de Bruijn HW, Beintema JJ. Eosinophil derived neurotoxin (EDN) levels in commercial human urinary preparations of glycoprotein hormones. Eur J Obstet Gynecol Reprod Biol 1999;82:111—3.

[51] Birken S, Krichevsky A, O'Connor J, Schlatterer J, Cole L, Kardana A, Canfield R. Development and characterization of antibodies to a nicked and hyperglycosylated form of hCG from a choriocarcinoma patient: generation of antibodies that differentiate between pregnancy hCG and choriocarcinoma hCG. Endocrine 1999;10:137—44.

[52] Valmu L, Alfthan H, Hotakainen K, Birken S, Stenman UH. Site-specific glycan analysis of human chorionic gonadotropin beta-subunit from malignancies and pregnancy by liquid chromatography-electrospray mass spectrometry. Glycobiology 2006;16: 1207—18.

The role of the free β-subunit of human chorionic gonadotropin in human malignancy

4.4

Snega M. Sinnappan, Robert C. Baxter, Deborah J. Marsh

hCGβ in primary human malignancy

According to the World Health Organization (WHO), cancer is the second leading cause of mortality worldwide [1]. The lack of specific symptoms, diagnostic tools, and biomarkers in some cancers can lead to diagnosis at a late stage when treatment can be difficult. Thus identification of new specific biomarkers for early detection and monitoring of disease, as well as the development of new therapeutic strategies, is pivotal to combating cancer.

The monomeric β-subunit of hCG (hCGβ), but not the heterodimer, is predominantly elevated in nontrophoblastic epithelial cancers [2,3], including bladder [4,5], cervical [6], and pancreatic [7] cancers and is often a hallmark of aggressive and metastatic disease with poor clinical outcomes (Table 4.4.1) [2,8−10]. High hCGβ levels have also been associated with tumors which are resistant to radiotherapy [11] and chemotherapy [12]. Monitoring the level of hCGβ as a biomarker for prognosis, relapse, and therapeutic response has been well established in trophoblastic cancers and germline tumors [2,13−15]. This chapter focuses on hCGβ in nontrophoblastic cancers, specifically its functional role, and its value as a biomarker and therapeutic target.

Ovarian cancer

Vartiainen and colleagues showed that elevated levels of hCGβ in patients with ovarian cancer correlated with the stage of the disease and poor survival outcomes. They found that elevated hCGβ occurred in 82% of patients with stage IV disease compared with 12% with stage I [16]. Another study, also by Vartiainen et al., found that the combination of elevated hCGβ levels and p53 expression was a strong prognostic marker in patients with serous ovarian cancer [17]. Specifically, the 5-year survival for patients with either elevated serum hCGβ levels or aberrant p53 expression was 44% but only 14% in patients who had both elevated hCGβ levels and

Table 4.4.1 Ectopic hCG/hCGβ profiles on various nontrophoblastic cancers.

Cancer type	% Expression of hCGβ (cohort size)	Tissue type	Outcomes
Ovarian			
	33% (N = 173)	Serum	Strong association between high levels of hCGβ and poor survival outcomes of patients with serous epithelial ovarian cancer (SEOC) [17].
	29% (N = 146)	Serum	The frequency of hCGβ elevation correlated with the stage of SEOC: 12% in stage I and 82% in stage IV [16].
	41% (N = 27)	Serum and ascites	The ratio of hCG/hCGβ levels was found to be elevated in serum and ascites fluids of patients with SEOC [18].
	67% (N = 123) 68% (N = 156)	Serum Tissue	Higher levels of hCG were detected in malignant tumors (SEOC and mucinous carcinoma) compared with benign tumors. In mucinous carcinomas, expression of hCG was significantly higher at stage III compared with stage I [63].
Bladder			
	47% (N = 38)	Serum	hCGβ levels potential indicator of malignant potential and aggression [31].
	38% (N = 86)	Tissue	hCGβ was associated with tumor grade, stage, and poor patient outcome [34].
	29% (N = 100)	Tissue	hCGβ in tumor tissue negatively correlated to response of patients to radiotherapy treatment [35].
Head and neck			
	12% (N = 16)	Tissue	hCGβ indicator of tumor aggression in mucoepidermoid carcinoma, adenoid cystic carcinoma [32].
	64% (N = 45)	Tissue	hCGβ in oral squamous cell carcinomas correlated with tumor grade [64].
Prostrate			
	15% (N = 80)	Tissue	hCGβ was indicative of poor prognosis; however, this was independent of tumor grade [9].

Table 4.4.1 Ectopic hCG/hCGβ profiles on various nontrophoblastic cancers.—*cont'd*

Cancer type	% Expression of hCGβ (cohort size)	Tissue type	Outcomes
Pancreatic			
	32% (N = 47)	Serum	Levels of hCGβ were indicative of malignant potential, aggression, and poor prognosis [31].
	42% (N = 36)	Serum	hCGβ levels were an indicator of high tumor aggression and poor patient outcomes [30].
Colorectal			
	36% (N = 136)	Tissue	hCGβ correlated with poor prognosis of early stage colorectal cancer patients [38].
	43% (N = 60)	Tissue	Presence of hCGβ may be involved in tumor invasion [39].
Cervical			
	33% (N = 45)	hCGβcf in urine	Elevated hCGβcf levels were indicative of poor survival outcomes for patients with cervical carcinomas [6].
Renal			
	20% (N = 177)	Serum	The concentration of hCGβ negatively correlated with patient survival [10,65].

aberrant p53 expression. The 5-year survival outcome for patients with normal hCGβ and p53 expression was 82%.

The value of hCGβ in monitoring disease progression in ovarian cancer is not well established. Grossman et al. have shown that the ratio of hCG/hCGβ correlated with tumor burden in a 47-year-old patient with ovarian cancer who had undergone chemotherapy followed by surgical debulking [18]. The patient received chemotherapy for 12 weeks during which time there was no response and hCG/hCGβ levels were elevated. Following tumor excision at 12 weeks, there was a significant drop in the level of hCG/hCGβ; however, this level increased following relapse of the disease.

Cervical cancer

A study by Crawford et al. had a different approach for the detection of hCGβ in patients with primary cervical carcinoma [6]. Specifically, a metabolic product of hCGβ, the β-core fragment (hCGβcf) was detected in urine samples. Samples were taken from 57 patients with early primary cervical carcinoma and 42 patients with recurrent disease. Results from the study showed that the 4-year survival outcome for hCGβcf negative women was 79% compared with only 14% of women who were hCGβcf positive.

The groups were then further divided into stages of presentation: early (stage 1) and late stage (stage 2 and more advanced) and survival outcomes were determined on the basis of disease stage and hCGβcf expression. The groups were hCGβcf positive/early, hCGβcf positive/late, hCGβcf negative/early, and hCGcβ negative/late. The 4-year survival for the hCGβcf negative/early group was the highest compared with all other groups.

These data suggest that hCGβ (hCGβcf) can be detected by a less invasive method (compared with serum or tissue extraction) in urine, as well as also being a prognostic biomarker for women with primary cervical carcinoma.

Breast cancer

Compared with the cancers discussed thus far, the effect of hCG and ectopic hCGβ on breast cancer is paradoxical, as the dimer and monomer appear to have opposing effects. Specifically, hCG seems to reduce the risk of developing breast cancer, while ectopic hCGβ is associated with aggravated progression of the cancer [19,20]. A number of studies have observed that biological conditions leading to exposure to high levels of hCG are associated with reduced risk of developing breast cancer, including conditions such as pregnancy [21−23] and hCG-induced weight loss treatment [21,24]. This apparently protective effect of hCG on breast cancer has led to proposal of the use of hCG as a treatment to reduce the risk of breast cancer [24]. However, the relationship between pregnancy and breast cancer is contentious as studies have also shown that pregnancy can in fact increase the risk of breast cancer [25]. These conflicting observations could be due to the difficulty of detecting malignant masses in the breast during pregnancy and lactation [25−27]. The cancer may have developed either prior to or during pregnancy—a chicken or egg scenario.

Elevated hCGβ on the other hand seems to be associated with metastatic breast cancer [28]. Furthermore, in vitro data generated by Sengodan et al. suggests that BRCA1 in breast cancer cell lines may regulate hCGβ expression [29]. Mutant BRCA1 or the absence of this protein seems to upregulate hCGβ. This study also suggests that hCGβ can induce migration and invasion, as well as proliferation, of mutant BRCA1 breast cancer cell lines through the interaction of hCGβ with the TGFβII receptor.

Small cell lung cancer

Szturmowicz et al. aimed to determine whether the level of hCGβ in the serum of patients with small cell lung cancer could be used as a prognostic factor or to reclassify the cancer into different subtypes [12]. They found that serum levels of hCGβ were elevated in 21 of 156 patients (14%) which correlated with poor survival outcomes (5% compared with 21% 2-year survival). Interestingly, 73% of patients with normal levels of hCGβ responded to chemotherapy, compared with 48% of patients with elevated hCGβ levels. These data suggest that hCGβ could be involved in resistance to chemotherapy in this tumor type.

Pancreatic cancer

Syrigos et al. compared the levels of hCGβ in serum of 36 patients newly diagnosed with exocrine pancreatic adenocarcinoma with 12 patients with chronic pancreatitis and 21 healthy individuals [30]. hCGβ was elevated in serum of 15 of the 36 (>40%) newly diagnosed pancreatic cancer patients versus only one of 12 patients (8%) with chronic pancreatitis. Healthy, nonpregnant individuals did not express hCGβ. This study also found cancer patients who were hCGβ positive had lower survival outcomes compared with patients who were hCGβ negative. These results suggest that serum hCGβ levels could be a prognostic biomarker of exocrine pancreatic adenocarcinoma. Another study showed similar results, with 32% ($N = 47$) of pancreatic cancer patients demonstrating elevated hCGβ, correlating with increased tumor aggression and poor patient outcomes [31].

Head and neck cancer

Meda et al. found that 12.5% of 16 tumors from patients with salivary gland cancer (mucoepidermoid carcinoma and adenoid cystic carcinoma) expressed hCGβ. In this study, the rate of hCGβ expression was an indicator of tumor aggression [32]. A case study in a female patient with sinonasal teratocarcinosarcoma (SNTCS) showed that serum hCGβ could be used to monitor tumor response to radiation therapy (RT). Specifically, hCGβ levels decreased post RT [33].

Bladder cancer

Expression of hCGβ has been shown in both tumor tissue and serum of patients with bladder cancer and is a possible indicator of malignant potential, aggression, tumor grade, stage, and poor patient outcome [34,35]. Interestingly, in a study that involved 100 patients with urothelial carcinoma, expression of hCGβ in tumor tissue negatively correlated with response of patients to RT [35].

A case study involving a woman with urothelial cancer demonstrated that the level of hCGβ in serum could be used to monitor the response of the patient to treatment [36]. High levels of hCGβ were observed at initial presentation, relapse, and metastasis. Decreased levels of hCGβ were indicative of a positive response toward treatment, which included initial transurethral resection of bladder tumor and intra-vesical immunotherapy with the live attenuated strain of *Mycobacterium bovis* Bacillus Calmette-Guérin (BCG) and subsequent chemotherapy with gentamicin and cisplatin.

Colorectal cancer

Bowel or colorectal cancer (CRC) is the third highest cause of cancer death in the world. The 5-year survival of patients diagnosed at an early stage can be above 90%, dwindling to as low as 10% when diagnosed at an advanced stage [37]. Studies have shown almost 40% of patients with CRC are hCGβ positive [38,39] and that this is an indicator of poor prognosis for both early [38] and late stage [40] CRC patients.

Insights into hCGβ function from cancer models

The hCGβ subunit alone cannot interact with its LHCG receptor, thus hCGβ was originally thought to have no functional biological role; however, a number of studies have shown evidence of its biological activity in nontrophoblastic cancers, with effects observed on proliferation, apoptosis, and malignant transformation. Fig. 4.4.1 describes the potential biological activity of hCGβ in nontrophoblastic cancers.

Cell proliferation

Gillott et al. observed that exogenous hCGβ could promote proliferation of the bladder cancer cell lines T24, SCaBER, RT112, and 5637 in a dose-dependent manner shown by the tetrazolium salt reduction assay (MTT) [41]. T24 cells secreted the least amount of hCGβ but showed the highest proliferative response to exogenous hCGβ. This group also showed that the proliferative effect of hCGβ could be reversed with the addition of anti-hCGβ antiserum in a dose-dependent manner. Additionally, the antiserum could only inhibit cell growth in bladder cancer cell lines that produced endogenous hCGβ [41]. Other studies, however, have shown that hCGβ expression does not have an effect on cell proliferation, e.g., in epithelial ovarian cancer [42] and colorectal cell lines [38]. These findings suggest that the effect of hCGβ on cell proliferation is likely dependent on cell type.

Cell apoptosis

hCGβ has been shown to be involved in preventing apoptosis in some cancer cell lines [43,44]. Janowaska et al. showed that downregulation of hCGβ in the cervical carcinoma cell line HeLa caused an increase in the population of cells undergoing apoptosis (shown by cell cycle analysis) [44]. Butler et al. found additional evidence

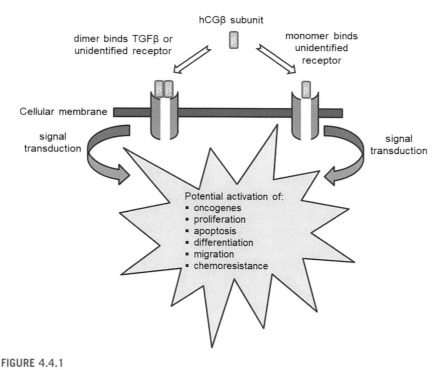

hCGβ subunit

dimer binds TGFβ or
unidentified receptor

monomer binds
unidentified
receptor

Cellular membrane

signal
transduction

signal
transduction

Potential activation of:
- oncogenes
- proliferation
- apoptosis
- differentiation
- migration
- chemoresistance

FIGURE 4.4.1

Potential biological activity of hCGβ in nontrophoblastic cancers.

in support of the antiapoptotic role of hCGβ by showing that exogenous hCGβ reversed the apoptotic effects of TGF-β1 in a dose-dependent manner in bladder cancer cell lines [43]. They proposed that due to the structural similarity between hCGβ and TGFβ, hCGβ may be competing with dimeric TGFβ for the TGFβ receptor. This is a plausible theory, given that it has been found that like some members of the cysteine knot family, hCGβ can form homodimers which are required for receptor interaction [45]. Therefore, even if hCGβ cannot interact alone with the LHCGR, it may be able to participate in cellular processes by binding to an alternative receptor.

Cell migration and invasion

Wu et al. showed that overexpression of hCGβ in prostate carcinoma cell lines caused a change in cellular morphology which increased migratory characteristics in these cells [46]. Cell morphology changed from rounded to more elongated shapes with increased cellular protrusions, decreased E-cadherin expression, and increased migration and invasion through matrigel. A successive paper from Wu and colleagues showed that activation of ERK1/2 and subsequent upregulation of matrix metalloproteinase-2 (MMP-2) was the mechanism by which hCGβ induced invasion and migration in the prostate cancer cell line DU145 [47]. They also demonstrated that hCGβ could increase motility of the human glioblastoma cell line U87MG by the same mechanism [48]. A recent in vivo study by Wu et al. on a nude mouse orthotopic ovarian model showed that overexpression of hCGβ in epithelial ovarian cancer cell lines could induce metastasis of the cells from their site of injection (ovaries) to parts of the peritoneum. They also showed that hCGβ potentially activated the ERK/MMP2 signaling pathway and was independent of the presence of LH and LHCGR [42]. Li et al. showed that overexpression of hCGβ in colorectal cancer cell line models increased the metastatic potential of these cells, both in vitro and in vivo [38].

Malignant transformation

Whether hCGβ is a driver of cancer progression or can actually transform normal cells into malignant cells was studied by Guo et al. [49]. This study showed that overexpression of hCGβ in ovarian surface epithelial (OSE) cells caused an increase in proliferation, anchorage independent growth, and a decrease in apoptosis by mechanisms that increased prosurvival proteins such as Bcl-X_L, as well as a decrease in the proapoptotic protein phospho-Bad. They also found that xenografts of these transformed cells were tumorigenic in nude mice.

Singh et al. showed that mice expressing hCGβ inoculated with Lewis lung carcinoma cell lines had an increase in tumor incidence and volume compared to nontransgenic mice. Examination of tumors extracted from the transgenic mice also showed increased expression of a number of factors including survivin, tumor necrosis factor (TNF-α), and vascular endothelial growth factor (VEGF), which are considered to be drivers of tumorigenesis [50].

hCGβ in chemoresistance and as a therapeutic target

Development of resistance to chemotherapeutic drugs is a factor for poor survival outcomes of many cancer patients [51]. This section focuses on the association of ectopic hCGβ with chemoresistance and opportunities for targeted immunotherapy.

Modeling chemoresistance

Berman et al. found that xenografts of small cell bronchial carcinoma which expressed hCGβ were resistant to the chemotherapeutic drug cyclophosphamide [52]. They studied xenografts of tumors established from patients with small cell lung cancer which had differing responsiveness to the chemotherapeutic drug cyclophosphamide. One chemosensitive xenograft (HX78) which was never exposed to cyclophosphamide was made resistant by repeated exposures to the drug. These investigators found that when the xenografts were maintained in culture, the cyclophosphamide-resistant line HX78Cy produced up to five times more hCGβ (detected in the media by radioimmunoassay) compared with the parental chemosensitive line (HX78) [53]. This suggests that the levels of secreted hCGβ could be linked to chemoresistance.

hCGβ-targeted immunotherapy in cancer therapy

The potential tumorigenic role of ectopic hCGβ in nontrophoblastic tumors has prompted consideration of hCGβ as a therapeutic target. A contraceptive vaccine known as CTP37-DT which is composed of synthetic peptides derived from the C-terminal peptide (CTP) of hCGβ conjugated to the diphtheria toxoid (DT) has been investigated for the treatment of hCGβ-producing cancers. The CTP sequence (CTP37) is specific to hCGβ and does not cross-react with LH [54,55]. CTP37-DT triggers an immune response resulting in the production of anti-hCGβ antibodies, thereby neutralizing hCGβ, and subsequently its activity [56,57].

An in vitro study by Butler et al. showed that hCGβ antisera derived from mice inoculated with CTP37 had an antiapoptotic effect on hCGβ-producing bladder cancer cells [58]. Results of clinical trials headed by Moulton et al. on the use of CTP37-DT in the treatment in patients with advanced colorectal cancer have shown promise [59]. Patients who produced anti-hCGβ antibody titers above the median value post-treatment had increased survival rates [59]. This group also showed the CTP37-DT (under the brand name Avicine) could trigger the production of two antibodies toward two distinct epitopes within the peptide. Colorectal cancer patients who produced both antibodies showed increased survival rates [60].

Research into immunotoxins, based on antibodies against hCG/hCGβ, is ongoing. Talwar's group developed a recombinant anti-hCG antibody (PiPP) and conjugated it to the toxin curcumin (diferuloylmethane) [61]. In vitro data showed that this PiPP-curcumin immunotoxin was effective in killing hCGβ expressing MOLT-4 (leukemia) and U-937 cells lines (lymphoma), as well as leukocytes from acute myeloid leukemia (AML) patients. However, due to the instability of the conjugate, the group developed an improved recombinant PiPP (scPiPP) conjugated to a portion of pseudomonas exotoxin A (PE38). In vitro data showed that scPiPP-PE38 had a cytotoxic effect on not just MOLT-4 and U-937 cell lines but also on the hCGβ expressing lung carcinoma cell line A549 [62].

Conclusions

Expression of ectopic hCGβ by various nontrophoblastic cancers highlights the potential of hCGβ as a biomarker for diagnosis, management, and patient outcomes. Experimental evidence shows that hCGβ may have a biological role in proliferation, migration, differentiation, and activation of oncogenic factors in some cancer cells. These findings position hCGβ as a target for immunotherapy for certain malignancies, including those presenting at an advanced stage with poor patient survival outcomes.

Acknowledgments

SMS was the recipient of a National Health and Medical Research Council (NHMRC) Dora Lush scholarship.

References

[1] World Health Organisation. Cancer. 2018. https://wwwwhoint/cancer/en/.

[2] Stenman U-H, Alfthan H, Hotakainen K. Human chorionic gonadotropin in cancer. Clin Biochem 2004;37(7):549−61.

[3] Iles RK, Delves PJ, Butler SA. Does hCG or hCGβ play a role in cancer cell biology? Mol Cell Endocrinol 2010;329(1−2):62−70.

[4] Iles RK, Persad R, Trivedi M, Sharma KB, Dickinson A, Smith P, et al. Urinary concentration of human chorionic gonadotrophin and its fragments as a prognostic marker in bladder cancer. Br J Urol 1996;77(1):61−9.

[5] Halim AB, Barakat M, el-Zayat AM, Daw M, el-Ahmady O. Urinary beta-HCG in benign and malignant urinary tract diseases. Dis Markers 1995;12(2):109−15.

[6] Crawford RA, Iles RK, Carter PG, Caldwell CJ, Shepherd JH, Chard T. The prognostic significance of beta human chorionic gonadotrophin and its metabolites in women with cervical carcinoma. J Clin Pathol 1998;51(9):685−8.

[7] Louhimo J, Alfthan H, Stenman UH, Haglund C. Serum HCG beta and CA 72-4 are stronger prognostic factors than CEA, CA 19-9 and CA 242 in pancreatic cancer. Oncology 2004;66(2):126−31.

[8] Acevedo HF, Hartsock RJ. Metastatic phenotype correlates with high expression of membrane-associated complete beta-human chorionic gonadotropin in vivo. Cancer 1996;78(11):2388−99.

[9] Sheaff MT, Martin JE, Badenoch DF, Baithun SI. Beta hCG as a prognostic marker in adenocarcinoma of the prostate. J Clin Pathol 1996;49(4):329−32.

[10] Hotakainen K, Ljungberg B, Paju A, Rasmuson T, Alfthan H, Stenman UH. The free beta-subunit of human chorionic gonadotropin as a prognostic factor in renal cell carcinoma. Br J Canc 2002;86(2):185−9.

[11] Jenkins BJ, Martin JE, Baithun SI, Zuk RJ, Oliver RT, Blandy JP. Prediction of response to radiotherapy in invasive bladder cancer. Br J Urol 1990;65(4):345−8.

[12] Szturmowicz M, Wiatr E, Sakowicz A, Slodkowska J, Roszkowski K, Filipecki S, et al. The role of human chorionic gonadotropin beta subunit elevation in small-cell lung cancer patients. J Cancer Res Clin Oncol 1995;121(5):309−12.

[13] Newlands ES. The management of recurrent and drug-resistant gestational trophoblastic neoplasia (GTN). Best Pract Res Clin Obstet Gynaecol 2003;17(6):905−23.

[14] Utsuki S, Oka H, Tanaka S, Tanizaki Y, Fujii K. Long-term outcome of intracranial germinoma with hCG elevation in cerebrospinal fluid but not in serum. Acta Neurochir 2002;144(11):1151−4.

[15] Bagshawe KD. Choriocarcinoma. A model for tumour markers. Acta Oncol 1992;31(1):99−106.

[16] Vartiainen J, Lehtovirta P, Finne P, Stenman UH, Alfthan H. Preoperative serum concentration of hCGβ as a prognostic factor in ovarian cancer. Int J Cancer 2001;95(5):313−6.

[17] Vartiainen J, Lassus H, Lehtovirta P, Finne P, Alfthan H, Butzow R, et al. Combination of serum hCG beta and p53 tissue expression defines distinct subgroups of serous ovarian carcinoma. Int J Cancer 2008;122(9):2125−9.

[18] Grossmann M, Hoermann R, Gocze PM, Ott M, Berger P, Mann K. Measurement of human chorionic gonadotropin-related immunoreactivity in serum, ascites and tumour cysts of patients with gynaecologic malignancies. Eur J Clin Investig 1995;25(11): 867−73.

[19] Schüler-Toprak S, Treeck O, Ortmann O. Human chorionic gonadotropin and breast cancer. Int J Mol Sci 2017;18(7):1587.

[20] Schuler S, Ponnath M, Engel J, Ortmann O. Ovarian epithelial tumors and reproductive factors: a systematic review. Arch Gynecol Obstet 2013;287(6):1187−204.

[21] Russo IH, Russo J. Pregnancy-induced changes in breast cancer risk. J Mammary Gland Biol Neoplasia 2011;16(3):221−33.

[22] Lukanova A, Andersson R, Wulff M, Zeleniuch-Jacquotte A, Grankvist K, Dossus L, et al. Human chorionic gonadotropin and alpha-fetoprotein concentrations in pregnancy and maternal risk of breast cancer: a nested case-control study. Am J Epidemiol 2008; 168(11):1284−91.

[23] Toniolo P, Grankvist K, Wulff M, Chen T, Johansson R, Schock H, et al. Human chorionic gonadotropin in pregnancy and maternal risk of breast cancer. Cancer Res 2010; 70(17):6779−86.

[24] Bernstein L, Hanisch R, Sullivan-Halley J, Ross RK. Treatment with human chorionic gonadotropin and risk of breast cancer. Cancer Epidemiol Biomark Prev 1995;4(5): 437−40.

[25] Stensheim H, Møller B, van Dijk T, Fosså SD. Cause-specific survival for women diagnosed with cancer during pregnancy or lactation: a registry-based cohort study. J Clin Oncol 2009;27(1):45−51.

[26] Eisenstein M. Pregnancy: delivery from breast cancer. Nature 2012;485:S54.

[27] Petrek J, Seltzer V. Breast cancer in pregnant and postpartum women. J Obstet Gynaecol Can 2003;25(11):944−50.

[28] Hoon DS, Sarantou T, Doi F, Chi DD, Kuo C, Conrad AJ, et al. Detection of metastatic breast cancer by beta-hCG polymerase chain reaction. Int J Cancer 1996;69(5):369−74.

[29] Sengodan SK, Nadhan R, Nair RS, Hemalatha SK, Somasundaram V, Sushama RR, et al. BRCA1 regulation on β-hCG: a mechanism for tumorigenicity in BRCA1 defective breast cancer. Oncogenesis 2017;6:e376.

[30] Syrigos KN, Fyssas I, Konstandoulakis MM, Harrington KJ, Papadopoulos S, Milingos N, et al. Beta human chorionic gonadotropin concentrations in serum of patients with pancreatic adenocarcinoma. Gut 1998;42(1):88−91.

[31] Marcillac I, Troalen F, Bidart JM, Ghillani P, Ribrag V, Escudier B, et al. Free human chorionic gonadotropin beta subunit in gonadal and nongonadal neoplasms. Cancer Res 1992;52(14):3901−7.

[32] Meda S, Reginald BA, Reddy BS. Immunohistochemical study of the expression of human chorionic gonadotropin-beta in salivary gland tumors. J Cancer Res Ther 2018; 14(5):952−6.

[33] Weinberg BD, Newell KL, Wang F. A case of a Beta-human chorionic gonadotropin secreting sinonasal teratocarcinosarcoma. J Neurol Surg Rep 2014;75(1):e103−7.

[34] Venyo AK, Herring D, Greenwood H, Maloney DJ. The expression of beta human chorionic gonadotrophin (β-HCG) in human urothelial carcinoma. Pan Afr Med J 2010;7: 20.

[35] Martin JE, Jenkins BJ, Zuk RJ, Oliver RT, Baithun SI. Human chorionic gonadotrophin expression and histological findings as predictors of response to radiotherapy in carcinoma of the bladder. Virchows Arch A Pathol Anat Histopathol 1989;414(3):273−7.

[36] Malkhasyan K, Deshpande HA, Adeniran AJ, Colberg JW, Petrylak DP. The use of serum hCG as a marker of tumor progression and of the response of metastatic urothelial cancer to systemic chemotherapy. Oncology 2013;27(10):1028. 30.

[37] Brenner H, Kloor M, Pox CP. Colorectal cancer. Lancet 2014;383(9927):1490−502.

[38] Li J, Yin M, Song W, Cui F, Wang W, Wang S, et al. B subunit of human chorionic gonadotropin promotes tumor invasion and predicts poor prognosis of early-stage colorectal cancer. Cell Physiol Biochem 2018;45(1):237−49.

[39] Buckley CH, Fox H. An immunohistochemical study of the significance of HCG secretion by large bowel adenocarcinomata. J Clin Pathol 1979;32(4):368−72.

[40] Yamaguchi A, Ishida T, Nishimura G, Kumaki T, Katoh M, Kosaka T, et al. Human chorionic gonadotropin in colorectal cancer and its relationship to prognosis. Br J Canc 1989;60(3):382−4.

[41] Gillott DJ, Iles RK, Chard T. The effects of beta-human chorionic gonadotrophin on the in vitro growth of bladder cancer cell lines. Br J Canc 1996;73(3):323−6.

[42] Wu W, Gao H, Li X, Peng S, Yu J, Liu N, et al. beta-hCG promotes epithelial ovarian cancer metastasis through ERK/MMP2 signaling pathway. Cell Cycle 2018:1−14.

[43] Butler SA, Ikram MS, Mathieu S, Iles RK. The increase in bladder carcinoma cell population induced by the free beta subunit of human chorionic gonadotrophin is a result of an anti-apoptosis effect and not cell proliferation. Br J Canc 2000;82(9):1553−6.

[44] Jankowska A, Gunderson SI, Andrusiewicz M, Burczynska B, Szczerba A, Jarmolowski A, et al. Reduction of human chorionic gonadotropin beta subunit expression by modified U1 snRNA caused apoptosis in cervical cancer cells. Mol Cancer 2008;7:26.

[45] Butler SA, Laidler P, Porter JR, Kicman AT, Chard T, Cowan DA, et al. The beta-subunit of human chorionic gonadotropin exists as a homodimer. J Mol Endocrinol 1999;22(2):185−92.

[46] Wu W, Walker AM. Human chorionic gonadotropin beta (HCGbeta) down-regulates E-cadherin and promotes human prostate carcinoma cell migration and invasion. Cancer 2006;106(1):68−78.

[47] Li Z, Li C, Du L, Zhou Y, Wu W. Human chorionic gonadotropin beta induces migration and invasion via activating ERK1/2 and MMP-2 in human prostate cancer DU145 cells. PLoS One 2013;8(2):e54592.

[48] Li Z, Du L, Li C, Wu W. Human chorionic gonadotropin beta induces cell motility via ERK1/2 and MMP-2 activation in human glioblastoma U87MG cells. J Neuro Oncol 2013;111(3):237−44.

[49] Guo X, Liu G, Schauer IG, Yang G, Mercado-Uribe I, Yang F, et al. Overexpression of the beta subunit of human chorionic gonadotropin promotes the transformation of human ovarian epithelial cells and ovarian tumorigenesis. Am J Pathol 2011;179(3):1385−93.

[50] Singh P, Sarkar M, Agrawal U, Huhtaniemi I, Pal R. The transgenic expression of the β-subunit of human chorionic gonadotropin influences the growth of implanted tumor cells. Oncotarget 2018;9(78):34670−80.

[51] Zheng H-C. The molecular mechanisms of chemoresistance in cancers. Oncotarget 2017;8(35):59950−64.

[52] Berman R, Steel GG. Induced and inherent resistance to alkylating agents in human small-cell bronchial carcinoma xenografts. Br J Canc 1984;49(4):431–6.

[53] Berman R, Gusterson B, Steel GG. Resistance to alkylating agents and tumour differentiation in xenografts of small cell lung cancer. Br J Canc 1985;51(5):653–8.

[54] Thanavala YM, Hay FC, Stevens VC. Affinity, cross-reactivity and biological effectiveness of rabbit antibodies against a synthetic 37 amino acid C-terminal peptide of human chorionic gonadotrophin. Clin Exp Immunol 1980;39(1):112–8.

[55] Naz RK, Gupta SK, Gupta JC, Vyas HK, Talwar GP. Recent advances in contraceptive vaccine development: a mini-review. Hum Reprod 2005;20(12):3271–83.

[56] Talwar GP, Vyas HK, Purswani S, Gupta JC. Gonadotropin-releasing hormone/human chorionic gonadotropin beta based recombinant antibodies and vaccines. J Reprod Immunol 2009;83(1–2):158–63.

[57] Talwar GP, Singh O, Pal R, Chatterjee N, Sahai P, Dhall K, et al. A vaccine that prevents pregnancy in women. Proc Natl Acad Sci USA 1994;91(18):8532–6.

[58] Butler SA, Staite EM, Iles RK. Reduction of bladder cancer cell growth in response to hCGβ CTP37 vaccinated mouse serum. Oncol Res 2003;14(2):93–100.

[59] Moulton HM, Yoshihara PH, Mason DH, Iversen PL, Triozzi PL. Active specific immunotherapy with a beta-human chorionic gonadotropin peptide vaccine in patients with metastatic colorectal cancer: antibody response is associated with improved survival. Clin Cancer Res 2002;8(7):2044–51.

[60] Iversen PL, Mourich DV, Moulton HM. Monoclonal antibodies to two epitopes of beta-human chorionic gonadotropin for the treatment of cancer. Curr Opin Mol Ther 2003;5(2):156–60.

[61] Vyas HK, Pal R, Vishwakarma R, Lohiya NK, Talwar GP. Selective killing of leukemia and lymphoma cells ectopically expressing hCGbeta by a conjugate of curcumin with an antibody against hCGbeta subunit. Oncology 2009;76(2):101–11.

[62] Nand KN, Gupta JC, Panda AK, Jain SK. Development of a recombinant hCG-specific single chain immunotoxin cytotoxic to hCG expressing cancer cells. Protein Expr Purif 2015;106:10–7.

[63] Lenhard M, Tsvilina A, Schumacher L, Kupka M, Ditsch N, Mayr D, et al. Human chorionic gonadotropin and its relation to grade, stage and patient survival in ovarian cancer. BMC Canc 2012;12:2.

[64] Bhalang K, Kafrawy AH, Miles DA. Immunohistochemical study of the expression of human chorionic gonadotropin-β in oral squamous cell carcinoma. Cancer 1999;85(4):757–62.

[65] Hotakainen K, Lintula S, Ljungberg B, Finne P, Paju A, Stenman U-H, et al. Expression of human chorionic gonadotropin β-subunit type I genes predicts adverse outcome in renal cell carcinoma. J Mol Diagn 2006;8(5):598–603.

hCG and gestational trophoblastic diseases: hydatidiform mole and choriocarcinoma

4.5

Laurence A. Cole

Hydatidiform mole—introduction

A hydatidiform mole or molar pregnancy is an abnormal pregnancy characterized by the abnormal growth of pregnancy, seen as abnormal trophoblasts.

There are two types of molar pregnancy, complete molar pregnancy and partial molar pregnancy. In a complete molar pregnancy, the tissue is swollen and appears as fluid-filled trophoblast tissue cysts. There is also no formation of fetal tissue. In a partial molar pregnancy, there may be normal placental tissue along with some abnormal placental tissue. There may be formation of some fetal tissue, but it is never able to survive and is usually miscarried early in the pregnancy.

In a complete molar pregnancy, an anucleate oocyte without maternal chromosomes is fertilized by two sperm, where all of the genetic material comes from the father. It can also in some cases be fertilized by just one sperm, and the chromosome set duplicated. In a partial molar pregnancy, a normal oocyte is fertilized by two sperm. As a result the embryo has 69 chromosomes instead of 46. Approximately 1 in every 1000 pregnancies is a molar pregnancy.

A molar pregnancy is more likely in women older than 36 or younger than 20 years of age. If you have had one molar pregnancy, you are more likely to have another, odds are 1 in 100.

A complete hydatidiform mole can be invasive or malignant, with the mass of tissue increasing rapidly and chemotherapy is needed. Similarly, half of cases of choriocarcinoma derive from pregnancy and half from complete hydatidiform mole cases.

Molar pregnancies

The B152 hyperglycosylated hCG test is useful in predicting complete mole cases that are becoming invasive and may need chemotherapy to resolve an invasive mole (Table 4.5.1).

100 Years of Human Chorionic Gonadotropin. https://doi.org/10.1016/B978-0-12-820050-6.00025-4

Table 4.5.1 B152 hyperglycosylated hCG test in predicting complete hydatidiform mole that are becoming invasive.

Total hCG test mIU/mL	Hyperglycosylated hCG mIU/mL	% Hyperglycosylated hCG
Complete hydatidiform mole		
24	1.01	4.2%
62	0.3	0.5%
83	0.3	0.4%
121	0.51	0.4%
127	1.44	1.1%
174	0.3	0.2%
386	2.67	0.7%
455	2.67	0.6%
619	0.3	0.0%
653	2.67	0.4%
735	3.31	0.4%
737	2.35	0.3%
746	1.92	0.3%
869	1.44	0.2%
897	1.55	0.2%
1122	1.33	0.1%
1160	0.59	0.1%
1356	4.37	0.3%
1596	1.81	0.1%
2416	16	0.7%
4080	26	0.6%
4750	42	0.9%
4890	71	1.5%
11,600	65	0.6%
14,740	762	5.2%
15,358	187	1.2%
16,317	160	1.0%
16,698	633	3.8%
18,810	758	4.0%
22,540	125	0.6%
24,160	1789	7.4%
30,255	355	1.2%
33,000	1532	4.6%
35,860	1964	5.5%
40,800	2904	7.1%
40,810	1611	3.9%
54,450	2593	4.8%

Table 4.5.1 B152 hyperglycosylated hCG test in predicting complete hydatidiform mole that are becoming invasive.—*cont'd*

	Total hCG test mIU/mL	Hyperglycosylated hCG mIU/mL	% Hyperglycosylated hCG
	64,680	1650	2.6%
	225,400	13,787	6.1%
Average	17,783	796	1.89%
SD	37,579	2247	2.1%

Complete hydatidiform mole. Invasive disease

	521	17.17	3.30%
	522	4.16	0.80%
	642	5.23	0.81%
	700	6.61	0.94%
	774	2.24	0.29%
	882	5.33	0.60%
	1445	2.99	0.21%
	1486	2.88	0.19%
	1981	22.67	1.14%
	2171	13.33	0.61%
	2364	48.53	2.05%
	2662	13.60	0.51%
	3316	12.00	0.36%
	3577	29.07	0.81%
	4059	35.47	0.87%
	5720	46.93	0.82%
	6149	68.80	1.12%
	9461	113	1.20%
	9580	110	1.15%
	11,490	145	1.26%
	12,710	282	2.22%
	15,092	192	1.27%
	15,170	173	1.14%
	20,020	2161	10.8%
	35,770	3197	8.9%
	36,818	418	1.14%
	48,900	7861	16.1%
	55,504	434	0.78%
	61,490	7568	12.3%
	109,056	1226	1.12%
	134,200	5893	4.4%
	154,650	1413	0.91%

Continued

Table 4.5.1 B152 hyperglycosylated hCG test in predicting complete hydatidiform mole that are becoming invasive.—*cont'd*

	Total hCG test mIU/mL	Hyperglycosylated hCG mIU/mL	% Hyperglycosylated hCG
	163,170	17,600	10.8%
	193,991	3680	1.90%
	302,550	39,013	12.9%
	313,500	115,500	36.8%
	369,600	14,929	4.0%
	573,100	142,214	24.8%
	652,300	33,786	5.2%
Average	85,566	10,212	4.53%
SD	156,125	29,416	0.076

As shown, the average hyperglycosylated hCG in the invasive disease group is 10,212, while in the noninvasive disease group, is 171 mIU/mL. Looking at hyperglycosylated hCG as a percentage of total hCG, the average is 4.53% in the invasive disease group and just 1.89% in the noninvasive disease group.

Second, it is noticed from the table of carbohydrate content on hCG that the percentages of triantennary oligosaccharides on complete hydatidiform mole case β-subunit is considerably raised over that of pregnancy, hCG, GGG, and GGGF, heading toward a choriocarcinoma status (Table 4.5.2). The six pregnancy samples of hCG are 5.4%, 10.8%, 10.4%, 17.7%, 21.6%, and 16.5% triantennary; the three hydatidiform mole cases were 18.2%, 32.0%, and 30.0% triantennary; and the five choriocarcinoma cases were 67.0%, 60.0%, 45.3%, 47.1%, and 42.9% triantennary. It is our understanding that triantennary hCG is a marker of extravillous cytotrophoblast invasive cells (see below under choriocarcinoma).

Introduction—choriocarcinoma

Choriocarcinoma is a very rare cancer, occurring at a rate of 1 in 30,000 pregnancies. While occurring seldomly in the United States, the incidence is much common in China and far eastern nations. Choriocarcinoma was first discovered in Germany by Hans Chiari [1], then by Max Saenger in Germany [2], and by Felix Marchand in Germany [3]. The problem was that they guessed at that time that it was malignant cancer, in that it behaved like lung cancer and other cancers, invading and growing all over the body, with secondary metastases in the lung and brain. Hans Chiari, Max Saenger, Felix Marchand nor any physician or scientist since has ever demonstrated that choriocarcinoma, like all proven cancers is actually a cancer by showing any

Table 4.5.2 The oligosaccharide content of hCG (1−12).

	α-Subunit N-linked oligosaccharides (%)							β-Subunit N-linked oligosaccharides (%)							O-linked oligosaccharides (%)		
	GM	GGF	GGM	GG	GGGF	GGG	Sialic acid pmol/pmol	GM	GGF	GGM	GG	GGGF	GGG	Sialic acid pmol/pmol	Type 1	Type 2	Sialic acid pmol/pmol
Pregnancy																	
CR127 pool	48.0	8.9	0	38.4	0	4.8	1.50	3.6	56.3	0	34.7	5.4	0	1.91	81.5	18.5	1.32
CR129 pool	49.7	3.1	0	37.8	0	9.4	1.47	2.2	59.3	0	27.7	10.8	0	2.01	84.4	15.6	1.25
Individual P3	53.8	7.3		36.4	2.6	0	1.76	6.5	44.3	0	38.9	8.3	2.1	2.00	87.7	12.3	1.62
Individual P7	40.7	7.9	0	37.1	14.3	0	1.70	4.4	54.9	0	23.0	13.2	4.5	2.32	81.0	19.0	1.02
Individual P8	41.5	7.3	0	41.1	10.1	0	1.73	1.9	51.9	0	24.6	17.4	4.2	2.06	87.5	12.5	1.46
Individual P9	61.9	9.4	0	29.2	0	0	na	8.8	38.2	0	36.4	12.1	4.4	2.03	84.6	15.4	0.88
Hydatidiform mole																	
Individual M1	43.4	16.7	0	32.3	3.6	3.9	1.32	5.5	57.2	0	19.1	16.5	1.7	2.1	88.9	11.1	0.45
Individual M2	53.1	4.4	0	36.6	0	5.9	1.38	6.9	38.4	0	22.6	20.9	11.1	2.1	61.9	38.1	0.80
Individual M4	35.7	0	0	54.6	0.5	9.2	1.39	8.1	22.8	0	39.0	18.5	11.5	2.66	80.3	19.7	0.98
Choriocarcinoma																	
Individual C1	38.5	16.0	3.6	18.9	6.2	16.7	1.70	6.8	14.8	0	14.8	52.2	11.4	2.37	33.4	66.6	0.52
Individual C2	56.6	24.2	3.7	5.7	0	9.8	1.36	5.9	23.4	0	22.6	38.0	10.1	1.82	52.1	47.9	1.14
Individual C3	71.1	19.1	2.2	4.9	0	2.9	1.06	16.4	23.8	0	11.7	33.6	14.5	2.36	11.8	88.2	0.97
Individual C5	74.8	18.2	2.3	3.5	0	1.2	0.92	15.9	31.9	0	4.4	42.7	5.1	2.19	0	103	1.15
Individual C7	56.5	20.3	5.1	8.0		4.3	0.98	10.9	24.4	9.1	7.5	35.2	12.9	1.60	31.9	68.1	1.05

transformation in the root cytotrophoblast cell or any major change between normal cytotrophoblast cells and choriocarcinoma cells.

Hyperglycosylated hCG is the root of all or most cancers, cells become transformed and start to produce hyperglycosylated hCG and its β-subunit. This generates malignancy in cancer cells, driving cell growth and invasion and blocking apoptosis [4,5]. The problem is that cytotrophoblast cells, the root cells of choriocarcinoma, naturally produce hyperglycosylated hCG and its free β-subunit as trophoblast cells. Here we look carefully at the structure of the hCG produced in normal pregnancy, produced by pregnancy, by extravillous cytotrophoblast, and by choriocarcinoma and the invasion potential trophoblast cells and choriocarcinoma cells and the invasion potential of hyperglycosylated hCG produced by these same cells and investigate whether choriocarcinoma truly is a cancer as suggested.

Results and discussion

I examined the carbohydrate structure of hCG (Table 4.5.2). This was determined for pregnancy hC hydatidiform mole hCG and choriocarcinoma hCG as published previously [6] (Table 4.5.2). Antibody B152 has been shown to only bind hyperglycosylated hCG or its β-subunit, or to only bind dimeric molecules with a type 2 O-linked oligosaccharide and monomeric β-subunit with type 2 O-linked oligosaccharides (Table 4.5.3). Of the six normal pregnancy samples, they contained

Table 4.5.3 The proportion of hCG detected by the B152 hyperglycosylated hCG assay.

Sample	B152 assay as a percentage of total hCG (siemens immulite assay)	Percentage type 2 O-linked oligosaccharides from Table 4.5.1
CR127 pooled pregnancy hCG	7.5%	5.4%
CR129 pooled pregnancy hCG	12.0%	10.8%
Individual P3 pregnancy hCG	9.4%	12.3%
Individual P7 pregnancy hCG	17.5%	19.0%
Individual P8 pregnancy hCG	12.7%	12.5%
Individual P9 pregnancy hCG	17.5%	15.4%
Individual M1 hydatidiform mole hCG	11.4%	11.1%
Individual M2 hydatidiform mole hCG	37.3%	38.1%
Individual M4 hydatidiform mole hCG	25.0%	19.7%
Individual C1 choriocarcinoma hCG	70%	66.6%
Individual C2 choriocarcinoma hCG	32%	47.9%
Individual C3 choriocarcinoma hCG	87%	88.2%
Individual C5 choriocarcinoma hCG	108%	103%
Individual C7 choriocarcinoma hCG	64%	68.1%

7.5%, 12.0%, 9.4%, 17.5%, 12.7%, and 17.5% B152 immunoreactivity or hyperglycosylated hCG (Table 4.5.2). Of the five choriocarcinoma samples, they contained 70%, 32%, 87%, 108%, and 64% B152 immunoreactivity or hyperglycosylated hCG (Table 4.5.3).

Recombinant hCG was pure 100% hormone hCG. It contained only type 1 O-linked oligosaccharides. This was concluded to be a marker of the hormone hCG. As shown in Table 4.5.2, the six pregnancy samples contained 81.5%, 84.4%. 87.7%, 81.0%, 87.5%, and 84.6% hormone hCG (Table 4.5.2), and the five chorio-carcinoma samples contained 33.4%, 52.1%, 11.8%, 0%, and 31.9% hormone hCG.

Multiple authors have reported that there are two distinct kinds of cytotropho-blast cells, normal cytotrophoblast cell, and invasive extravillous cytotrophoblast cells [7−13]. Extravillous cytotrophoblast cells are the invasive cell of blastocyst implantation [14] and hemochorial placentation deep implantation of pregnancy [15,16], and are the cells that link hemochorial placentation to the uterus that accumulate as invasive extravillous cytotrophoblast cells in the second and third trimesters of pregnancy [15,16].

Percoll-density centrifugation sorted term cytotrophoblast primary cells are a model of extravillous cytotrophoblast cells, and ACH-3P cells are a model of first trimester pregnancy cells [17]. As found, the percentage triantennary oligosaccha-rides on first trimester ACH-3P cell hCG matches that on first trimester pregnancy cells, 12.3% versus 5.4%, 10.8%, 10.4%, 17.7%, 21.6%, and 16.5% (Table 4.5.2), while the percentage produced by term cytotrophoblast primary cells (extravillous cytotrophoblast cells) is 48.0% versus 63.6%. 48.1%, 48.1%, 47.8%, and 48.1%, closely matches the percentage produced by choriocarcinoma cells.

Similarly, in a study of trophoblast cell invasion, capability in Matrigel basement membrane chambers, or of cell invasion capability, the invasion capability of Jar and JEG-3 choriocarcinoma cell lines was $48 \pm 11\%$ and $49 \pm 10\%$ (Table 4.5.4), while the invasion capability of extravillous cytotrophoblast cells (term cytotrophoblast primary cells) was $40 \pm 10\%$. The invasion capability of first trimester pregnancy ACH-3P cells was just $12 \pm 2.4\%$. Once again, choriocarcinoma matches extravil-lous cytotrophoblast cells, just as choriocarcinoma triantennary content on hCG matched that on extravillous cytotrophoblast hCG.

Table 4.5.4 Proportion of invasive cells. Penetration of Matrigel basement membrane chambers. Mean $\pm$ SD of quadruplicate determinations.

Penetration of Matrigel membranes (%)	Mean ± SD
ACH-3P first trimester trophoblast cell line	$12 \pm 2.4\%$
Extravillous cytotrophoblast (fresh term cytotrophoblast primary cells)	$40 \pm 10\%$
Jar choriocarcinoma cell line	$49 \pm 10\%$
JEG-3 choriocarcinoma cell line	$48 \pm 11\%$

It is concluded that choriocarcinoma triantennary oligosaccharides on hCG match pregnancy invasive extravillous cytotrophoblast hCG, just as the invasion potency of choriocarcinoma-matched pregnancy invasive extravillous cytotrophoblast cell invasion potency. It is inferred that choriocarcinoma cells are just invasive extravillous cytotrophoblast cells and nothing more.

The invasive extravillous cytotrophoblast cells are the root cells from which choriocarcinoma arises. This study shows that choriocarcinoma derives from invasive extravillous cytotrophoblast cells to start with. These are the highly invasive cells of pregnancy, the cells which promote invasion and deep implantation in pregnancy [14−16]. It simply invades the uterus, lung, and brain as pregnancy extravillous cytotrophoblast, and nothing else. Nobody has ever seen any evidence that choriocarcinoma transforms in any way, it does not, it is simply pregnancy extravillous cytotrophoblast tissue.

Women with choriocarcinoma do not need to be told that they have a cancer. They have a pregnancy disorder. It should be renamed, invasive extravillous cytotrophoblast disease or IECD.

References

[1] Chiari H. Uber drei Falle von primarem kacino in findus und corpus des uterus. Med Jahrb 1877;7:364−7.

[2] Saenger M. Deciduoma malignum. Zbl Gyak 1889;167:537.

[3] Marchand FJ. Uber die sogenannten "decidualen" geshwulskeim im anshluss an nor − male geburt, abort, blasenmole und extrauterineschwanggerahaft. Monatsschr Geburtshilfe Gynakol 1895;1:419−38.

[4] Cole LA. Hyperglycosylated hCG drives malignancy in most or all human cancers: tying all research together. J Anal Oncol 2018;7:14−21.

[5] Cole LA. Hyperglycosylated hCG and its ß-subunit drives malignancy. J Anal Oncol 2018 (in press).

[6] Elliott MM, Kardana A, Lustbader JW, Cole LA. Carbohydrate and peptide structure of the α - and ß-subunits of human chorionic gonadotropin from normal and aberrant pregnancy and choriocarcinoma. Endocrine 1997;7:15−32.

[7] Tetugu BP, Adachi K, Schlitt JM, Ezahi T, Schust DJ, Roberts RM, Schulz LC. Comparison of extravillous trophoblast cells derived from human embryonic stem cells and from first trimester placentas. Placenta 2013;34:436−543.

[8] DaSilva-Arnold S, James JL, Al-Khan A, Zamudio S, Illsey NR. Differentiation of first trimester cytotrophoblast to extravillous trophoblast involves and epithelial-mesenchymal transition. Placenta 2015;36:1412−8.

[9] Leach RE, Kilburn B, Wang J, Liu Z, Romero R, Armant DR. Heparin-binding EGF-like growth factor regulates human extravillous cytotrophoblast development during conversion to the invasive phenotype. Dev Biol 2004;266:223−37.

[10] LaMaca HL, Dash PR, Vishnuthevan K, Harvey E, Sullivan DE, Morris CA, Whitley G. Epidermal growth factor-stimulated extravillous cytotrophoblast motility is mediated by activation of PI3-K, Akt and both p38 and p42/44 mitogen-activated protein kinases. Hum Reprod 2008;23:1733−41.

[11] Naruse K, Innes BA, Bulmer JA, Robson SC, Searle RF, Lash GE. Secretion of cytokines by villous cytotrophoblast and extravillous trophoblast in the first trimester of human pregnancy. J Reprod Immunol 2010;86:148—50.

[12] Wong BS, Lam KK, Lee CL, Wong VH, Lam MP, Chu IK, Yeung WS, Chiu PC. Adrenomedullin enhances invasion of human extravillous cytotrophoblast-derived cell lines by regulation of urokinase plasminogen activator expression and S-nitrosylation. Biol Reprod 2013;88:1—11.

[13] Bandeira CL, Borbely AU, Francisco RPV, Schultz R, Zugaib M, Bevilacqua E. Tumorigenic factor CRIPTO-1 is immunolocalized in extravillous cytotrophoblast in placenta creta. Biomed Res Int 2014;2014:893856.

[14] Evans J. Hyperglycosylated hCG: a unique human implantation and invasion factor. Am J Reprod Immunol 2016;75:333—40.

[15] Cole LA, Brennan MC, Hsu C-D, Bahado-Singh R, Kingston JM. Hyperglycosylated hCG drives deep implantation in pregnancy causing preeclampsia and gestational hypertension. In: Cole LA, Butler SA, editors. 100 years of hCG. Elsevier; 2019 (in press).

[16] Cole LA. hCG and hyperglycosylated hCG. In: Nicholson R, editor. Promoters of villous placenta and hemochorial placentation. Placenta: functions, development and disease. Nova Publishers; 2013. p. 155—66.

[17] Hiden U, Wadsack C, Prutsch N, Gauster M, Weiss U, Frank HG, Schmitz U, Fast-Hirsch C, Hengstschläger M, Pötgens A, Rüben A, Knöfler M, Haslinger P, Huppertz B, Bilban M, Kaufmann P, Desoye G. The first trimester human trophoblast cell line ACH-3P: a novel tool to study autocrine/paracrine regulatory loops of human trophoblast subpopulations–TNF-alpha stimulates MMP15 expression. BMC Dev Biol 2007;7:137.

Immunotherapy of advanced stage, invariably drug-resistant cancers expressing ectopically hCG

4.6

G.P. Talwar, Jagdish C. Gupta, Hemant K. Vyas, Shilpi Puruswani, R.S. Kabeer

Human chorionic gonadotropin and its expression in terminal cancers

Human chorionic gonadotropin (hCG) is normally made by the early embryo soon after fertilization of the egg [1]. It plays a vital role in the implantation of embryos and in sustenance of pregnancy. Neither nonpregnant females, nor healthy males make this hormone. However, a number of publications have appeared in literature reporting the unexpected synthesis and secretion of hCG by advanced stage cancers in both males and females. Almost all types of cancers, such as lung cancer [2], bladder carcinoma [3,4], pancreatic carcinoma [5,6], breast cancer [7], cervical carcinoma [8,9], oral cancers [10,11], head and neck cancers [12], prostate cancer [13], renal carcinoma [14], colon adenocarcinoma [15], gastric carcinoma [16,17], vulva/vaginal cancers [18,19], secrete hCG. Invariably the expression of hCG/subunits takes place at an advanced stage of cancer. The prognosis of such cancers is poor with adverse survival of the patients carrying the β-hCG expressing cancers than the patients suffering from the same type of cancers but not expressing hCG or its subunits [20]. It appears that the dedifferentiation of cells goes to a stage that they become like embryonic cells, thereby expressing proteins such as β-hCG and carcinoembryonic antigen. hCG is a promoter of invasiveness and angiogenesis [21].

Moab PiPP for immunotherapy of hCG positive cancers

Cancers are treatable at early stages by surgery, radiation, and drugs. However, a stage arises when these become resistant to all available drugs which leads to the death of the patient, and nothing else can be done. Immunotherapy by employing specific monoclonal antibodies targeting the diseased cells offers an attractive mode of therapy of such cancers. It was pertinent to inquire whether a monoclonal

100 Years of Human Chorionic Gonadotropin. https://doi.org/10.1016/B978-0-12-820050-6.00026-6

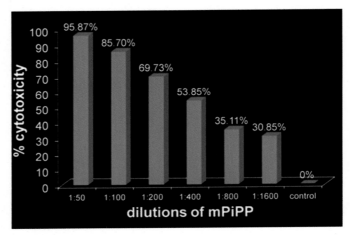

FIGURE 4.6.1

Dose-dependent cytotoxicity exercised by a monoclonal anti-hCG antibody cPiPP on A549 lung cancer cells [23].

antibody PiPP developed by us, many years back, exercised any action on the growth and multiplication of hCG expressing cancer cells. Moab PiPP ($Ka = 3 \times 10^{-10}$ M) has high affinity and specificity for hCG [22].

Recapitulated below are observations on A549 lung cancer cells. Indeed, the antibody in the presence of Complement exercised dose-dependent cytotoxicity on these cancer cells in vitro (Fig. 4.6.1) [23]. In nude mice, the growth of ChaGo lung cancer is blocked in proportion to the antibodies injected [24]. Similar observations have been made on colorectal cancer cells (CCL-253). These cells also express hCG, and anti-hCG antibodies kill these cells in the presence of Complement in vitro [25]. Also, in nude mice implanted with CCL-253 colorectal cancer cells, administration of anti-hCG antibodies caused a significant reduction in tumor uptake, and all treated animals with anti-hCG antibodies survived in contrast to the mortality of control animals [25].

Moab PiPP for homing and targeted delivery of safe anticancerous compounds to cancer cells

Antibodies have the ability to "home" specifically to discrete epitopes on the antigen, be these on membranes of cells or elsewhere. Could PiPP be employed to deliver radiations or a "drug" directly to the cancer cells? Fig. 4.6.2 is a body scan of a nude mouse. The mouse was infected in hind left limb by JEG-3 tumor cells which also express hCG. Injection of ^{131}I-anti-hCG monoclonal antibody led antibodies to location of the tumor and not everywhere else (Fig. 4.6.2A). An

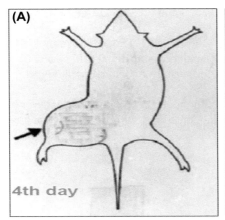
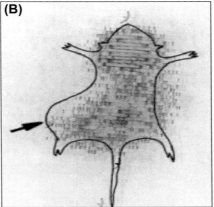

FIGURE 4.6.2

Whole body scan of JEG-3 tumor is localized by the ^{131}I-anti-hCG monoclonal antibody. (Panel A) and ^{131}I-irrelevant monoclonal after 4 days (Panel B) [26].

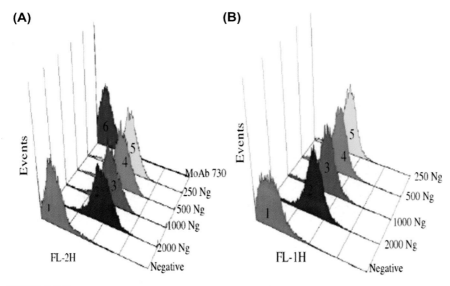

FIGURE 4.6.3

Reactivity of (A) anti-α-hCG (P22376) and (B) anti-β-hCG (cPiPP) antibodies with MOLT-4 cells. FACS analysis was carried out at indicated antibody concentrations. In each case, 80%–91% cells show binding with these antibodies. Histogram in both (A) and (B) shows fluorescence of cells without antibody. A non-hCG-reactive monoclonal antibody (MoAb 730) demonstrated a lack of recognition (Histogram 6) in (A) [27].

irrelevant monoclonal antibody labeled with [131]iodine did not go to the tumor, but was spread all over the body (Fig. 4.6.2B).

MOLT-4 cells express ectopically both α and β hCG. This is shown by a FACS conducted with a monoclonal against α-hCG and the monoclonal PiPP reactive with β-hCG. Fig. 4.6.3 shows the findings. An irrelevant monoclonal antibody did not react with MOLT-4 cells.

MOLT-4 cells express hCG but anti-hCG antibodies do not kill these cells with or without Complement, even though the antibodies bind with the cells. We linked

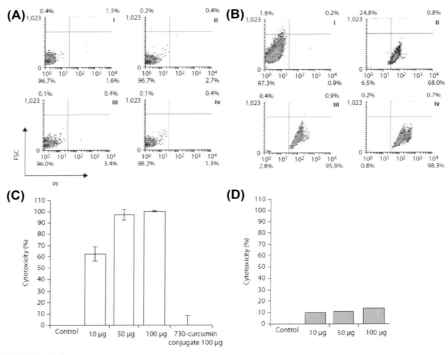

FIGURE 4.6.4

Cytotoxic effect of cPiPP-curcumin on MOLT-4 cells. (A) 0.1 million cells were cultured with RPMI 1640 supplemented with (I) 0 μg, (II) 10 μg, (III) 50 μg, and (IV) 100 μg/mL of the antibody equivalent for 48 h. FACS analysis of cells was carried out after staining with propidium iodide. (B) Cytotoxic effect of cPiPP-curcumin conjugate on MOLT-4 cells by FACS analysis of PI-stained cells at (I) 0 μg, (II) 10 μg, (III) 50 μg, and (IV) 100 μg/mL. Percentages of dead cells appearing in right lower quadrant were 0.9%, 68%, 96%, and 98.3%, respectively. (C) The cytotoxic effect of the immunoconjugate was confirmed by trypan blue exclusion assay. Curcumin conjugated to an irrelevant antibody (MoAb 730) was devoid of cytotoxicity on MOLT-4 cells. (D) Lack of cytotoxic action of cPiPP-curcumin conjugate on PBMCs bearing CD13 marker of an AML patient (R.D.) [30].

curcumin (diferuloyl methane), the active principle of *Curcuma longa*, with cPiPP (mouse-human chimeric antibody against hCG). This was achieved by creating an amino linker on terminal hydroxyl group of curcumin, which was condensed with carboxylic acid of acidic amino acids of the antibody. It may be stated that curcumin has anti-inflammatory and anticancerous properties [28]. It is totally nontoxic and fully safe. Phase I clinical trials showed that amounts taken up to 8 g per day orally were well tolerated and caused no side effects of any type in humans [29]. While cPiPP, the anti-hCG antibody, did not kill any MOLT-4 cell (Fig. 4.6.4A), the same cells incubated with cPiPP-curcumin conjugate were killed in proportion to the dose of the conjugate, reaching 98.3% at 100 µg concentration of the conjugate (Fig. 4.6.4B,C). The antibody-curcumin conjugate itself was not cytotoxic. It did not exercise any cytotoxicity on peripheral blood mononuclear cells (PBMCs) of a normal healthy donor (Figs. 4.6.4D and 4.6.5) [30].

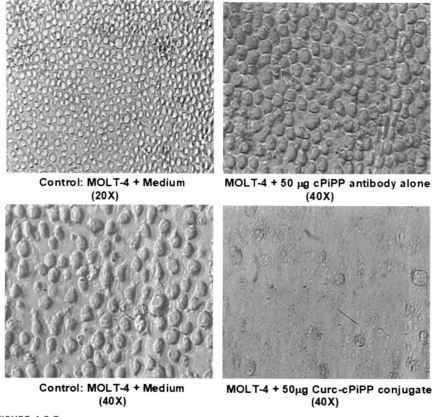

FIGURE 4.6.5

Photomicrograph of MOLT-4 cells after incubation with cPiPP alone and cPiPP-curcumin conjugate. Cells incubated in culture medium are used as control [26].

The cytotoxic action of cPiPP-curcumin was not only exercised on MOLT-4 cells but also on U-937 lymphoma cells killing at saturating dose of the conjugate the entire lot of cells expressing hCG ectopically. Thus employing "homing" antibodies to deliver curcumin acted as a magic bullet killing the target cancer cells. It may be stated that curcumin is a potent inhibitor of Stat 3, which plays a pivotal role in tumor growth, invasion, and metastasis of many cancers [31].

Thus PiPP is a broad-spectrum monoclonal antibody which can be of potential utility in immunotherapy of a wide range of hCG expressing cancers such as colon cancer, hepatocellular carcinoma, pancreatic and bladder cancers besides T-lymphoblastic leukemia, histiocytic lymphoma, and lung cancer.

These observations are highly interesting and demand further work on various cancers reported to make hCG ectopically. We do have a good vaccine against hCG as reported in Chapter 3.7. The high-affinity mouse antibody PiPP was converted into a mouse-human chimeric antibody and expressed as a recombinant protein in plants [32]. Work is in progress in our lab to humanize fully this antibody for eventual use in humans, thereby minimizing the side effects associated with mouse antibodies in humans.

Acknowledgments

The work reviewed in this chapter received research grants from the Departments of Biotechnology, Govt. of India and the Indian Council of Medical Research.

References

[1] Fishel SB, Edwards RG, Evans CJ. Human chorionic gonadotropin secreted by preimplantation embryos cultured in vitro. Science 1984;223:816—8.

[2] Yokotani T, Koizumi T, Taniguchi R, Nakagawa T, Isobe T, et al. Expression of alpha and beta genes of human chorionic gonadotropin in lung cancer. Int J Cancer 1997; 71(4):539—44.

[3] Iles RK, Persad R, Trivedi M, Sharma KB, Dickinson A, et al. Urinary concentration of human chorionic gonadotrophin and its fragments as a prognostic marker in bladder cancer. Br J Urol 1996;77(1):61—9.

[4] Nishimura R, Koizumi T, Morisue K, Yamanaka N, Lalwani R, et al. Expression and secretion of the beta subunit of human chorionic gonadotropin by bladder carcinoma in vivo and in vitro. Cancer Res 1995;55(7):1479—84.

[5] Syrigos KN, Fyssas I, Konstandoulakis MM, Harrington KJ, Papadopoulos S, et al. Beta human chorionic gonadotropin concentrations in serum of patients with pancreatic adenocarcinoma. Gut 1998;42(1):88—91.

[6] Alfthan H, Haglund C, Roberts P, Stenman UH. Elevation of free beta subunit of human choriogonadotropin and core beta fragment of human choriogonadotropin in the serum and urine of patients with malignant pancreatic and biliary disease. Cancer Res 1992; 52(17):4628—33.

[7] Bièche I, Lazar V, Noguès C, Poynard T, Giovangrandi Y, et al. Prognostic value of chorionic gonadotropin beta gene transcripts in human breast carcinoma. Clin Cancer Res 1998;4(3):671—6.

[8] Crawford RA, Iles RK, Carter PG, Caldwell CJ, Shepherd JH, et al. The prognostic significance of beta human chorionic gonadotrophin and its metabolites in women with cervical carcinoma. J Clin Pathol 1998;51(9):685—8.

[9] Grossmann M, Hoermann R, Gocze PM, Ott M, Berger P, et al. Measurement of human chorionic gonadotropin-related immunoreactivity in serum, ascites and tumour cysts of patients with gynaecologic malignancies. Eur J Clin Investig 1995;25(11):867—73.

[10] Hedström J, Grenman R, Ramsay H, Finne P, Lundin J, et al. Concentration of free hCGbeta subunit in serum as a prognostic marker for squamous-cell carcinoma of the oral cavity and oropharynx. Int J Cancer 1999;84(5):525—8.

[11] Bhalang K, Kafrawy AH, Miles DA. Immunohistochemical study of the expression of human chorionic gonadotropin-beta in oral squamous cell carcinoma. Cancer 1999; 85(4):757—62.

[12] Scholl PD, Jurco S, Austin JR. Ectopic production of beta-HCG by a maxillary squamous cell carcinoma. Head Neck 1997;19(8):701—5.

[13] Sheaff MT, Martin JE, Badenoch DF, Baithun SI. Beta hCG as a prognostic marker in adenocarcinoma of the prostate. J Clin Pathol 1996;49(4):329—32.

[14] Jiang Y, Zeng F, Xiao C, Liu J. Expression of beta-human chorionic gonadotropin genes in renal cell cancer and benign renal disease tissues. J Huazhong Univ Sci Technolog Med Sci 2003;23(3):291—3.

[15] Lundin M, Nordling S, Carpelan-Holmstrom M, Louhimo J, Alfthan H, et al. A comparison of serum and tissue hCG beta as prognostic markers in colorectal cancer. Anticancer Res 2000;20(6D):4949—51.

[16] Rau B, Below C, Liebrich W, von Schilling C, Schlag PM. Significance of serum b-hCG as a tumor marker for stomach carcinoma. Langenbecks Arch Chir 1995;380: 359—64.

[17] Louhimo J, Nordling S, Alfthan H, von Boguslawski K, Stenman UH, et al. Specific staining of human chorionic gonadotropin beta in benign and malignant gastrointestinal tissues with monoclonal antibodies. Histopathology 2001;38(5):418—24.

[18] de Bruijn HW, ten Hoor KA, Krans M, van der Zee AG. Rising serum values of beta-subunit human chorionic gonadotrophin (hCG) in patients with progressive vulvar carcinomas. Br J Canc 1997;75(8):1217—8.

[19] Carter PG, Iles RK, Neven P, Ind TE, Shepherd JH, et al. Measurement of urinary beta core fragment of human chorionic gonadotrophin in women with vulvovaginal malignancy and its prognostic significance. Br J Canc 1995;71(2):350—3.

[20] Hotakainen K, Ljungberg B, Paju A, Rasmuson T, Alfthan H, et al. The free beta-subunit of human chorionic gonadotropin as a prognostic factor in renal cell carcinoma. Br J Canc 2002;86(2):185—9.

[21] Zygmunt M, Herr F, Keller-Schoenwetter S, Kunzi-Rapp K, Münstedt K, et al. Characterization of human chorionic gonadotropin as a novel angiogenic factor. J Clin Endocrinol Metab 2002;87(11):5290—6.

[22] Gupta SK, Talwar GP. Development of hybridomas secreting anti-human chorionic gonadotropin antibodies. Indian J Exp Biol 1980;18:1361—5.

[23] Talwar GP, Rulli SB, Vyas H, Purswani S, Kabeer RS, et al. Making of a unique birth control vaccine against hCG with additional potential of therapy of advanced stage cancers and prevention of obesity and insulin resistance. J Cell Sci Ther 2014;5:159.

[24] Kumar S, Talwar GP, Biswas DK. Necrosis and inhibition of growth of human lung tumor by anti-alpha-human chorionic gonadotropin antibody. J Natl Cancer Inst 1992;84: 42–7.

[25] Khare P, Singh O, Jain SK, Javed S, Pal R. Inhibitory effect of antibodies against human chorionic gonadotropin on the growth of colorectal tumour cells. Indian J Biochem Biophys 2012;49(2):92–6.

[26] Talwar GP, Puruswani S, Vyas HK. Immunological approaches against human chorionic gonadotropin for control of fertility and advanced stage cancers expressing ectopically hCG. In: Kumar A, Rao CV, Chaturvedi PK, editors. Gonadal and nongonadal action of gonadotropins. New Delhi: Narosa Publishing House; 2010. p. 183–96.

[27] Kabeer RS, Pal R, Talwar GP. Human acute lymphoblastic leukemia cells make human pregnancy hormone hCG and expose it on the membrane: a case for using recombinant antibody against hCG for selective delivery of drugs and/or radiations. Curr Sci 2005; 89(9):1571–6.

[28] Aggarwal BB, Kumar A, Bharti AC. Anticancer potential of curcumin: preclinical and clinical studies. Anticancer Res 2003;23:363–98.

[29] Cheng AL, Hsu CH, Lin JK, Hsu MM, Ho YF, et al. Phase I clinical trial of curcumin, a chemopreventive agent, in patients with high-risk or pre-malignant lesions. Anticancer Res 2001;21:2895–900.

[30] Vyas HK, Pal R, Vishwakarma R, Lohiya NK, Talwar GP. Selective killing of leukemia and lymphoma cells ectopically expressing hCGbeta by a conjugate of curcumin with an antibody against hCGbeta subunit. Oncology 2009;76(2):101–11.

[31] Kamran MZ, Patil P, Gude RP. Role of STAT3 in cancer metastasis and translational advances. BioMed Res Int 2013;2013. 421821.

[32] Kathuria S, Sriraman R, Nath R, Sack M, Pal R, Artsaenko O, Talwar GP, Finnern R. Efficacy of plant-produced recombinant antibodies against HCG. Hum Reprod 2002; 17(8):2054–61.

A potential cure for cancer

4.7

Laurence A. Cole

Introduction

This a review describing recent research on hCG and cancer, now ongoing, that hopefully will find a cure for all or most human cancers and advanced cancers and deadly cancers like pancreatic cancer. The research has been already published [1], most of the tables and figures presented are repeats, published with author approval [1].

hCG and cancer

The occurrence of hCG as a tumor marker has been extensively studied. The best test by far for hCG or hCGβ as a tumor marker is an assay of first morning urine using the antibody B204. It measures urine β-subunit, nicked β-subunit, nicked β-subunit missing the C-terminal peptide, and β-core fragment, or all the hCG and β-subunit serum degradation products as a tumor marker. The first study tested 91 trophoblastic cancers and 2167 nontrophoblastic cancers using the standard B204 immunometric assay. The assay has a 3.0 pmol/mL cutoff for cancer (Table 4.7.1). As shown, 91 of 91 (100%) trophoblastic cancers were detected, and just 949 of 2167 (44%) nontrophoblastic cancers were detected. A much more sensitive B204 assay was developed, using ^{125}I-iodinated tracer antibody, and 1/12,000 rather than 1/4000 capture antibody. Samples were incubated for 12 hours with B204 and 12 hours with radiolabeled tracer antibody. Using this assay had a cutoff for cancer of 0.1 pmol/mL 341 nontrophoblastic cancers were again tested using this sensitive assay. All, 341 of 341 (100%) had detectable levels pmol/mL of hCG, some with B204 immunoreactivity as low as 0.20 pmol/mL. From this one study, it appears that hCG is produced by all cancer with an extremely wide range varying from 0.20 pmol/mL (pancreatic cancer) to 22,000,000 pmol/mL (choriocarcinoma).

What forms of hCG are cancers producing? Immunoassay for free β-subunit (FBT11 assay), total hCG (Immulite 1000 assay), and B152 hCG (measures only hyperglycosylated hCG and extravillous cytotrophoblast hCG) were measured in

Table 4.7.1 Urine B204 assay (cancer cutoff 3.0 pmol/mL) and supersensitive B204 assay (cancer cutoff 0.1 pmol/mL), detects β-core fragment, free β-subunit, hyperglycosylated hCG free β-subunit, and nicked free β-subunit.

Source	Urine B204 assay Ultrasensitive assay, cutoff > 0.1 pmol/mL			Urine B204 assay Regular assay, cutoff >3 pmol/mL		
	#Cases	#Detected	Sensitivity	#Cases	#positive	sensitivity
A. Trophoblastic malignancies						
Choriocarcinoma				63	63	100%
Ovarian germ cell cancer				11	11	100%
Testicular germ cell cancer				17	17	100%
Total				**91**	**91**	**100%**
B. Nontrophoblastic malignancy						
Bladder cancer				140	62	44%
Breast cancer	130	130	100%	456	156	34%
Cervical cancer				410	197	48%
Colorectal cancer				80	29	36%
Endometrial cancer				233	103	44%
Gastric cancer				205	90	44%
Hepatic cancer				46	20	44%
Lung cancer	115	115	100%	154	38	25%
Intestinal cancer				17	8	47%
Lymphoma				41	13	32%
Ovarian cancer	56	56	100%	207	145	70%
Pancreatic cancer	40	40	100%	29	16	55%
Prostate cancer				12	9	75%
Renal cancer				66	32	48%
Uterine cancer				63	26	41%

Vulvar cancer	341			8	4	50%
Total	341	341	100%	2167	949	44%
C. Healthy						
NED, postcancer chemotherapy				33	2	6%
NED, postcancer surgery				21	1	5%
Healthy female, no cancer history				72	2	3%
Healthy male, no cancer history				28	1	4%
Total				**154**	**6**	**4%**
D. Benign disease						
Benign gynecological lesion, tumor				28	0	0%
Follicular ovarian cyst, benign				71	1	0%
Benign ovarian cyst, nonfunctional				26	0	0%
Cervical carcinoma in situ				12	0	0%
Cervical dyskaryosis				66	2	0%
Condyloma				30	0	0%
Endometriosis				16	1	0%
Myoma				27	3	0%
Total				**276**	**7**	**0%**

32 trophoblastic cancer cases and 52 nontrophoblastic cancer cases and Con A-Sepharose chromatography was carried out [1]. It became very clear that all (100%) of trophoblastic cancers, no exceptions, were producing extravillous cyto-trophoblastic hCG, and that all (100%) nontrophoblastic cancers, no exceptions, were producing extravillous cytotrophoblast hCG free β-subunit.

The structure of extravillous cytotrophoblast hCG is shown in Fig. 4.7.1. This structure is seemingly acting on the cancer cell transforming growth factor-β (TGFβ) receptor to control cancer cell biology [3–5].

Eight published articles showed that hCG β-subunit had a role is cancer cell growth, cancer cell invasion of adjacent cells, and blocked cancer cell apoptosis [3,6–12] (Table 4.7.2). I investigated extravillous cytotrophoblast hCG and free β-subunit action on 10 cancer cell lines (Table 4.7.3). As shown (Table 4.7.3), they promoted growth of cancers over 24 hours by 130%−172%. I concluded from this and the eight other studies (Table 4.7.2) that extravillous cytotrophoblast hCG and its free β-subunit promotes malignancy in all or most cancers. That is, it promotes cancer cell growth, cell cancer cell invasion of adjacent tissue, and blocks apoptosis in all or most cancers. It probably controls other cancer cell functions which are, as yet, not investigated.

Mouse monoclonal antibody was raised against C5 hCG [13] (see also Chapter 1.1). It was named B152 and shown to bind hyperglycosylated hCG and extravillous cytotrophoblast hCG [14] with type 2 O-linked oligosaccharides and not to bind the hormone hCG with type 1 O-linked oligosaccharides.

B152 antibody blocked growth in seven of seven cancer cell lines [1]. In nude mice transplanted with choriocarcinoma and cervical cancer it blocked malignancy (Fig. 4.7.2). This confirmed that extravillous cytotrophoblast hCG and its β-subunit were the malignancy factors in all or most cancer cells.

Nude mice, without an immune system and with apoptosis blocked by extravillous cytotrophoblast hCG and its free β-subunit, are used. In humans this would be a cure for cancer. Firstly, ridding the body of malignancy, and secondly with the immune system and apoptosis ridding the body of remnant cancer tissue. Unfortunately, this is not possible as human therapy and without a humanized antibody the immune system would reject the mouse protein.

In conclusion, extravillous cytotrophoblast hCG and its free β-subunit are produced by all cancers. Extravillous cytotrophoblast hCG and its free β-subunit control malignancy in all or most cancers; there may be exception, in this respect is the centerpiece of all or most cancers. A cure may be in the works removing extravillous cytotrophoblast hCG from all or most cancers.

Most oncology journals disregard an article on hCG and cancer in their journal, claiming that hCG is a pregnancy hormone and that its production by cancers is incidental, but the data suggest otherwise. Hopefully, within a year we will have confirmed these studies using new systems which are well tolerated in humans and have a potential therapy for clinical trials.

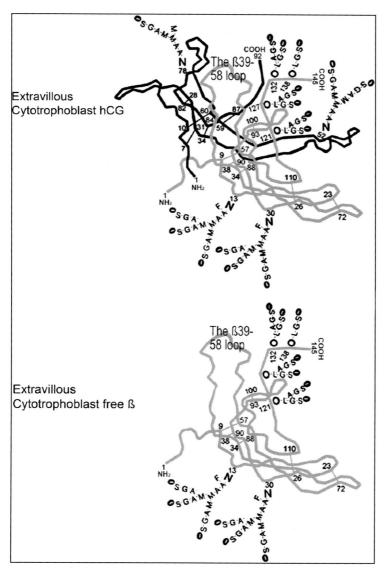

FIGURE 4.7.1

Structure of extravillous cytotrophoblast hCG and its free β-subunit. Shown using Butler modeling [2].

Table 4.7.2 Eight independent reports that hyperglycosylated hCG and hCG β-subunit promote cancer cell malignancy [1,3,6−12].

Year	Author	Cancer cell tested	Promotes cancer cell growth	Promotes cancer cell invasion	Blocks cancer cell apoptosis	References
1996	Gillott et al.	T24 Epithelial bladder cancer cell line	X		X	[6]
		SCaBER squamous bladder cancer cell line	X		X	
		RT112 bladder carcinoma cell line	X		X	
		5637 adherent bladder carcinoma cell line	X		X	
2000	Butler et al.	ScaBER squamous bladder cancer cell line	X		X	[3]
2002	Devi et al.	DU145 prostate carcinoma cells	X			[7]
2006	Cole et al.	Jar choriocarcinoma cell line	X	X		[8]
		JEG-III choriocarcinoma cell line	X	X		
2008	Jankowska et al.	12 patients with planoepithelial cervical cancer			X	[9]
		1 patient with glossy cell cervical cancer			X	
		1 patient with basaloid cell cervical cancer			X	
		1 patient with intraepithelial cervical cancer			X	

Year	Author	Sample				Reference
2008	Li et al.	15 patients with endometrial cancer			X	[10]
2011	Guo et al.	81 patients with uterine cervical cancer	X		X	[11]
		T29 ovarian epithelial carcinoma cell line	X		X	
		T80 ovarian epithelial carcinoma cell line	X		X	
		15 patients with ovarian carcinoma	X		X	
2018	Kawamata et al.	80 patients with colorectal cancer		X	X	[12]
		Caco-2 epithelial colorectal cancer		X	X	
		LoVo epithelial colorectal cancer		X	X	
		HCA-7 epithelial colorectal cancer		X	X	
		WiDr colorectal adenocarcinoma		X	X	
		T84 epithelial colorectal cancer		X	X	

Table 4.7.3 Promotion of cancer cell 24 hours growth at 70% confluency by C5 extravillous cytotrophoblast hCG.

Cells	Supplement added to culture fluid	% Effect on cell count	T Test
Jar choriocarcinoma	No additive	100% cell count after 24 hours	$P = .0123$
	C5 extravillous cytotrophoblast hCG 2 ng/mL	112% cell count after 24 hours	
	C5 extravillous cytotrophoblast hCG 20 ng/mL	130% cell count after 24 hours	
JEGIII choriocarcinoma	No additive	100% cell count after 24 hours	$P = .0018$
	C5 extravillous cytotrophoblast hCG 2 ng/mL	110% cell count after 24 hours	
	C5 extravillous cytotrophoblast hCG 20 ng/mL	128% cell count after 24 hours	
NTERA testicular germ cell	No additive	100% cell count after 24 hours	$P = .0018$
	C5 extravillous cytotrophoblast hCG 2 ng/mL	118% cell count after 24 hours	
	C5 extravillous cytotrophoblast hCG 20 ng/mL	132% cell count after 24 hours	
Hec-1-a endometrial adenocarcinoma	No additive	100% cell count after 24 hours	$P = .0021$
	C5 extravillous cytotrophoblast hCGβ 2 ng/mL	138% cell count after 24 hours	
	C5 extravillous cytotrophoblast hCGβ 20 ng/mL	166% cell count after 24h	
ScaBER squamous bladder cancer	No additive	100% cell count after 24 hours	$P = .010$
	C5 extravillous cytotrophoblast hCGβ 2 ng/mL	150% cell count after 24 hours	
	C5 extravillous cytotrophoblast hCGβ 20 ng/mL	156% cell count after 24h	
KLE endometrial adenocarcinoma	No additive	100% cell count after 24 hours	$P = .0.001$

Table 4.7.3 Promotion of cancer cell 24 hours growth at 70% confluency by C5 extravillous cytotrophoblast hCG.—cont'd

Cells	Supplement added to culture fluid	% Effect on cell count	T Test
	C5 extravillous cytotrophoblast hCGβ 2 ng/mL	117% cell count after 24 hours	
	C5 extravillous cytotrophoblast hCGβ 20 ng/mL	132% cell count after 24 hours	
T24 epithelial bladder carcinoma	No additive	100% cell count after 24 hours	$P = .011$
	C5 extravillous cytotrophoblast hCGβ 2 ng/mL	137% cell count after 24 hours	
	C5 extravillous cytotrophoblast hCGβ 20 ng/mL	148% cell count after 24 hours	
SK-MES-1 epithelial lung cancer	No additive	100% cell count after 24 hours	$P = .0001$
	C5 extravillous cytotrophoblast hCGβ 2 ng/mL	142% cell count after 24 hours	
	C5 extravillous cytotrophoblast hCGβ 20 ng/mL	172% cell count after 24 hours	
KM-H2 Hodgkin's lymphoma	No additive	100% cell count after 24 hours	$P = .022$
	C5 extravillous cytotrophoblast hCGβ 2 ng/mL	121% cell count after 24 hours	
	C5 extravillous cytotrophoblast hCGβ 20 ng/mL	139% cell count after 24 hours	
CaSki cervical carcinoma	No additive	100% cell count after 24 hours	$P = .010$
	C5 extravillous cytotrophoblast hCGβ 2 ng/mL	132% cell count after 24 hours	
	C5 extravillous cytotrophoblast hCGβ 20 ng/mL	146% cell count after 24 hours	

All experiments carried out in quadruplicate. Sixteen T75 flask of each cancer cell line were grown to approximately 70% confluent. Four flasks rejected to prevent 70% confluence imbalance, four flask used for 70% confluence cell count. No additive flask results (−70% count) considered as blank and subtracted from all results. In case of Jar choriocarcinoma cells, for instance, mean no additive result 100,360 cells, mean 70% confluency result 128,880 cells, blank = 128,880−100,360 = 28,520 cells, blank = 100%. 20 ng extravillous cytotrophoblast hCG mean result 158,540 cells, 158,540-blank = 130,020 cells, 130,020/100,360 × 100 = 130%.

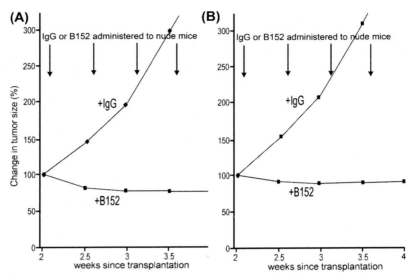

FIGURE 4.7.2

Nude mice transplanted with (A) choriocarcinoma or (B) cervical cancer. Cancer treated with nonspecific IgG or monoclonal antibody B152.

References

[1]   Cole LA. hCG and cancer. J Clin Endocrinol Metab 2019 (in press).

[2]   Cole LA. The minute structural difference between the hormone hCG and the autocrine hyperglycosylated hCG. J Glycobiol 2017;6:1000127.

[3]   Butler SA, Ikram MS, Mathieu S, Iles RK. The increase in bladder carcinoma cell population induced by the free beta subunit of hCG is a result of an anti-apoptosis effect and not cell proliferation. Br J Canc 2000;82:1553−6.

[4]   Berndt S, Blacher S, Munuat C, Detilleux J, Evain-Brion D, Noel A, Fournier T, Foidart JM. Hyperglycosylated human chorionic gonadotropin stimulates angiogenesis through TGF-ß receptor activation. FASEB J 2013;12:213686.

[5]   Ahmud F, Ghosh S, Sinha S, Joshi SD, Mehta VS, Sen E. TGF-ß-induced hCG-ß regulates redox homeostasis in glioma cells. Mol Cell Biochem 2015;399:105−12.

[6]   Gillott DJ, Iles RK, Chard T. The effects of beta-human chorionic gonadotrophin on the in vitro growth of bladder cancer cell lines. Br J Canc 1996;73:323−6.

[7]   Devi GR, Oldenkamp JR, London CA, Iversen PL. Inhibition of human chorionic ß-subunit modulates the mitogenetic effect of *c-myc* in human prostate cancer cells. Prostate 2002;53:200−310.

[8]   Cole LA, Dai D, Leslie KK, Butler SA, Kohorn EI. Gestational trophoblastic diseases: 1. Pathophysiology of hyperglycosylated hCG-regulated neoplasia. Gynecol Oncol 2006;102:144−9.

[9]   Jankowska A, Gunderson SI, Warchol JB. Reduction of hCGß subunit expression by modified U1 snRNA caused apoptosis in cervical cancer cells. Mol Cancer 2008;7:26−9.

[10] Li D, Wen X, Ghali L, Al-Shalabi F, Purkis P, et al. hCG β expression by cervical squamous carcinoma-in vivo histological association with tumour invasion and apoptosis. Histopathology 2008;53:147−55.

[11] Guo X, Liu G, Schauer IG, Yang G, Mercado-Uribe I, Yang F, Zhang S, He Y, Liu J. Overexpression of the β subunit of human chorionic gonadotropin promotes the transformation of human ovarian epithelial cells and ovarian tumorigenesis. Am J Pathol 2011;179:1385−93.

[12] Kawamaja F, Nishihara H, Homma S, et al. Chorionic gonadotropin-ß modulates epithelial-mesenchymal transition in colorectal carcinoma metastasis. Am J Pathol 2018;188:207−15.

[13] Birken S, Krichevsky A, O'Connor J, Schlatterer J, Cole LA, Kardana A, Canfield R. Development and characterization of antibodies to a nicked and hyperglycosylated form of hCG from a choriocarcinoma patient. Endocr J 1999;10:137−44.

[14] Cole LA. The carbohydrate structure of the hormone hCG, the autocrine hyperglycosylated hCG, and the extravillous cytotrophoblast hyperglycosylated hCG. J Glycobiol 2019;7 (in press).

Conclusion

Where has hCG research been? What is hCG research doing? Which direction will it go in the future?

5.1

Laurence A. Cole

Introduction

The history of the hormone hCG goes back 100 years to the early 20th century, to Aschner, Fellner, and Ascheim and Zondek [1−4], the first discoverers of the hormone. In 1912, Aschner successfully promoted the genital tract of guinea pigs with injections of water-soluble extracts of human placenta [1]. In 1913, Fellner successfully promoted ovulation in immature rabbits with saline extracts of human placenta [2]. In 1919, Hirose successfully induced ovulation and normal luteal function in immature rabbits by repeated injections of human placental tissue [3].

All of these studies show that there was a clear link between a placenta hormone and the female gonads [1−3]. In 1927, Ascheim and Zondek successfully demonstrated that pregnant women produce a gonad-stimulating molecule or hormone [4]. They showed that injecting this hormone into intact immature female mice let to follicular maturation, ovulation, and hemorrhaging into the ovarian stroma. Ascheim and Zondek used hCG to develop the first pregnancy test.

The realization around this time that the placenta was producing a molecule or a hormone that promoted ovarian progesterone production led researchers to coin the name human chorionic gonadotropin (hCG): Chorion comes from the Latin chordata meaning afterbirth; gonadotropin because the hormone was considered a gonad tropic molecule, or a stimulator of gonads (or ovary) steroid production.

I am far from sure, however, that the name hCG is still valid today. First, because the hormone and autocrine dealt with today are now know to be normally produced by cells other than placenta cells. Second, because the hormone and autocrine do not act primarily on gonad cells, they act primarily on the placenta in pregnancy.

Considering that it is now known to be both a hormone (hCG) and an autocrine (hyperglycosylated hCG), a general name like human pregnancy glycoprotein or human acidic stimulator might be more appropriate.

hCG is surely a master molecule in humans, its evolution directed and drove specifically the evolution of humans. It drives pregnancy and development in human fetuses, and drives and governs cancers in humans, effectively defining who will live and who will die.

The story of hCG has come a very long way on its 100 years of history, from the discovery of the hormone hCG [1—4] to the discovery that there are two forms of hCG, the hormone hCG and the autocrine hyperglycosylated hCG [5—8]. From the discovery of the gonadal hormone [1—4] to the discovery of the pregnancy hormone [9,10], and onto the discovery of the cancer promoter [6,11—14], hCG shows great promise in the future in the treatment and diagnosis of cancer and management of reproductive disorders [15,16].

Where has hCG research been?

Very clearly the hormone hCG's primary role is in the synthesis of hemochorial placentation, the very efficient fetal feeding system. This primary role was established by the showing that hCG physically drives four separate receptor-driven functions in hemochorial placentation.

First, it promotes maternal spiral arteries in the maternal uterus to extend their reach to hemochorial placentation [17—19]. Second, it promotes the growth of the uterine circulation to link hemochorial placentation with the fetus [20—22]. Third, hyperglycosylated hCG promotes the growth of the villous tissue or the core structure of hemochorial placentation [23—25], and finally, the hormone hCG drives the differentiation of villous cytotrophoblast cells to form the syncytiotrophoblast skin or fetal filtering skin that surround hemochorial placentation [26].

Hemochorial placentation is hCG's primary function. In fact, the evolution of chorionic gonadotropin in early primates introduced hemochorial placentation to primates. Chorionic gonadotropin—driven hemochorial placentation introduced a superefficient fetal feeding system that allowed brain growth to occur in primates permitting humans to develop [25,27—29].

For reasons not clearly understood, outside of the field of hCG research, it is somehow conceived that progesterone promotion in pregnancy is the principal function of hCG. Every obstetrics and gynecology textbook without exception, every medical textbook, and every biology book or lay book, makes this ridiculous claim for the function of hCG. Yes, from the 4th week of gestation to the 7th week of gestation, hCG takes over from luteinizing hormone (LH), the promotion of progesterone production by ovarian corpus luteal cells [9]. So what, this is a trivial role for hCG that partially came about because hCG evolved out of LH β-subunit and has biological similarity to LH. This is not construction of a superefficient fetal feeding system that permitted growth of the human brain [25,27—29].

Early research showed other major functions of hCG in pregnancy. hCG suppresses maternal macrophage action on fetal and placental tissues [30,31]. Other research showed that hCG suppressed myometrial contractions in response to a pregnancy and that hCG level had to diminish at term to give way to labor [32,33].

Ongoing research in the last 40 years with hCG showed that hCG bound a joint hCG/LH receptor, imposing all biological functions [34−36]. Other research showed that hCG was a dimeric glycoprotein hormone−like follicle stimulating hormone and LH [37], a hormone comprising an α- and β-subunit, 4 biantennary N-linked oligosaccharides, and 4 trisaccharide/tetrasaccharide O-linked oligosaccharides [5,7].

The three-dimensional structure of hCG was investigated by Wu et al. Lustbader et al., and Lapthorn et al. [38−40]. All were faced with the problems of a molecule that was 30% sugar by molecular weight. In order to make crystals of hCG they had to cleave all 8 carbohydrate side chains, cleave the C-terminal peptide off the β-subunit of hCG, and cleave other peptides from hCG [38−40]. The final crystals were made from β2-β111 of a 145 amino acid β-subunit, and α5-α89 of a 92 amino acid α-subunit, or from just 50% of the hCG molecule. Yes, we have a three-dimensional structure of a pseudo-hCG, but it is only half of the hCG molecule [38−40].

Stephen Butler, Ph.D., in England, like me, very frustrated with the limited structural data on hCG, used computers to make three-dimensional thermodynamic models of the hormone hCG and the autocrine hyperglycosylated hCG [41].

Other old research shows that hCG is produced by the fetus in pregnancy [42−44]. That fetal hCG is produced by the fetal liver and fetal kidney. That fetal hCG drives growth and development of fetal organs during pregnancy [42−44].

In summary, past research, 1912−97, has given us what hCG does, the receptor which the hormone hCG binds, the carbohydrate and amino acid composition of hCG, and the three-dimensional structure of a pseudo-hCG, or half of the hCG molecule.

What is hCG research doing?

Research in the last 20 years, 1997−2017, has very much changed hCG, changed this molecules' story, changed where hCG is going, and changed the whole future of this molecule. Everything started in 1997 with the discovery that hCG is not one molecule, a hormone, but rather is two separate molecules, the hormone hCG produced by syncytiotrophoblast cells and the autocrine hyperglycosylated hCG made by cytotrophoblast cells, two completely separate and totally independent molecules made by separate cells [5].

The α-subunit and the β-subunit gene make a 92 amino acid α-subunit and a 145 amino acid β-subunit. To this, four N-linked oligosaccharides are added, and 4 small O-linked oligosaccharides. Dependent solely on whether they are type 1 O-linked oligosaccharides (three to four sugars), or type 2 O-linked oligosaccharides (five to six sugars), you either have the hormone hCG, or the totally independent autocrine hyperglycosylated hCG [41].

Hyperglycosylated hCG is a malicious antagonist that acts on a transforming growth factor-β (TGFβ) receptor [6,41,45]. It is malicious in that it drives cell growth and cell to cell enzymatic invasion. Hyperglycosylated hCG drives blastocyst implantation into the uterus [24,46,47], the faulty implantation of failing pregnancies [8,24,46,47], and the deep implantation of hemochorial placentation [48,49]. Other new research, which is detailed below, shows that hyperglycosylated hCG, or just its free β-subunit, drives malignancy, or drives cancer, by all cancer cells [50,51], and drives invasion in ovulation, so that the oocyte reaches the fallopian tube [14].

As shown by the Stephen Butler Ph.D.'s three-dimensional models [41], the two molecules differ around their β-subunit C-terminal peptides, an area of the molecule that Wu, Lustbader, and Lapthorn did not model and claimed would not effect the three-dimensional structure of hCG [38−40]. Because of the type 1 O-linked oligosaccharides, the C-terminal peptide on the hormone hCG fold into loop β39-55 blocking nicking at β47-48. This does not happen on hyperglycosylated hCG. The end result is that the hyperglycosylated hCG is rapidly nicked and dissociated, the nicked free β-subunit is the antagonist of TGFβ. The hormone hCG, however, is blocked from nicking and only binds the LH/hCG receptor intact [41].

Multiple centers have now shown that "β-subunit" (β-subunit of hyperglycosylated hCG) drives malignancy functions in cancer cells, most notably blocks apoptosis, drives cancer all cell growth and all cancer cell invasion [11−15,52−54]. It has recently been concluded that this molecule drives malignancy or drives the root of cancer [15]. Carcinogenesis must involve activation of the hCG β-subunit gene [15].

Other research completed in the last 10 years show that the two forms of hCG drove human evolution [27−29]. The appearance of hemochorial placentation, driven by chorionic gonadotropin, and the advancement of hemochorial placentation, driven by the advancing acidity of chorionic gonadotropin, effectively drove the development of humans [27−29].

hCG, advancing from a single molecule into two molecules, and developing from the molecule that drives pregnancy on into the molecule that drove human evolution and the molecule that drives human cancers, has somehow become a master molecule or a supermolecule [16]. hCG, its inhibitors, and antibodies show great promise in the future, in the treatment and diagnosis of cancer, and in the management of reproductive and other disorders [15,16].

Which direction will it go in the future?

Laurence Cole, Ph.D., discovered hyperglycosylated hCG [5], determined the pertide and carbohydrate structures of the hormone hCG and the autocrine hyperglycosylated hCG, discovered hyperglycosylated hCG as the source of implantation and the cause of failing pregnancies [8,46,47], discovered hyperglycosylated hCG as the source of preeclampsia and deep implantation of pregnancy [24], and discovered hyperglycosylated hCG as the source of enzymatic ovulation [52]. Laurence also discovered hyperglycosylated hCG as the cancer malignancy agent [15] and hyperglycosylated hCG as what drives trophoblastic cancers [14].

Laurence Cole Ph.D. is 65 years old now and will be stepping down and retiring very shortly. The future of the hormone hCG and the autocrine hyperglycosylated hCG, will no longer have much to do with me. Other young scientists will be developing professorial careers like I did with hCG. I personally think that future science with hCG is extremely exciting and shows great promise for these future scientists.

I personally believe that the future of cancer research lies in hyperglycosylated hCG, in finding antagonists to hyperglycosylated hCG and its free β-subunit in blocking cancer at its root. The future in reproductive biology is in preventing pregnancy failures (spontaneous abortion, biochemical pregnancy, and ectopic pregnancy) and allowing all pregnancies to go to term [8,46,47]. Using hyperglycosylated hCG prevented preeclampsia and gestational hypertension [24], the biggest killers in pregnancy in the world and the causes of tens of thousands of deaths each year [24]. Research is showing that failure of ovulation and ovarian cysts may be due to shortage of hyperglycosylated hCG [52]. The development and use of hyperglycosylated hCG as a pharmaceutical may be invaluable.

This is all in the future promise of hCG which I will not see. I wish everybody luck with their research developments in the future and great promise.

Just to name some examples of research needing to be done urgently, possible research project of students working toward a Ph.D. or of postdoctoral fellows working toward a postdoctoral fellowship. We know that hyperglycosylated hCG is responsible for cancer mutagenesis [16]. We do not know and need to know how a radiation or chemical damage or mutation damaged cell signals for hCG β-subunit to be expressed. This is an important issue for cancer research and cancer treatment to be addressed.

References

[1] Aschner B. Ueber die function der hypophyse. Pflug Arch Gest Physiol 1912;146: 1—147.

[2] Fellner OO. Experimentelle untersuchungen uber die wirkung von gewebsextrakten aus der plazenta und den weiblichen sexualorganen auf das genital. Arch Gynakol 1913; 100:641.

[3] Hirose T. Experimentalle histologische studie zur genese corpus luteum. Mitt Med Fakultd Univ ZU 1919;23:63—70.

[4] Aschheim S, Zondek B. Das Hormon des hypophysenvorderlappens: testobjekt zum Nachweis des hormons. Klin Wochenschr 1927;6:248—52.

[5] Elliott MM, Kardana A, Lustbader JW, Cole LA. Carbohydrate and Peptide structure of the α- and ß-subunits of human chorionic gonadotropin from normal and aberrant pregnancy and choriocarcinoma. Endocrine 1997;7:15—32.

[6] Butler SA, Ikram MS, Mathieu S, Iles RK. The increase in bladder carcinoma cell population induced by the free beta subunit of hCG is a result of an anti-apoptosis effect and not cell proliferation. Br J Canc 2000;82:1553—6.

[7] Valmu L, Alfthan H, Hotakainen K, Birken S, Stenman UH. Site-specific glycan analysis of human chorionic gonadotropin beta-subunit from malignancies and pregnancy by liquid chromatography - electrospray mass spectrometry. Glycobiology 2006;16: 1207—18.

[8] Sasaki Y, Ladner DG, Cole LA. Hyperglycosylated hCG the source of pregnancy failures. Fertil Steril 2008;89. 1871-1786.

[9] Niswender GD. Molecular control of luteal secretion of progesterone. Reproduction 2002;123:333—9.

[10] Riss PA, Radivojevic K, Bieglmayer C. Serum progesterone and human chorionic gonadotropin in very early pregnancy: implications for clinical management. Eur J Obstet Gynecol Reprod Biol 1989;32:71—7.

[11] Iles RK. Ectopic hCGß expression by epithelial cancer: malignant behavior metastasis and inhibition of tumor cell apoptosis. Mol Cell Endocrinol 2007;260:264—70.

[12] Jankowska A, Gunderson SI, Warchol JB. Reduction of hCGß subunit expression by modified U1 snRNA caused apoptosis in cervical cancer cells. Mol Cancer 2008;7: 26—9.

[13] Li D, Wen X, Ghali L, Al-Shalabi F, Purkis P. hCG β expression by cervical squamous carcinoma-in vivo histological association with tumour invasion and apoptosis. Histopathology 2008;53:147—55.

[14] Cole LA, Butler SA. Hyperglycosylated hCG, hCGß and hyperglycosylated hCGß interchangeable cancer promoters. Molec Cellul Endcrinol 2012;349:232—8.

[15] Cole LA. Hyperglycosylated hCG and its free ß-subunit: the root causes of malignancy and cancer. J Molec Oncol Res 2017;1:53.

[16] Cole LA. Chorionic gonadotropin (CG) a human master molecule. Mol Cancer Res 2018 (in press).

[17] Lei ZM, Reshef E, Rao CV. The expression of human chorionic gonadotropin/luteinizing hormone receptors in human endometrial and myometrial blood vessels. J Clin Endocrinol Metab 1992;75:651—9.

[18] Zygmunt M, Herr F, Keller-Schoenwetter S, Kunzi-Rapp K, Munstedt K, Rao CV, Lang U, Preissner KT. Characterization of human chorionic gonadotropin as a novel angiogenic factor. J Clin Endocrinol Metab 2002;87:290—5296.

[19] Zygmunt M, Herr F, Munstedt K, Lang U, Liang OD. Angiogenesis and vasculogenesis in pregnancy. Eur J Obstet Gynecol Reprod Biol 2003;110:S10—8.

[20] Rao CV, Li X, Toth P, Lei ZM. Expression of epidermal growth factor, transforming growth factor-alpha and their common receptor genes in human umbilical cords. J Clin Endocrinol Metab 1995;80:1012—20.

[21] Rao CV, Li X, Toth P, Lei ZM, Cook VD. Novel expression of functional human chorionic gonadotropin/luteinizing hormone receptor in human umbilical cords. J Clin Endocrinol Metab 1993;77:1706—14.

[22] Wasowicz G, Derecka K, Stepien A, Pelliniemi L, Doboszynska T, Gawronska B, Ziecik AJ. Evidence for the presence of luteinizing hormone—chorionic gonadotrophin receptors in the pig umbilical cord. J Reprod Fertil 1999;117:1—9.

[23] Cole LA. hCG and hyperglycosylated hCG, promoters of villous placenta and hemochorial placentation. In: Nicholson R, editor. Placenta: functions, development and disease. Nova Publishers; 2013. p. 155—66.

[24] Cole LA, Khanlian SA, Kohorn EI. Evolution of the human brain, chorionic gonadotropin and hemochorial implantation of the placenta: origins of pregnancy failures, preeclampsia and choriocarcinoma. J Reprod Med 2008;53:449—557.

[25] Cole LA. hCG and hyperglycosylated hCG in the establishment and evolution of hemochorial placentation. J Reprod Immunol 2009;82:111—7.

[26] Shi QJ, Lei ZM, Rao CV, Lin J. Novel role of human chorionic gonadotropin in differentiation of human cytotrophoblasts. Endocrinology 1993;132:387—95.

[27] Cole LA. The evolution of the primate, hominid and human brain. Primatologia 2015;4: 100124.

[28] Cole LA. hCG and hyperglycosylated hCG in the establishment and evolution of hemochorial placentation. J Reprod Immunol 2009;82:112—8.

[29] Cole LA. The evolution of the primate, hominid and human brain. Primatology 2015;4: 1000124.

[30] Akoum A, Metz CN, Morin M. Marked increase in macrophage migration inhibitory factor synthesis and secretion in human endometrial cells in response to human chorionic gonadotropin hormone. J Clin Endocrinol Metab 2005;90:2904—10.

[31] Matsuura T, Sugimora M, Iwaki T, Ohashi R, Kanayama N, Nishira J. Anti-macrophage inhibitory factor antibody inhibits PMSG-hCG induced follicle growth and ovulation in mice. J Assist Reprod Genet 2002;19:491.

[32] Eta E, Ambrus G, Rao V. Direct regulation of human myometrial contractions by human chorionic gonadotropin. J Clin Endocrinol Metab 1994;79:1582—6.

[33] Doheny HC, Houlihan DD, Ravikumar N, Smith TJ, Morrison JJ. Human chorionic gonadotrophin relaxation of human pregnant myometrium and activation of the BKCa channel. J Clin Endocrinol Metab 2003;88:4310—5.

[34] Ascoli M, Fanelli F, Segaloff DL. The lutropin/choriogonadotropin receptor, a 2002 perspective. Endocr Rev 2002;23:141—74.

[35] Dufau ML. The luteinizing hormone receptor. Annu Rev Physiol 1998;60:461—96.

[36] Jiang X, Dias JA, He X. Structural biology of glycoprotein hormones and their receptors: insights to signaling. Mol Cell Endocrinol 2014;382:424—51.

[37] Fiddes JC, Goodman HM. The gene encoding the common alpha subunit of the four human glycoprotein hormones. J Mol Appl Genet 1982;1:3—18.

[38] Lustbader JW, Yarmush DL, Birken S, Puett D, Canfield R. The application of chemical studies of human chorionic gonadotropin to visualize is three-dimensional structure. Endocr Rev 2013;14:291—310.

[39] Wu H, Lusbader JW, Yee L, Canfield RE, Hendriickson WA. Structure of human chorionic gonadotropin at 2.6Å resolution from MAD analysis of the selenmethionyl protein. Structure 1994;2:545—58.

[40] Lapthorn AJ, Harris DC, Littlejohn A, Lustbader JW, Canfield RE, Machin KJ, Morgan FJ, Isaacs NW. Crystal structure of human chorionic gonadotropin. Nature 1994;369:455—62.

[41] Cole LA. The minute structural difference between the hormone hCG and the identical amino acid sequence TGFß autocrine hyperglycosylated hCG. Am J Obstet Gynecol 2018 (in press).

[42] Goldsmith PC, McGregor WG, Raymoure WJ, Kuhn RW, Jaffe RB. Cellular localization of chorionic gonadotropin in human fetal kidney and liver. J Clin Endocrinol Metab 1983;57:54—61.

[43] Abdallah MA, Lei ZM, Li X, Greenwold N, Nakajima ST, Jauniaux E, Rao CV. Human Fetal nongonadal tissues contain human chorionic gonadotropin/luteinizing hormone receptors. J Clin Endocrinol Metab 2004;89:952—6.

[44] McGregor WG, Raymoure WJ, Kuhn RW, Jaffe RB. Fetal tissues can synthesize a placental hormone. Evidence for chorionic gonadotropin β-subunit synthesis by human fetal kidney. J Clin Investig 1981;68:306—9.

[45] Berndt S, Blacher S, Munuat C, Detilleux J, Evain-Brion D, Noel A, Fournier T, Foidart JM. Hyperglycosylated human chorionic gonadotropin stimulates angiogenesis through TGF-ß receptor activation. FASEB J 2013;12:213686.

[46] Ahmud F, Ghosh S, Sinha S, Joshi SD, Mehta VS, Sen E. TGF-ß-induced hCG-ß regulates redox homeostasis in glioma cells. Molec Cellul Biochemist 2015;399:105—12.

[47] Cole LA. Blastocyst implantation and causes pregnancy failures. In: Cole LA, editor. Human chorionic gonadotropin (hCG). 3rd ed. New York: Elsevier; 2018.

[48] Cole LA. Hyperglycosylated hCG and pregnancy failures. J Reprod Immunol 2012;93: 119—22.

[49] Cole LA, Brennan MC, Hsu C-D, Bahado-Singh R, Kingston JM. Hyperglycosylated hCG, a sensitive screening test for preeclampsia and gestational hypertension. Am J Obstet Gynecol 2018 (in press).

[50] Bahado-Singh RO, Oz AU, Kingston JM, Shahabi S, Hsu CD, Cole LA. The role of hyperglycosylated hCG in trophoblast invasion and the prediction of subsequent preeclampsia. Prenat Diagn 2002;22:478—81.

[51] Cole LA. Hyperglycosylated hCG drives malignancy. J Molec Oncol Res 2017 (in press).

[52] Cole LA. Ovulation and hyperglycosylated hCG. Am J Obstet Gynecol 2018 (in press).

[53] Cole LA, Dai D, Leslie KK, Butler SA, Kohorn EI. Gestational trophoblastic diseases: 1. Pathophysiology of hyperglycosylated hCG-regulated neoplasia. Gynecol Oncol 2006;102:144—9.

[54] Hamade AL, Nakabayashi K, Sato A, Kiyoshi K, Takamatsu Y, Laoag-Fernandez JB, Ohara N, Maruo T. Transfection of antisense chorionic gonadotropin ß gene into choriocarcinoma cells suppresses the cell proliferation and induces apoptosis. J Clin Endocrinol Metab 2005;90:4873—9.

Index

323

Printed in the United States
By Bookmasters